YOGA:
CRITICAL
ALIGNMENT

YOGA: CRITICAL ALIGNMENT

Building a Strong, Flexible Practice
through Intelligent Sequencing
and Mindful Movement

GERT VAN LEEUWEN

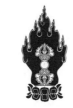

SHAMBHALA
Boston & London
2013

Shambhala Publications, Inc.
Horticultural Hall
300 Massachusetts Avenue
Boston, Massachusetts 02115
www.shambhala.com

English translation © 2013 Gert van Leeuwen, www.criticalalignment.nl.
© 2013 Uitgeverij Altamira, Haarlem, The Netherlands; a division of
the Gottmer Uitgeversgroep BV, www.altamira.nl.
Originally published in Dutch under the title: *Critical Alignment Yoga*, © 2009.
Design and illustrations by Zander Dekker, www.zanderdekker.com

9 8 7 6 5 4 3 2 1

FIRST EDITION
Printed in the United States of America

Distributed in the United States by Random House, Inc., and in Canada by Random House of Canada Ltd

LIBRARY OF CONGRESS CATALOGING-IN-PUBLICATION DATA
Leeuwen, Gert van.
Yoga: critical alignment: building a strong, flexible practice through intelligent sequencing and mindful movement / Gert van Leeuwen.
pages cm
ISBN 978-1-61180-063-0 (pbk.)
1. Hatha yoga. 2. Yoga. 3. Mind and body. I. Title.
RA781.7.L447 2013
613.7'046—dc23
2012047852

Contents

Preface

I first met my yoga teachers, Norman E. Sjoman and H. V. Dattatreya, thirty years ago. They came from Mysore, South India, and were teaching in Amsterdam in 1983. Although I had practiced yoga for many years prior, their classes were a turning point for me. Their approach was totally different from the yoga previously taught in the Netherlands in the 1980s. They were not hindered by traditions, nor did they flout a mystical approach. Their teaching was based on rational experience and research. They tested their anatomical knowledge and their theories of movement against modern scientific research, and they compared movement in yoga with other forms of movement.

The open-minded attitude they fostered allowed me to analyze other types of movement theories and inspired me to conscientiously refine my own knowledge of yoga exercises. My first project was the headstand, for which I developed a headstand bench. With the help of this bench and newly developed mobilization techniques for deeply penetrating the muscular structure of the body, I succeeded in restoring the alignment of the spinal column in a very precise way for people with upper-back complaints. As a result of this, my teacher, Norman Sjoman, suggested that I name this unique practice "Critical Alignment."

Since then the headstand project has been followed by a flood of other insights, which led to the development of an altogether new insight into yoga movement. As the alignment of body parts plays such an important role in this vision, I decided to use "Critical Alignment" as the name for my whole method. I have therefore named this book, in which the whole method is described, *Yoga: Critical Alignment.*

During the process of writing *Yoga: Critical Alignment,* I have developed many new ideas. These ideas have become welcome supplements to the method. I developed the concept of *connections* and was able to eliminate overly general descriptions such as "relaxation" or "space" in my teaching by articulating concrete steps toward accessing higher consciousness.

I believe it is important to link yoga to the circumstances and experiences of daily life. Much of our physical and mental stress is caused by our social and psychological landscape. I pay a lot of attention to the mutual relationship between the physical and psychological buildup of tension and show how yoga is able to break these patterns.

My vision for Critical Alignment has grown into a thick book with many illustrations. In fact, it has become a reference manual that is eminently suitable for experienced yoga students, teachers in training, and teachers. It is my hope that this information will be meaningful for serious beginners as well.

The concepts of Critical Alignment enrich other yoga styles and other related disciplines such as dance and massage therapy, and can be easily integrated into those practices. It has already been established from studies at the University of Amsterdam that this method has a superior application in physical therapy.

I hope that my book challenges the image of yoga as a static tradition to be strictly followed. Yoga should be approached as an open tradition which can be developed through study, creativity, and positive thinking.

Acknowledgments

Writing such an extensive book while continuing my busy practice as a teacher and therapist was an enormous effort. I could never have written this book without the help of a number of people close to me.

First, I want to mention Wijnand Geraerts. He transformed my practice-based thinking into the structure and shape that this book now represents. I thank him sincerely for the enormous amount of work and energy he has spent on both the Dutch and the English versions. I would also like to thank Monique Stoop for her final critical editing of the text. Furthermore I would like to thank my dear friend Heiltje van der Kroon for all the work she did and for her loving support, as well as for being a model, along with Kina Broekmans, for all the illustrations and pictures.

I would like to thank my publisher in the Netherlands, Chris van Gelderen, for the trust, patience, and freedom he gave me during the long period when I was writing the book. I want to thank Zander Dekker for his continuous support, his enthusiasm, and the skill with which he designed the illustrations and the layout. Further thanks go to Klaas Fopma for the photographs inside the book and Barend van Herpe for the cover photograph in the original Dutch edition.

I also want to thank Jacoline Norden and Selle Postma, who substituted for me in my classes when I was writing. I want to thank my friend Paul Braaksma for his support and all the students, teachers in training, and graduate teachers at my institute, Bharata Yoga. Over the years they have been the guinea pigs for me to test my ideas, and through their sometimes critical but positive responses, they have contributed to the making of my book.

A special word of thanks is due to Prof. C. V. Chandrasekhar for his many years of inspiration as my Bharata Natyam dance teacher. His strict yet open-minded way of teaching influenced my teaching of yoga.

Finally, I would like to thank Bert Mentink and Dick Bakker. They are practitioners of other disciplines, orthomanual medicine and cognitive behavior therapy, respectively, and working with them for many years has been very fruitful for the Critical Alignment method.

For the English edition I would first like to thank Lucie van Leeuwen. She spontaneously offered to translate my book into English and spent many hours on the first translation. I also want to thank Norman Sjoman, who not only edited the first translation but also gave valuable feedback on the text. Being a Sanskrit scholar and the author of a number of books, including *The Yoga Tradition of the Mysore Palace* and *Yoga Touchstone* (Black Lotus books), his comments on chapter 5 provided a new perspective for this part of the text. I also wish to thank John Abbott, Derk Sauer, and Ellen Verbeek for their support and their help to find an American publisher. Finally, I give special thanks to Shambhala Publications, who was willing to publish this substantial volume on yoga.

Part One

Critical Alignment
and the Tradition

In this first section, I present a general outline of the Critical Alignment concept, along with a short explanation of yoga traditions. The foundations of Critical Alignment are formed from two of the most important of these traditions: the asana system and the meditative/philosophical system. By joining these two disciplines into one system, I have developed a new concept in modern yoga—Critical Alignment.

I

CRITICAL ALIGNMENT IN THE MODERN YOGA TRADITION

1.1   Introduction

India has a long tradition of philosophy and meditation. Yoga is at the very center of these traditions as it is part of the basic practice of every philosophical system and meditation tradition. This chapter highlights the disciplines and the people who have been important to the development of the yoga system and sources of inspiration for the Critical Alignment concept.

You could say that yoga consists of two main disciplines: one is a meditative/philosophical discipline, and one works with particular physical exercises (the asanas). This is an oversimplification, but it clarifies my argument. The physical tradition of yoga is not very old historically; no ancient manuscripts that refer to the precise practice of asanas have been found. This is not true for the meditative/philosophical history that, with some effort, can be traced back to ancient texts, including that of Patanjali (allegedly from around 150 B.C.E.). This chapter illustrates how Critical Alignment has united both disciplines and, in doing so, initiated a unique practice within yoga today that has the potential to transform the way we practice.

1.2   Meditation and philosophy in yoga

Yoga is one of six traditional disciplines of Indian philosophy and is best described as a meditative/philosophical system. The oldest of the six disciplines and the most important for yoga is the *Samkhya* philosophy. Samkhya is a dualistic philosophy that assumes two primeval forces are at work in the universe—namely, *purusa* (consciousness) and *prakrti* (material existence). The enormous complexity and diversity of the universe is derived from the interaction of these two forces. Samkhya bases its conclusions about the universe purely and simply on logical thinking; thus, in contrast to many religions, it does not call on revelation to support its insights.

Today, the Samkhya philosophy and the yoga philosophy are closely connected, and the yoga philosophy recognizes the existence of the primal forces of purusa and prakrti. There are, however, essential differences:

- Yoga, for example, recognizes the existence of a God, although belief in God is not necessary to reach liberation.
- Yoga recognizes unique physical and moral practices that have been embraced by Samkhya and are also adopted in various formats by other Indian philosophical systems.

References to yoga in the Upanishads and other very old texts indicate that yoga probably has a long tradition. Most of the information on the meditative/philosophical aspect of yoga came from Patanjali, who presented it as a spiritual discipline. He has been a great influence and deserves a brief introduction.

Patanjali and the eight limbs of yoga

Patanjali is the author of the Yoga Sutras, a collection of short aphorisms that address different subjects, such as the essence of yoga, the results you can expect from a consistent meditation practice, and the practical methods you should follow to achieve these results. However, no prominent schools have actually practiced yoga as it is described in the Yoga Sutras, so it can be considered a dead tradition.

The Sutras are short and powerful and lend themselves easily to interpretation. They have been explained by many commentators in numerous ways and from various spiritual viewpoints. The first classical interpretation was by Vyasa (around 600 c.e.). His commentary has long been the standard interpretation.

Patanjali gives the following definition of yoga in the second sutra[1]:

Yoga is the restraint of the movements of the mind.

This can be interpreted as "the yoga practitioner can concentrate completely on one thing." It does not refer to the restraint of *all* movements of the mind. There is, however, a form of concentration in which even that one thing disappears and we meditate on what lies beyond. This metaphysical concept is an extension of breathing and meditation. For this sort of meditation, the level of concentration has to be extremely focused and held for a long time. Vyasa describes this sort of concentration in the Yoga Sutras as follows: "If the subject on which the meditator concentrates slowly fades but is followed by the same thought, and this process repeats itself, even during sleep, then it is yogic meditation."

What makes the Yoga Sutras interesting is that they make this seemingly unattainable goal possible. Patanjali also states that we should not concentrate on the end result but enjoy the path itself.

The second *pada* (chapter) of the Sutras gives the physical means to this ultimate concentration—the eightfold path, or the eight limbs of yoga. The practice of asanas is the third limb of the eightfold path and is preceded by *yamas* and *niyamas*, which provide a practical guide to living that can be compared to the moral rules of all religions. Following the *asanas* are *pranayama* (breathing exercises), *pratyahara* (withdrawal of the senses), *dharana* (concentration), *dhyana* (meditation), and *samadhi* (enlightenment). The Sanskrit scholar and yoga practitioner Norman E. Sjoman is an authority on the

Yoga Sutras and interprets Patanjali's definition of the word *samadhi* as "when you see only that object (the mind) being, as it were, empty."[2]

This definition can be compared to that already mentioned from the second Sutra, so we could say that yoga, according to Patanjali, is the same as samadhi. Patanjali gives a new meaning to the word *yoga*. Before this time, *yoga* had always been defined as "union," referring to the union of the individual soul with the universal soul. When we examine the definition of *samadhi* in more detail, we can see that Patanjali is actually referring to the acquisition of knowledge. Here is a simple example.

Imagine three people watching a girl walk down the opposite side of the street. Each of these people—the mother, the boyfriend with whom she just broke up, and the best friend with whom she is going on vacation—have their own thoughts about the girl. In other words, they have all added their own "I" element to their observations. The girl is certainly not seen as she really is but through the tinted glasses of personal feelings, memories, and so on that color each watcher's observation. According to the definition of *samadhi,* the object (in this case, the girl) should not be colored by the "I" element; it should be observed as it really is. This is only possible through meditation.

1.3   Asana in yoga

It is often claimed that the yoga poses used today come from an ancient tradition, but little is known about the development of asanas through the ages. Only limited information can be found prior to 1400 c.e., and what is available is very fragmented. Texts from between 1400 and 1800 c.e. describe asanas such as Hathapradipika by Svatmarama (fifteenth century). Unfortunately, these texts are cursory. For example, the instructions for Paschimottanasana (see chapter 10.5, number 6) read as follows: "Stretch both legs straight like sticks on the floor. Hold the toes with both hands. Let the forehead rest on the knees. . . . This is the most important pose of all the asanas. It directs the course of the breath along the back or spine, stimulates the digestive fire, contracts the stomach, and gives the practitioner good health." Although these instructions are interesting to read, they are unsuitable as a guide for teaching. What adjustments would I offer if a student experienced pain in her lower back or became breathless during Paschimottanasana?

It is a source of confusion that all physical forms of yoga are now called Hatha Yoga. Hatha Yoga is actually an independent tradition that focuses on the awakening of *kundalini,* a form of physical energy that can be awakened with the help of special exercises and breathing techniques. *Hatha Yoga* (Rider & Company, 1951), written by Theos Bernard, describes in detail the terms that must be fulfilled in order to awaken kundalini. Practitioners must be able to stand on their head for three hours, sit in Padmasana for three hours, and be able to hold their breath for one hour.

The only manuscript describing just the asanas is from the period between 1811 and 1868. It contains drawings of poses and was found in the palace library of Mysore. This document is also unsuitable for teaching purposes, because of the way the descriptions of the asanas can be hard to follow and are not very logical.[3]

In this book, I have limited myself to the developments in the yoga tradition from South India in the twentieth century. This tradition, through its lineage of teachers, has made the primary contribution to the modern asana tradition, which is closely related to ideas in Critical Alignment.

The first teacher I want to discuss is Krishnamacariar. He was affiliated with the palace of Mysore in the 1930s and taught the maharaja's family both simple and difficult asanas without any sort of system or preparation. The poses were not divided into the related groups we know today from Pattabhi Jois, the founder of Ashtanga Yoga, and B. K. S. Iyengar, the founder of Iyengar Yoga (both of whom were Krishnamacariar's students). Krishnamacariar was a unique source of knowledge and inspiration. It seems that under his guidance, gymnastic and even military exercises were incorporated into the asana system.[4]

Pattabhi Jois and B. K. S. Iyengar both organized poses into groups or sequences. Pattabhi Jois created three groups, consisting of series of primary, intermediate, and advanced asanas. He inserted groups of movement (*vinyasas*) between individual asanas that he learned from Krishnamacariar. The movements can be quite complicated, especially in the advanced series. There is also a special breathing technique that accompanies the movements called Ujjayi breath. These series are strenuous and take approximately two hours of continuous movement per series. Power yoga, the popular style of yoga, is based on this system.

B. K. S. Iyengar shaped the series into groups of physiologically related asanas: specifically, standing poses, forward bends, backbends, twists, balance poses, and inversions. He excluded the vinyasas and brought Ujjayi breath and other techniques under the umbrella of pranayama. He also held the poses for longer periods of time. All this led to a greater precision, which allowed the asanas to penetrate the body deeply and achieve beneficial effects. Iyengar is well known in the West, partly through his book, *Light on Yoga,* which has had a huge circulation.

1.4 Critical Alignment and modern asana

Critical Alignment stems from this aforementioned modern yoga tradition and is closely related to the system developed by Iyengar. This means, among other things, that it uses the same grouping of asanas and that the poses are held for long periods of time.

Critical Alignment, however, goes further. It recognizes the importance of chains of movement where small movements are fluidly passed on through the relevant body parts to create larger movements. It emphasizes the essential role of the postural muscles in larger movements (see chapter 2.2 for an explanation of postural and movement muscles).

To reach the postural muscles and the skeletal areas they serve, Critical Alignment introduces different innovations. First, the grouping of the asanas has been refined to include subgroups so that precise penetration, literally, to bone level is possible (see part 4). With respect to this, Critical Alignment introduces a detailed description of connections between body parts that are crucial for transferring smaller movements from which the asanas are built (see part 3). Furthermore, the upper back should ideally be straight (see chapter 2). All of this has important implications for the practice of asanas.

Regarding the meditative/philosophical aspect of yoga, as a teacher, I have been more motivated by the Yoga Sutras than by the Hatha Yoga tradition. I am especially inspired by Patanjali's statement that we should not color our perceptions with our "I" components but should see situations and people as they really are. This point of view is valuable for practicing yoga. By returning you to a situation in which you can see yourself as you truly are, assuming that body and mind are one, the bodywork done in yoga attains far-reaching significance. Yoga exercises serve not only to make you feel fitter, but they become a way of experiencing yourself through your body—that is, objectively, without the filter of your "I" component.

Patanjali gives the following instruction for practicing asanas[5]:

Relax the effort and meditate on the endless.

This sutra is understood by many modern schools to mean that the effort should come first, that the movement must be complete before the muscles can relax. This results in teaching methods where the movement is produced through willpower; the (superficial) large movement muscles are used primarily, and the (deeper) postural muscles are relatively inactive.

Critical Alignment, on the other hand, works with the original meaning of this sutra and states that the effort should be relaxed. This occurs by relaxing the movement muscles prior to the movement, so the postural muscles get the opportunity to produce the movement from a place of relaxation. Rather than forcing movement through willpower, relaxation is associated with terms like *relaxed breathing, pressure, right balance,* and *total awareness.* As I will explain in the following chapters, the superficial movement muscles are particularly sensitive to tension and stress.

During performance of the asanas, Critical Alignment emphasizes the development of total attention. It is total attention, together with breathing, that makes it possible to view stiffness in the movement chains objectively for what it really is: tension resulting from psychological and social pressures that lead to a stagnation of energy and limit free movement. This objective observation of ourselves allows us to release tension and return to an earlier, free, and open—feeling effortless, with no trace of muscular tension—state of moving (see chapter 5 for examples).

Critical Alignment also emphasizes the spiritual side of practicing asanas. Practice not only serves a therapeutic goal, but it establishes balance in the body, so the body becomes open and subtle, and free energy can circulate. We can experience a total awareness during asana practice that gives us an acute feeling of being in the here and now.

This is how Critical Alignment unites the meditative/philosophical and the asana disciplines of yoga so they cannot exist independently of each other; they are completely intertwined. That is why Critical Alignment has an entirely new place within the modern yoga world and is essential for revitalizing contemporary yoga practice.

Part Two

The Foundations of
Critical Alignment

In the previous chapter, I illustrated how the meditative/philosophical limb and the asana limb of the yoga system are united within Critical Alignment. In this part, I will expand on certain aspects of this concept to give it more substance. I will emphasize the following points:

1. Ordinary body movements and asanas (chapter 2)

The theory of movement chains is central to the concept of Critical Alignment, which explains in a simple way how ordinary, daily movements are carried out and how they can cause physical problems. In a movement chain, relevant body parts pass along smaller movements to each other in order to achieve movement. Both the postural and movement muscles have leading roles here. When these muscles work together in harmony, movement is open, fluid, and light. When their cooperation is disturbed (mostly through a stiffening of the movement muscles), then restrictions develop in the movement chains. These restrictions can lead to serious problems.

Movement chains are also important in the performance of asanas, but there are clear differences between asana movements and ordinary movements. In Critical Alignment, relaxation of the movement muscles is central, because this relaxation makes it possible to pass on smaller movements at the skeletal level. This is not necessary in ordinary movement. Through the relaxation of the movement muscles and the passing along of smaller movements, yoga practice can be used successfully to release restrictions in the movement chains.

2. Habitual movements and consciousness (chapters 3 and 4)

We all develop unique postural and movement patterns during our lives. These patterns frequently lead to a serious degeneration in range of motion and can be so harmful that they lead to malformations of the skeleton. Habitual patterns are caused by the body's reaction to social and psychological influences, which include ambition, motivations, and stress. Critical Alignment shows how these distorted movement patterns can be resolved, allowing your body to return to an open, light balance by practicing asanas in a correct manner with total attention. Through attentive practice, you can come face-to-face with your ambitions and other motivations and with the stress that is an inevitable part of such ambitions. This mental attitude of awareness allows you to create space in your body by remaining passive and not trying to change the situation. Total attention ensures that ambition and stress slowly lose their grip on your body. This leads to the possibility of returning to a better balance within the chains of movement, which supports deeper awareness.

3. The interaction between the body, thought, and emotions and the realization of total attention (chapter 5)

One of the first steps in developing awareness is confronting personal ambitions and mental stress while practicing yoga poses. Total attention is necessary to deal with this confrontation; otherwise, you will remain unaware of the ambitions and stress. Total attention can only arise when the body and mind become relaxed through correct balance in asanas. It is not so much a question of cooperation between mind and body as it is a union of the body intelligence with the mental intelligence through which a new form of consciousness can be realized. Openness, relaxation, and a feeling of space in the body and mind are typical of this consciousness. This makes it possible to trancend the limited "I" consciousness and become aware of the here and now. Thus, we enter the area of meditation and spirituality, and our yoga practice becomes a spiritual discipline.

2

INTRODUCTION TO MOVEMENT CHAINS

2.1   Introduction

Almost everyone experiences diminishing mobility during their lives. This is a gradual process, but it can also be instantaneous, as in the case of an accident or injury. Mobility is dependent on the flexibility of the joints and the spinal column and on the ease of movement in the muscles that support them. These factors are inseparable: if muscles are stiff, they cannot move the joints with ease; if the joints are stiff, the muscles cannot perform their function adequately.

For many, this is the beginning of a negative spiral that develops gradually over the years and does not disappear spontaneously. We may become progressively stiffer. In the long term, this stiffness can become so serious that it becomes a threat to our health. Most people do not want to fall into this situation, and it is preventable. Indeed, yoga is gaining in popularity worldwide because it can help with prevention. Yoga focuses on keeping the body flexible, on supple movement and all that this encompasses.

These days, everyone has an idea of how movement occurs. The following simplified description of movement is widely documented: the central nervous system activates the muscles via the nerves; the muscles move certain parts of the skeleton, creating a complete movement. My theory is that this is only half the story. For example, it explains how bad posture can cause a pinched nerve whereby certain muscles cannot function properly and walking becomes difficult (as discussed in chapter 4).

But movement encompasses much more. Through simple observation, it is obvious that the entire body is involved, not just a few discrete parts. For example, when done well, walking involves not only the legs but also the arms and the torso; there is a suppleness and "swing." All the separate parts of the body work harmoniously together to form a fluid movement. Similarly, if there is stiffness in a certain area, this is mirrored throughout the body and results in an unnatural, forced manner of movement.

Yoga is often wrongly seen as being static. A yoga pose necessarily involves movement. Complex movements must be initiated to achieve an end position. What occurs during these movements dictates the appearance of the end pose. The entire body is involved with maneuvering into an asana, just as it is in walking. Therefore, it is crucial to pay close attention not only to the final pose but to the movements leading up to it.

This chapter explores how parts of the body communicate with each other, forming (movement) chains in which small movements are passed along, making open, free movement possible. The concept of movement chains is applied to both ordinary, everyday movements and to yoga practice. Ordinary daily movements are compared to those done in yoga to show clearly that yoga done in accordance with the Critical Alignment method can be used to recover healthy alignment of the skeleton and natural ease of movement.

2.2 Ordinary movements such as walking and lifting evolve through movement chains, while postural and movement muscles work together to pass small movements through the body.

Ordinary movements such as walking and lifting seem simple, but if we look closely, they are complex. Many processes and structures are involved at many levels in the body. These include the simple molecules that provide electrical currents to the nerves, which in turn stimulate the muscles; the complete muscular system that controls the skeleton; the complex brain systems that plan movements and integrate and initiate the muscular system; and finally, the total movement with all its inherent behavioral patterns. With the exception of the last point, we know a lot about these processes. However, it is still largely unknown how the different body parts work together to form a fluid, complete movement.

Movement chains

Total movement occurs automatically as small movements are passed on through a chain of linked body parts. Critical Alignment is based on the understanding that *movement chains* are the foundation of larger movements. This concept explains, in a simple way, how different body parts work together to create movement, taking into account gravity, correct balance, and body weight. Furthermore, the concept of movement chains clearly shows how problems that manifest in one part of the body can originate in an entirely different part, which is called *referred pain*.

For example, an upper back that is bent and stiff—creating a roadblock in that part of the movement chain—can lead to shoulder and neck problems in people who sit a lot, while those who stand may develop lower back problems. This occurs regularly, but it is not recognized by most therapeutic systems. In this chapter, the concept of movement chains is applied to ordinary movements and then to yoga movements. Critical Alignment makes use of the movement chains to practice yoga in an entirely new way.

In concepts formulated by L. Busquet,[1] ordinary, daily movements such as walking and lifting are made up of smaller movements that are passed along via the *chaines musculaires* (literally, "muscle chains") from one part of the body to another. The term *muscle chains* clearly places emphasis on the muscles, thereby indicating Busquet's background in physiotherapy. It is my opinion that structures other than muscles are also important for the generation of movement. Therefore, I prefer a term that emphasizes that broader involvement: *movement chains*.

Getting up from a chair is an example of a movement chain in everyday life. The head initiates the chain by first moving forward and upward. Movement is then passed along to the neck. The neck passes it to the upper back, the upper back to the lower back, and so on, until the complete movement of "getting up from a chair" occurs. This description is not entirely accurate, as it would mean that we rise like a puppet pulled on a string. We are also pushed up by muscles in the lower back, legs, and trunk, and we constantly adjust our posture so we do not lose our balance. This shows that there are two components in action: one that drives the movement and another that controls posture and balance. Movement physiology is a profession that categorizes two types of muscles with characteristics that correspond with the postural and movement muscles.

Postural muscles

The postural muscles lie deep within the body, primarily in the midline of the torso and limbs. The muscles around the spine and the joints belong to this category as well (figure 2.2-1). The muscles that are important for the stability of the lower back and pelvis—the diaphragm, the transverse abdominals, the pelvic floor, and the deeper postural muscles of the lower back that form the "inner tube" (or column)—are postural muscles. The lower back muscles are called the inner tube because they resemble the inner tube of a car tire. Together, they form a hollow, cylindrical structure that wraps around the front of the body behind the stomach muscles and against and around the spine in the back of the body. The diaphragm is the top, and the pelvic floor

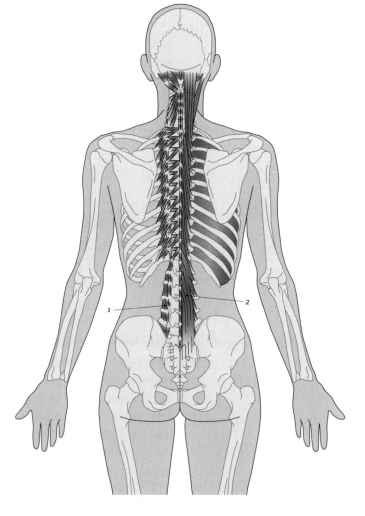

2.2-1

Back view of the skeleton showing the postural muscles of the spinal column
1. Left of the spinal column: small postural muscles
2. Right of the spinal column: large postural muscles

is the base. When a car tire is full of air, it is strong and flexible. The same principle applies to the inner tube, which is full of viscera (the intestines, liver, pancreas, and so on) instead of air and is also strong and flexible.

The body's main center of gravity is located in the inner tube, in the area above the pelvic floor and just under the navel. The most important function of the inner tube is stabilizing the body's balance through muscles that prevent the vertebrae in the lower back from stiffening. These muscles allow the vertebrae to move freely and, if used properly, keep them in the correct position.

Postural muscles can be activated for long periods of time without negative consequences and without causing stiffness. They are perfectly suited for coordinating our balance during long-term static use—for example, when sitting for hours at the computer or while practicing yoga. Even during long hours of sitting, they can maintain the flexibility of the spine and the joints of the shoulders, pelvis, and limbs.

Movement muscles

The biceps, triceps, deltoids, trapezius, glutei, quadriceps, and calf muscles are all movement muscles. Such muscles are generally located near the surface of the body in the torso, arms, and legs. They can only be used for relatively short periods of time, then they must relax. This clearly distinguishes them from the postural muscles. Movement muscles are better suited for short-term, repetitive movements of the torso and limbs such as lifting, walking, working out at the gym, or playing sports.

The postural muscles form the infrastructure of the body's posture and movement. However, because movement is not possible without the movement muscles, intensive interaction between postural and movement muscles is necessary for fluid movement. Walking, if done correctly, is a good example of this interaction. Here, the inner tube is responsible for upright posture and the suppleness (swing) of the lower back. The muscles of the lower back do not stiffen as they do when we walk in a stiff, careful way because we have back pain. At the same time, the movement muscles of the trunk, arms, and legs ensure that there is a rhythmic pattern to the forward movement.

2.3 Distorted interaction between postural and movement muscles leads to restrictions in movement chains and other physical problems.

Unfortunately, the interaction between postural and movement muscles is seldom ideal. Sooner or later, this interaction becomes distorted and can lead to problems such as a stiff, stooped upper back that develops from being hunched over a computer; an overly hollow or flattened, tense lower back, which we may develop when we consciously or unconsciously rotate our pelvis in a certain direction without understanding the consequences for the spine itself; or misaligned and rotated spinal column and ribs. This can arise from repetition of unbalanced movements during sports or work. Even stiff shoulders, hips, and knees indicate a distortion in the cooperation between the postural and movement muscles. These distortions are mostly caused by habits linked to preferential postures and habitual movements (which receive extensive attention in chapter 3).

Diagram 1

Tension in movement muscles

↓

Atrophied movement muscles

↓

Immobility

↓

Vicious circle exacerbating immobility

↓

Obstruction of movement chains

↓

Movement compensation

↓

Onset of problems in other parts of the movement chain(s)

The effects of distortions in movement chains are often disastrous. Following is a sequence of events bound together through a cause-and-effect relationship that leads to malformations in the body. Diagram 1 will help you keep track of the sequence of events.

The first phase is stiffness due to the prolonged activation of movement muscles in a tense, cramped manner. As these muscles are not meant to be activated for long periods of time, the body has to adapt to this unnatural situation. The muscles gradually stiffen, and this stiffening ultimately afflicts the overall structure. Even during sleep, these muscles cannot relax. It is interesting to note that stiffening in a bent upper back does not always mean that the muscles shorten. Static use of the upper back muscles causes them to lengthen and stiffen. Such compensations can offer a short-term solution, but in the long run, they lead to the next phase in a downward spiral. In the places where the body compensates, there is a negative effect on the postural muscles with serious consequences.

The postural muscles cannot perform their functions adequately, because the stiffened movement muscles hold the skeleton and joints in an iron grip. This leads to the next phase, in which the postural muscles slowly begin to atrophy. But the negative spiral has not yet reached its lowest point.

The debilitated functioning of both the movement and, subsequently, postural muscles causes poor alignment and malformations of the skeleton that lead to a loss of mobility in the spinal column and joints. The feeling of inflexibility persists.

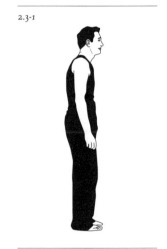

2.3-1

You would hope that, having reached this low point, the negative developments would stop, but the opposite is true: the situation gets steadily worse, and a vicious circle is created. The stiffening and malformations of the skeleton have further negative effects on the local postural and movement muscles, which become even stiffer and harder. This exacerbates the problem, causing the skeleton to stiffen further and deform accordingly. This is clearly visible during the aging process; the curvatures of the spine become more obvious with the passing years.

At that point, the movement chains become clear. The loss of mobility in a certain area of the body means there is an obstruction in one or more movement chains. To grasp the seriousness of the situation, it is necessary to understand the consequences of these obstructions. Remember, movement chains pass along smaller movements from one part of the body to another, making larger movements such as walking and lifting possible. Thus, if one part of a chain is blocked, movement cannot be passed along adequately to parts of the body further along the chain. There is a serious danger that large movements can only be done poorly, if at all. Nevertheless, the body will do everything to avoid total immobility. This causes even more problems in parts further along the movement chain.

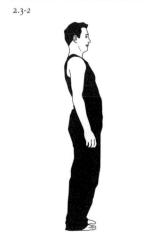

2.3-2

A common example of this is the stiff, lower back that frequently develops as a reaction to the stiffening and bending of the upper back. The problems that develop in other areas are caused because more work is done by fewer vertebrae, thereby increasing the chance of overload. We can again use the example of rising from a chair. When we stand up, the movement should be passed along from the head through the neck to the upper back. If this doesn't happen because the upper back is stiff, the movement will get "hung up" in the neck (see figure 2.3-1), or the lower back will compensate by curving inward (see figure 2.3-2) to achieve an upright body posture. Both the neck and the lower back become susceptible to overload. This leads to the adoption of cramped and abnormal postures in areas around the blockage. The same pattern of cause and effect repeats in contiguous parts of the body. It begins with a cramping and stiffening of the movement muscles and results in the gradual weakening of the postural muscles and eventual malformations of the skeleton.

2.4 The yoga practices of Critical Alignment are aimed at the skeleton; they are based on principles that differ from ordinary movements.

2.4.1 In Critical Alignment, smaller movements in movement chains are passed through the midline of the body by the free movement of the skeleton.

The basic foundation of Critical Alignment is that the large movements in both yoga and ordinary movements are the result of smaller movements that are passed on via movement chains. However, the similarity of yoga and everyday movements ends here. The main difference between them becomes clear when we practice yoga. The first step is relaxing the movement muscles, something that does not apply to ordinary movements. This step is followed by others that lead to the transfer of movement at the skeletal level. This does not apply to ordinary movements either. To clarify this, I will give a broad description of relevant points for practicing yoga according to the principles of Critical Alignment. This will be followed by a plan for practicing the asanas.

As soon as the movement muscles relax, movement comes under the control of the postural muscles. The midline of the trunk and limbs coordinate the execution of yoga poses. Because the movement muscles of the trunk and limbs are relaxed, movement can only occur through the midline, where the postural muscles and skeletal parts (vertebrae and joints) are located. In other words, the midline starts to function as a power line that processes movement.

The skeleton and postural muscles primarily ensure that the front/back and right/left sides of the body remain in balance. This guarantees free movement of the breath, which allows for the further development of relaxation (discussed in detail in chapter 5). With the help of the postural muscles and skeleton, small movements can be transferred from one body part to another via the midline (power line). The relaxation of the movement muscles increases the mobility of the vertebrae and joints so they can join in the chain of movement. This cannot occur if the movement of the joints or vertebrae is blocked by tensed movement muscles. With relaxation, the work is spread equally through the deeper layers of muscle, and the use of less muscle increases the total ease of movement.

The small movements are surprisingly minute. In the spinal column, which is the most important structure for transferring movement, movements pass from vertebra to vertebra by only one to a few centimeters. If the spine is stiff, more and more vertebrae get tangled together. They are not malformed, but they are held together by rigid muscles. If these muscles are released, the vertebrae can be mobilized. In a stiff spine, large segments of the back move as fused units, because the mobility of individual vertebrae is lost. When this happens, patterns of movement develop whereby only five or six vertebrae (of the twenty-four) can be used actively. As the spine can move in two opposing directions (toward the head and toward the pelvis), small movements can also be passed along in opposite directions toward neighboring vertebrae. The net result is that small movements in the upper back are directed toward the feeling of extending the crown, while on the other end, the tailbone or sit bones feel extended. In this way, the body part at each end of the spine (the pelvis and the head) can make optimal use of gravity, because pressure is applied through the weight of the body. When practicing asanas, this pressure is used to mobilize joints and vertebrae (see the three illustrations in figure 2.4.1-1).

The person in figure 2.4.1-1a habitually works with a bent lower back. This lack of extension is compensated for in the neck, which collapses and becomes concave. The same applies when standing: the body hangs forward, the lower back is not straight, and the neck remains concave (figure 2.4.1-1b). In a yoga exercise, this lack of extension becomes painfully obvious (figure 2.4.1-1c). The extra strain on the back that is caused by this position accentuates the habitual use of the back. The neck becomes even more concave, and the lower back gets rounder. The result is that the extremities of the spine cannot be stretched any longer. The lower back prevents the movement from reaching the hips, because it is too convex; the neck prevents the movement from reaching the crown, because it is too concave. The back does not discharge tension but accumulates it. (This will be explained further in chapter 2.4.2 in the examples of asanas.)

Critical Alignment focuses on the spine because it is here that the most important structures and tissues for movement are found: the vertebrae and discs, the postural muscles around the spine, and the nerves that leave the spine and innervate (control and provide information to) the muscles and their blood vessels.

When the spinal column functions well, the extremities—the shoulders and arms, and the pelvis and legs—also function well. If the spinal column does not function well, then the extremities will also suffer. (This is covered in more detail in chapters 4 and 6.)

Protocol: relaxation, movement, and strength and coordination

Critical Alignment makes use of the aforementioned protocol. It is a practical guideline that is applied during yoga practice. Critical Alignment starts with the relaxation of the movement muscles and ends with balancing the skeleton. There are three essential steps for breaking an existing faulty structure and replacing it with better posture.

The first step, relaxation, is aimed at actively relaxing the movement muscles. This is an important stage and is clearly different from the passive relaxation that is achieved through massage. During physiotherapy, the muscles are initially relaxed via massage and then subjected to exercise; that is, they tighten. The approach of Critical Alignment is fundamentally different.

In Critical Alignment, the movement muscles are relaxed by using gravity—specifically, the weight of the body or body part. If necessary, this pressure can be achieved by using yoga props (see chapter 2.5). When practicing yoga, the weight of the body is brought, via the power line, to the area of the movement chain where the stiff postural muscles and joints are located. This is where relaxation must develop. Breathing plays an important part here. For example, in Trikonasana, the weight of the upper body is transferred via the power line of the spine to the pelvis, and this pressure can be used to release stiffness around the hips, hamstrings, and lower back. The movement muscles

2.4.1-1a

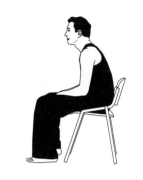

2.4.1-1b

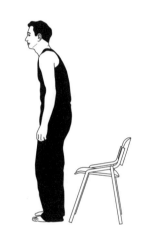

2.4.1-1c

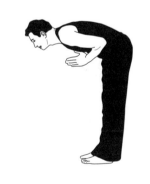

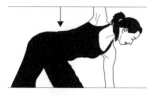

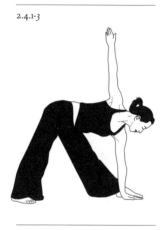

on the side of the lower back play an important role here (see the arrow in figure 2.4.1-2). Relaxation can only happen if the weight of the body is used to loosen the muscles in the said areas. In Trikonasana, we also have to *stretch*. The hamstrings must lengthen to achieve a free movement in the upper body (figure 2.4.1-3).

There are two possibilities for relaxation:

1. Conscious relaxation of muscles around a joint or vertebra, so that it can move more freely, allowing the postural muscles to take over
2. Stretching of stiff movement muscles

The power line changes in different yoga poses. This is determined by the areas where relaxation must develop. During Sirsasana on the headstand bench, for example, relaxation means freeing the movement of the upper back. That is why the body weight must be guided via the lower back through the power line (spinal column) to the upper back (figure 2.4.1-4). The movement muscles of the stomach have an important role here (see chapter 6). If these muscles are not controlled properly, the natural curve of the lower back will collapse, trapping the movement instead of transporting the body's weight to the area between the shoulder blades.

When doing this exercise for the first time, almost everybody ends up with a bent upper back as they bring their hips over their head (figure 2.4.1-5), because the back is very strong in this position. The superficial movement muscles maintain the bent upper back and are hard at work over the entire width of the back. The pressure of body weight (figure 2.4.1-6) in this area can also be supported by relaxing the local movement muscles, after which the back can straighten (figure 2.4.1-7). The straighter the back, the less effort that is required by the superficial movement muscles. This process will be examined in detail in the discussion of the asanas.

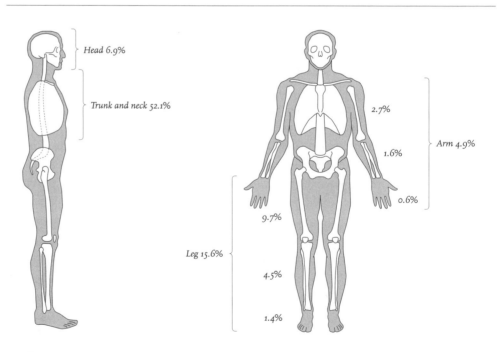

2.4.1-6 Weight of body parts as a percentage of total body weight

Breathing plays an important part when the body confronts tension; both the exhalation and the inhalation have specific roles. The exhalation is aimed at the muscles and structures that must relax. The inhalation is directed toward achieving a free and open feeling in the entire body.

During inhalation, we literally connect our body to the space we are in. This teaches us to move with a feeling of openness that is as light and transparent as the space around us. For this to happen, we need open and passive attention—an attention that closely follows the inhalation and exhalation and the associated relaxation—paired with technically correct movement. This is difficult, as the places that must relax to achieve free movement are often painful and sore. The body never chooses pain, instead following the path of least resistance and inevitably moving around pain. When practicing yoga, we search for this resistance. This can only occur when we consciously go along with the process, relaxing the body and calmly and deliberately guiding it to the heart of painful places.

The second step for replacing a faulty structure is movement that is directed toward the joints and vertebrae, including the intervertebral discs, to increase mobility. When the movement muscles are relaxed, the postural muscles are better able to do their work. They can move and allow parts of the skeleton to extend away from each other. Accordingly, movement can be brought, via the power line, from one part of the body to another. This movement ensures that, in Sirsasana on the headstand bench, the vertebrae are stacked so little effort is needed to keep the body in balance.

The last step in achieving better movement, strength and coordination, is aimed at optimizing the function of the postural muscles. This means the strength and coordination of these muscles will be developed through regular practice and increased time spent on the asanas. Postural muscles that function optimally create a feeling of space and freedom in the body.

These three steps literally go down to the bone. The initial goal is to create alignment and mobility at the skeletal level. Ultimately, the goal is to create a connection between all parts of the body, so that it comes into a dynamic yet relaxed and open balance. Critical Alignment always applies the three steps together and in this order. This is the basic requirement for breaking habitual movement patterns and creating the possibility of free movement.

Other therapies that treat physical problems have fewer steps and different interpretations. Physiotherapists, chiropractors, and massage therapists, for example, only use the steps of relaxation and movement. The problem with omitting the strength and coordination step is that the client is treated passively, so there is almost no change to posture and movement. The body is not invited to learn new patterns. Other physical therapies only use the steps of movement and strength and coordination. These therapies are often directed toward the movement muscles, so they increase the chance of stiffness and immobility.

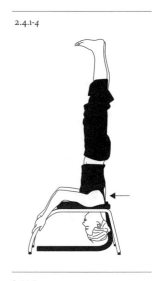

2.4.1-4

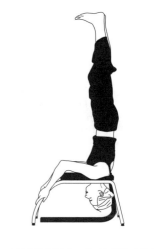

2.4.1-5

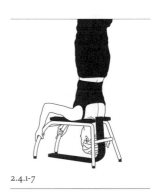

2.4.1-7

2.4.2 *The movement chains of yoga asanas have diverse functions*

Yoga comprises a richly diverse group of some six hundred asanas.[2] Modern yoga practice makes use of approximately two hundred poses, more than a hundred of which are described in this book. The asanas can be used for realigning the body and alleviating

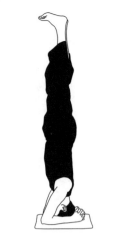

many of the complaints that originate from a poorly functioning skeleton. The large variety of asanas means that, in principle, there is also a rich variety of movement chains. (This aspect becomes clear in chapter 6, where the building blocks of movement chains are discussed.)

The differences between asanas ultimately depend on the differences in the movement chains involved. In addition, the different use of gravity (in the weight of the body and the limbs) noticeably increases the diversity. Ustrasana (Camel Pose; see chapter 11.3, number 4) and Dhanurasana (Bow Pose; see chapter 11.3, number 5) are structurally similar to each other, but the different use of gravity makes them two very different exercises.

Besides gravity and the postural muscles, certain movement muscles also play a role. To give you an idea of the complexity involved, the following examples illustrate asanas that are different because of these considerations. Each pose has its own dynamic that is typical for a larger group of asanas. Sirsasana (Headstand; figure 2.4.2-1) is a good example of the inversions group of serene asanas in which the body is stacked and in balance. A second group includes Utthita Trikonasana (Extended Triangle Pose; figure 2.4.2-2); in this group, the upper body is brought out of the midline, and the lower back is the axis for the completion of the asana. Standing poses, forward bends, and some twists also belong in this group. Finally, there is a group of asanas that are particularly dynamic, such as balancing poses and backbends, especially Viparita Chakrasana (Backward Turning Wheel; figure 2.4.2-3a-i).

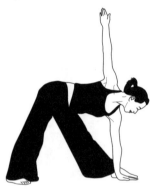

In the interest of clarity, the descriptions are kept simple. The three steps of the protocol and the dynamics of the end poses are indicated, as is the use of gravity or the pressure of body weight. For more detailed descriptions, see chapter 8.2, various numbers, for Sirsasana; chapter 9.3, number 8, for Utthita Trikonasana; and chapter 11.4, number 9, for Viparita Chakrasana.

Sirsasana

In the starting position (figure 2.4.2-4a), the upper back between the shoulder blades is relaxed by directing the breath there (first step: relaxation). Then the legs are raised above the pelvis (figure 2.4.2-4b), and their weight is passed along to the midline between the shoulder blades. This area of the spine can bear the pressure because the movement

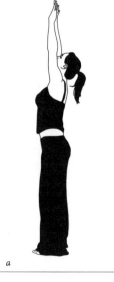

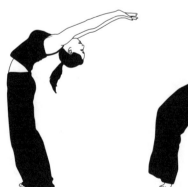

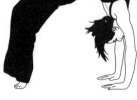

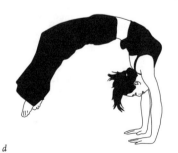

a   b   c   d

muscles are relaxed. The midline functions here as a power line. The spine can then use this body pressure to stretch and pass along movement (second step: movement).

This movement goes simultaneously in opposite directions, toward both the head and the lower back. By moving the ribs toward the stomach, these movements and the power line in the spine are strengthened. The result is that the spine, pelvis, and legs move closer toward ideal "stacking" and into increasingly subtle balance. Initially, this can feel unstable, which is a sign that the coordination and strength of the postural muscles is being built up (third step: strength and coordination). Sirsasana can now develop into a dynamic and meditative end pose. Slow, deep breathing ensures that an increasingly deeper level of relaxation can be achieved in the movement muscles so that the postural muscles become more important. This is better for the stability of the body and permits an experience of lightness and tranquillity.

In my experience, the upper back is straight if it is carrying the weight of the body in a relaxed manner. This counts not only for Sirsasana, but also for seated and standing poses. As I will show later in this book, an upper back that is straight has far-reaching consequences for the alignment of the entire body. Furthermore, I have observed that the upper back often adopts a straight position when it relaxes, which contradicts many medical sources that claim the upper back should be bent.

Utthita Trikonasana

In this asana, the upper body actively moves away from the vertical midline, and it is necessary to activate certain movement muscles constantly to use gravity to achieve extension and pass the movement along. To start, the upper body is placed in position (figure 2.4.2-5). By relaxing the lower back, the inner tube is activated (first step: relaxation). The upper body is then turned sideways, toward the floor (figure 2.4.2-6). This movement is initiated and controlled by the lower back's postural and movement muscles. Thus, the lower back is stretched, and movement passes via the power line along the spine toward the pelvis and hips and in the opposite direction toward the upper back, neck, and head. If the leg that receives this movement does so correctly, it will transfer the movement on to the hip (step two: movement). This, together with the contraction of the movement muscles found on the left (or right) side of the lower back, places the upper body parallel with the floor via the power line along the spine. Thus,

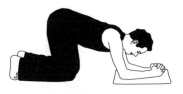

2.4.2-4a

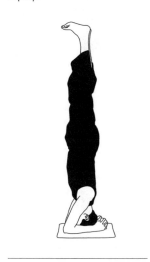

2.4.2-4b

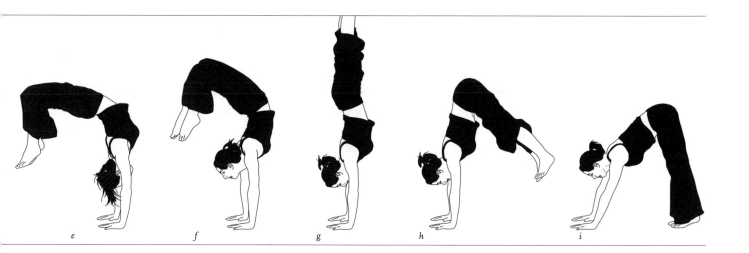

e f g h i

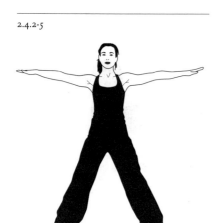

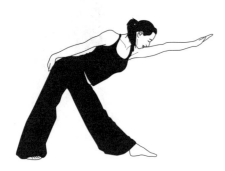

both the leg and the lower back push the hip away in a powerful yet relaxed manner (step three: strength and coordination). This intensifies the power line along the spine and leads to a dynamic pose where, despite the fact that the force of gravity has to be neutralized constantly, the relaxation of the lower back, hip, and hamstrings can be increased. The resulting physical experience of lightness and tranquillity can be intensified through conscious inhalation.

Viparita Chakrasana

This asana is all about movement and has no static end position. The passage of movement must be coordinated from the power line along the spine. If it is carried out in this manner, it is a spectacular example of lightness and tranquillity in movement. Correct balance between the two gravity points is very important for the ideal execution of this asana. The secondary gravity point of the spine, which is the heart area, must be placed precisely above the main gravity point that lies in the pelvis (see also chapter 6). Both points are totally dependent on the mobility of the spine, but especially that of the lower back, as this is the last part of the movement chain. If the lower back keeps its mobility, the sternum (or breastbone) remains aloft, free, and relaxed, and the movement is directed downward, where it leaves the spine and is passed along to the legs, which then make the jump. This free and open position of the spine and sternum depends on good balance with body weight being borne on the front of the heels. The crucial point in the movement is breaking the fall. The action of the hands touching the floor should result in the sternum moving past the arms, as in figure 2.4.2-7 (first step: relaxation). This movement of the gravity point ensures that hardly any strength is necessary to continue the movement. By moving the head toward the back of the neck, together with a light jump with the feet, the rest of the body follows automatically, as shown in figure 2.4.2-8a (second step: movement). The shifting of the gravity point in the chest must be compensated for in the arms and later on, during movement, through the stomach muscles, as seen in figure 2.4.2-8b (third step: strength and coordination), which guide the body into Adho Mukha Vrksasana (Handstand).

Many people find practicing yoga asanas difficult. This is understandable when you look at the complexity of the movements. Many requirements must be met, as we have seen. The most important of these are: application of the three steps of the protocol (relaxation, movement, and strength and coordination); the right application of the breath, gravity, and vibrancy in the final pose; and the right balance between movement and postural muscles.

Everyday activities are also complicated when we look at them in detail, but we do not feel they are difficult, because we generally act on automatic pilot (see also chapter 3). That is simply not possible when practicing yoga. Yoga movements must be done slowly and consciously, so the steps are achieved in the right sequence and with the correct interactions. If our attention is lost, fast and tense movements are completed on automatic pilot, just as in everyday activities. Thus, the movements are affected by mindless preferences that the body has developed over the years. The right kind of attention is crucial for practicing yoga; it is a passive and open attention that does not attempt to keep everything under control. Trying to control everything activates the movement muscles, which is not helpful during yoga. It is not the purpose of movement in yoga.

2.5 Critical Alignment, with props and manual mobilization techniques, can break through movement restrictions and restore mobility.

Everyday activities such as walking, bending, and playing sports are nearly always carried out automatically and, therefore, without awareness. This is why they are susceptible to such factors as stress; habits; desires; and other, often unconscious urges. This leads to the development of preferential movements that become so strong that blockages occur in the movement chains. After that, serious problems can develop in the body.

Considering that normal daily movements are closely allied to automatisms, they are a definite factor in causing movement problems. Therefore, it seems wrong to assume that normal daily movements are a good basis for the treatment of these complaints. But this is exactly what is done in physiotherapy. It is my contention that serious recovery must initially be found at a deeper level; namely, the skeletal level. It is here that alignment and mobility are lost. When they are recovered, there is a good chance that mobility will return to the rest of the body. Critical Alignment focuses on the skeleton and is therefore well suited to treat complaints and problems related to movement.

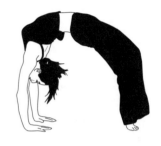

2.4.2-7

To understand how Critical Alignment can resolve these problems, it is useful to look at two types of students. The first group has mild complaints, such as a general stiffness and/or specific problems that have not yet led to blockages in the movement chains with their associated immobility. The second group has succumbed to immobility due to blockages.

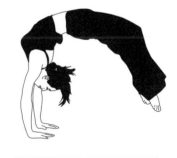

2.4.2-8a

The protocol of Critical Alignment can be applied to both groups to recover the skeleton's alignment and extension and the body's mobility. The first group can perform the different steps of the protocol independently—albeit with regular instruction from a teacher and, if need be, with the use of the props and mobilization techniques. This is not possible for the second group. These students will not be able to relax the movement muscles on their own, because their body is extremely cramped in certain places. Body weight that is directed to those places will not be accepted and cannot be used to extend and move the skeleton via the power line. (Some places are so tight that the vertebrae do not move anymore, even when we want to move them through the coordination of our own body weight.) The confrontation with tension in these places is therefore doomed to fail. But it is possible to reach the skeleton passively by using props and mobilization techniques.

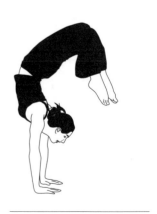

2.4.2-8b

These props and techniques are especially advantageous for people who cannot break through habitual movement patterns on their own, because they no longer know how a certain body part should move naturally. Because of the tension that has built up, they are no longer aware of these areas and their ability to feel the relevant body part is largely lost. Props give precise support and pressure to the areas that are stiff so they can be "felt" again, allowing contact to be restored. Thus, a passive confrontation with the tension can be made. The props function, in a way, as suppliers of body weight, so the postural muscles and the skeletal parts they serve can be reached. The props used in Critical Alignment have been designed to alleviate the tension in the body without disturbing balance and coordination, so the mobility of specific body parts can be increased.

Frequently used props

The *headstand bench* (figure 2.5-1) is one of the most important props and is mainly used for Sirsasana. The following section includes an example of how to use the headstand bench when dealing with a bent upper back.

The *backbender* (figure 2.5-2) is used for mobilizing the upper back, usually with a rubber strip, described later.

The *roll*, which is 20 inches wide and 4 to 6 inches thick (figure 2.5-3), is used under the upper or lower back during prone poses. A rolled-up felt mat works well.

A *rubber strip* measuring 40 inches long, 2 inches wide, and 1 inches deep (figure 2.5-4) is ideal for supporting (parts of) the spine in prone positions.

A *belt* (figure 2.5-5) is often used in exercises, including Sarvangasana (Shoulderstand).

A *shoulderstand block* (figure 2.5-6) is used in many other exercises besides Sarvangasana.

A sticky *yoga mat* (figure 2.5-7) is placed on the floor beneath you during all the exercises.

Application of the props and mobilization techniques

Teachers regularly use props in combination with mobilization techniques. This is the preferred way for achieving relaxation. The mobilization techniques infer that the student (through the breath and by actively interacting with the teacher) can learn new ways of moving. It is important that the student use a specific breathing pattern during this interaction; otherwise, the mobilization turns into manipulation, and the process of learning stops. The teacher then takes over all initiative, and the student remains passive, which is customary in certain therapies. This is not the case in Critical Alignment; the student must actively learn the new way of moving, or it will not make an imprint.

The application of props and mobilization techniques are shown in the following example, which continues the earlier description of the bent upper back. A bent upper back means there is a blockage in the movement chain that connects the neck with the pelvis. According to physical therapists and doctors who deal with movement therapy, there are hardly any treatment possibilities to recover this connection. Accordingly, I

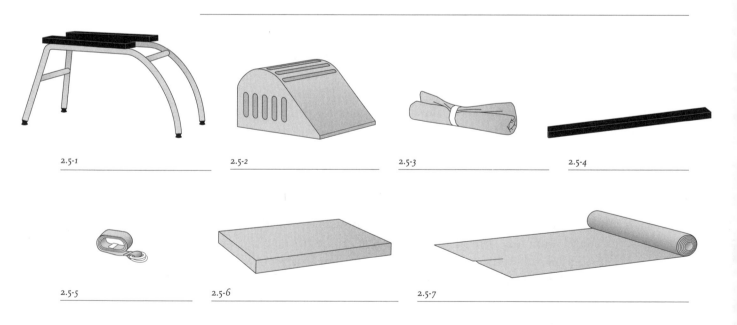

2.5-1   2.5-2   2.5-3   2.5-4

2.5-5   2.5-6   2.5-7

began experimenting with Sirsasana in the headstand bench and developed a method to mobilize the upper back.[3] If you have a bent upper back and do a normal Headstand, with your head on the floor, you would use your back in the same way as you do when standing erect. That is, your shoulders would be pulled up and forward, leading to an enormous amount of tension in your neck (see the arrow in figure 2.5-8). If you could lessen the tension in your neck by lifting your neck and shoulders, your lower back would compensate for the curvature in your upper back (see the arrow in figure 2.5-9).

The first advantage of the headstand bench is that it supports the shoulders, relieving the pressure on the neck and head while retaining the benefits of Sirsasana, namely a good connection between the neck and pelvis. The second advantage is that nearly everybody is able to absorb the teacher's corrections immediately. When you have a stiff, bent upper back, stand on the headstand bench (see figure 2.5-10), and allow your back to relax, you will immediately lose your balance and fall over backward. This is because the lower part of the curvature in the back (illustrated by the arrow) is moving downward. To prevent you from falling, the teacher stands in front of you and asks you to lean your legs on his back (figure 2.5-11). Here, a large part of your body weight is supported by the teacher, and the lowest part of the curvature in your upper back can be shifted into an upward position (illustrated by the arrow).

You can now use gravity to your back's advantage by sending your exhalations into that area and allowing your spine to sink in. Thanks to gravity and the teacher's support, you do not fall backward, and when you relax your muscles, your back will actually become straighter.

The first step of the process, relaxation, is actually the most tenuous part of the entire process. Some students understand immediately what is meant when they are asked to send their breath to the place where pressure is applied in order to lessen the muscle tension, while other students must search for a long time. When the muscle tension lessens, the teacher guides the student's body weight to the place where the pressure is applied in the hope that the relaxed body structure will carry the weight.

The second step, movement, is where the body weight is slowly brought back to the shoulders, taking care that muscle tension does not return. Ultimately, the spine will become much straighter and be able to carry the body's weight in a relaxed manner (see figures 2.5-12 and 2.5-13). This is an extremely interesting moment therapeutically,

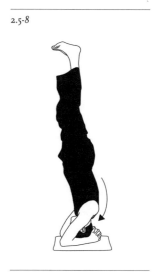

2.5-8

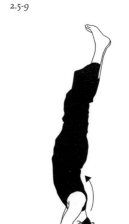

2.5-9

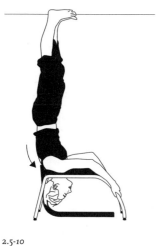

2.5-10

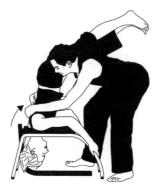

2.5-11

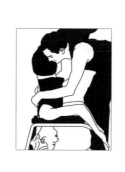

2.5-12

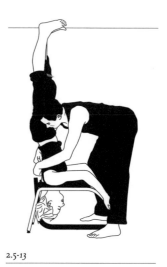

2.5-13

because the "established reflex" is broken, a process that the teacher can easily feel. The established reflex is connected with preferred postures (both of these terms are discussed in chapter 3).

The third and final step, strength and coordination, is where the pose, which initially feels unstable, eventually becomes more and more tranquil. With time, the body is able to achieve these movements alone, without help from outside. When the exercises can finally be done independently, a breakthrough can be made with essential coordination exercises. Gradually, the new movements will become part of normal daily movements.

2.6   The healing effects of Critical Alignment are twofold: therapeutic and meditative.

The practice of asanas is intriguing because it works in two ways: therapeutic and meditative. *Therapeutic* should be understood here in its broadest sense. It involves not only the treatment of serious problems but also simple body exercises. I will say only a few words about this here, but I will return to this topic in later chapters.

It is essential that both therapeutic and meditative aspects should be addressed when practicing asanas. This has to do with the fact that yoga has a strong physical foundation with excellent techniques to keep the body in good condition and is well suited to treating movement problems. Simultaneously, yoga has a level of difficulty that requires a meditative approach.

The physical and meditative aspects of yoga asanas are intimately intertwined and dependent on each other. When practiced correctly, there is a balance between the two, but it is a fragile balance that can easily tip either way. The important effects of yoga are not confined to the classroom or studio setting; they are taken out of the studio into daily life. In this way, the principles of movement can be applied to normal activities, and consequently, the relationship with the body in daily life becomes of vital importance. This also applies to the confrontation with the self. (I will come back to this in chapters 3 and 6.)

2.6.1   *Critical Alignment restores interaction between postural and movement muscles and, through this, the relationship with the body.*

For the serious practitioner, Critical Alignment will not be an easy road—certainly not in the beginning—because the practice of Critical Alignment actively seeks limitations in movement and thereafter creates a confrontation with tension and immobility at the deepest level. This technique breaks the vicious circle that results in increasing stiffness and deformation of the skeleton by restoring skeletal alignment and, with that, the coordination of the movement and postural muscles. This generally has a positive effect on your relationship with your body, and you can derive interesting insights from it.

The first insight directs your attention to how movement happens and how and why problems can develop. With this knowledge, it is possible to use the principles of yoga exercises in normal everyday movements. The lower back is, for example, always bent slightly inward in Critical Alignment. Even though some asanas work with a bent back, there is always a dynamic movement inward. This principle can easily be applied to such daily activities as sitting, lifting, and so on, which can alleviate problems when done with attention.

The second insight is that if the body is able to move freely, the feeling of physical oppression disappears. Instead, a positive feeling of lightness develops, as if energy is circulating freely, causing the tension to disappear. The dissolution of tension is an important step on the road to recovering your relationship with your body. When tension builds in certain areas, the sensitivity and therefore your relationship with your body is lost. The practice of asanas is often initially painful, but this becomes manageable, especially when you experience a feeling of space (that is, the circulation of energy) when muscle tension is transformed to relaxation (see also chapter 6).

2.6.2 A relationship with the body is a prerequisite for an experience of the self.

A deeper confrontation is possible as a result of your recovered relationship with your body. Freely circulating energy is synonymous with space in the body. This energy is the bearer of an all-embracing attention that makes it possible to experience yourself and your environment in an objective way. You can see your body, with all its problems as well as your intentions and emotions, with dispassion and without judgment. By relaxing and opening yourself, you can finally experience the deep feeling of harmony and freedom that is a part of yourself—or more specifically, your Self. (I will come back to this subject in chapter 6.)

3

EMBRACING THE TOTAL
EXPERIENCE OF MOVEMENT

3.1 Introduction

3.2 Habitual postures and movements are created in childhood and shaped by ambitions, motivations, and stress.

3.3 Critical Alignment can stop the negative effects of habitual posture and movement patterns and restore the total experience of movement.

3.1 Introduction

Nearly everyone's skeleton is straight and aligned at birth, but as we get older, we tend to get stiff and bent. These bends, twists, and malformations occur slowly and disturb our naturally free balance and movement. Later in this chapter, I will explain in more detail why this occurs.

The imbalance, which is initially the result of a malfunction of the muscles, causes unhealthy postural and movement patterns to develop. Some muscles shorten permanently from constant tension and then pull specific parts of the skeleton closer together. Other muscles lengthen, creating excessive space in different areas. Because of this, we see irregularities in posture like a difference in the height of the left and right shoulder or the left and right side of the pelvis. This is a sign that the balance of the entire body, not just that of the shoulders or pelvis, is disturbed, even though it may be difficult to see from the outside.

When muscles shorten permanently, there is no chance of spontaneous lengthening during relaxation. The shortening is maintained during the day and remains even during sleep. This results in all sorts of movement constraints.

Yoga, practiced following the guidelines of Critical Alignment, can recover the original balance and agility of the body. The yoga exercises focus on mobility, strength, and relaxation through which the muscles can regain their balance. That is, stiff muscles can relax, and weak muscles can be stimulated. Recovery of muscular balance has a healing effect on the skeleton, which increases flexibility and reclaims natural balance in posture. Therefore, recovery from the skeletal malformations and imbalances described in this chapter is possible in most cases.

We all develop our own postural and movement patterns; I call these patterns *habitual postures or movements*. An example of a habitual posture is always leaning on one leg when standing for a long time. This can lead to tension in the lower back, hip, and sacroiliac joint on the side that bears the weight.

When we move our bodies with a goal in mind (for example, when vacuuming), our goal is achieved through willpower. However, *how* the movement is done is primarily unconscious. We are so conditioned that we seem "forced" to perform sequences of habitual postures and movements unconsciously and repeatedly over the years. We always hold a vacuum cleaner with the same hand in front and, because of that, continuously twist our shoulders and back the same way, place the same leg forward, and so on. If we try to change this habit, it feels uncomfortable, maybe even painful, and the body always chooses to avoid discomfort and pain.

All these habitual movements have been documented by manual therapists and can be diagnosed through mobility tests. The preferred leg, preferred arm, and even the preferred eye can be diagnosed. As these patterns are very stubborn and can lead to many problems, an entire chapter (chapter 4) is devoted to them.

Because yoga exercises are done symmetrically, habitual postures and movements are easy to notice, and the differences between left and right become obvious. Critical Alignment shows how these old patterns can be broken so that new patterns can be learned—or how faulty patterns that have developed can be dissolved and how we can return our body to its original balance. It is more about unlearning than learning.

Correct balance leads to freedom of movement and the possibility of deep relaxation during rest. Freedom of movement creates positive feelings in the body: lightness, openness, and sensitivity. Restricted movement leads to poor body consciousness. The body becomes less sensitive to the positive feelings in the body, which is why we rely more on thinking. This leads to such statements as, "I think I feel good." Feelings that should be experienced directly through the body are reduced to mental processes; we experience feeling in our head instead of our body.

3.2   Habitual postures and movements are created in childhood and shaped by ambitions, motivations, and stress.

There are great differences between the movements of children and those of adults. Children's movements are free, spontaneous, and open and are directed toward the exploration of their surroundings. In contrast, the movement of adults is often automatic and habitual and tends to shut us off from the outside world and from ourselves. Small children are much more flexible than adults and can easily accomplish all kinds of movements. They can, for example, constantly bend their backs during a game or sport, but they never develop a cramped pose and can easily straighten up when needed. Adults lose a lot of flexibility. Most adults have a diminished potential for movement, and most of the movements are ingrained and habitual.

The change in the quality of movement, from the open movements of childhood to the habitual movements of adulthood, starts early. School plays an important role here, as children *must* learn. In school, they are constantly evaluated on their achievements. This causes stress and causes them to develop ambitions, aspirations, fears, competition, and so on to deal with their environment. If these tactics fail, then all sorts of new strategies are created to cope with this unnatural pressure.

Children are made to sit for much of the day bent over books and this, in combination with the obligation to perform, can slowly cause the back to stiffen. This is the first step in the conditioning. Understandably, these obligations, ambitions, and pressures are all coupled with a tense posture and strained breathing.

The shift from the exploratory, open movement of young children to the controlling behavior of adults occurs slowly and may be unavoidable. Besides school, many social and psychological situations trigger this gradual change and stimulate the process of conditioning. A child's own ambitions also play a role, as do problematic situations, such as the imitation of idols and leaders of the group to which the child belongs. These situations are often combined with tension. Surprisingly, this also applies to playing sports—certainly to the competitive aspects, as we will see shortly.

Adulthood is really no different than our schooldays. The circumstances change and become the grown-up pressures of gainful employment, personal and professional rivalry, relationship problems, and so on. These stressful situations strengthen the already established conditioning caused by tension arising from fear, uncertainty, ambition, and desires, which further reinforces habitual movements. Frequent repetition of these movements ensures that they become ingrained patterns—our habitual postures and movements. Particular stress situations cause particular cramped movement patterns that can become so strong that cramped postures are adopted even during relaxation. People regularly pull up their shoulders and tighten all sorts of muscles when they are "relaxing," such as when watching a movie or socializing with friends.

Our friends and family recognize us from a distance because of our characteristic posture and movement. In the morning, when we get out of bed and support our body weight, all sorts of muscle chains are activated that return us to our characteristic posture. This phenomenon is known as the *postural reflex*. We often feel the most "at home" in our habitual postures and experience other movements as unusual, strange, or painful. Our habitual postures may even give us a strong feeling of identity, a feeling of "this is who I am." This is why movement therapies that are based on corrections during standing or sitting have such a difficult time breaking through flawed habits. Our immediate reaction to them is, "This is not me." Critical Alignment breaks through this process by using yoga exercises that constantly move our bodies into poses we don't use in our daily lives. Thus, we do not make any connection between them and our personal identity. This makes change less threatening.

At first, it seems strange that habitual posture and movement take on such a personal character. You would think that it would only be about the stiff upper back or the excessive lordosis many people experience, and that everyone would have similar conditions. This would imply that there are hardly any individual differences from one person to the next. However, at least one factor helps to determine the individual characteristics of habitual postures and movements, and that factor concerns the movement potential we inherit at birth. Consider physique and dexterity, as well as the strength and flexibility of bones, muscles, tendons, and connective tissue: these are all factors that differ from person to person. They are responsible for the differences that exist between people in their predisposition toward certain sports and other movement systems like dance, tai chi, and Hatha Yoga. They are also responsible for the differences in people's normal movements, such as walking, bending, cycling, and so on. Ingrained habitual movements, combined with inherited movement potential, lead to individual differences in habitual postures and movements.

Yoga exercises often confront your habitual postures and movements and thus your personal ambitions. As these usually have a long history, it means that you are confronted with your past in the form of stiffness and pain. However, yoga is not about psychoanalyzing your past. On the contrary, it is all about seeing yourself in the here and now and not walking away, even when the perceived image of yourself is difficult to accept.

Finally, I want to discuss two issues that have an important role in the development of habitual postures and movements—namely, stress and sports. I emphasize stress because it is prevalent and common. It is also partly responsible for the transformation of haphazardly developed habitual postures and movements into compulsive habits.

I have chosen to focus on sports and exercise because many people think that exercise is always healthy. It is my experience that participation in sports plays an important role in the development of habitual postures and movements.

Stress

Here, I want to discuss the development of *chronic* stress, which plays a major role in the development of habitual postures and movements. Chronic stress can develop relatively quickly as the result of an intense emotional event, such as losing a loved one or being involved in a car accident. However, chronic stress most often occurs slowly as the result of stressful situations that accumulate over the years. The psychological and social developments mentioned earlier also play an important role. The following explanation clarifies how "normal" stressful situations can, over time, lead to chronic stress. Let's start with a simple example to illustrate what sorts of situations cause the body to release stress hormones and what the effects are.

Imagine, you are crossing the street without looking both ways. Suddenly you hear a horn blasting and the screech of tires. A car manages to stop just before hitting you. Your adrenal glands immediately release a large amount of stress hormones into your blood. These hormones have two important effects. One is on your brain; this ensures that you experience a feeling of acute danger that forces you to run. The other is on your liver, which frees an enormous amount of glucose into your blood. Glucose provides the energy necessary to run for your life. Running away ensures that these sugars are used within a short period of time, so your blood sugar can return to normal levels. A similar situation occurs with the stress hormones that were released via the adrenal glands into the blood; running away causes the levels of these hormones to drop so that blood levels return to normal, and the stress is alleviated. This is called *stress release*. With this release, the body and mind can return to a relaxed state if the situation stays normal.

However, what happens to this stress when you are not able to neutralize it through vigorous physical activity? And what if a new stressful situation occurs when you are still in the previous stress response? For example, imagine you are totally stressed and working toward an important deadline; as soon as you have met that deadline, another is already looming, and you have no time to go for a brisk walk. In this situation, the sugars and hormones that have been released into your system cannot be neutralized. Tension remains high in your body and mind. When the next stressful situation arises on top of those already present, the stress hormones in the blood becomes more concentrated. If this cycle is repeated, the stress becomes steadily worse. At a certain point, it crosses a threshold and becomes chronic.

Chronic stress is common in our society and can lead to serious psychological and physical problems, such as burnout and depression. At school, at work, and at home, we are constantly confronted with stress in the form of irritations and arguments caused by our desire to achieve, demanding bosses, too many deadlines, poor working conditions, and/or emotional conflicts. All these situations result in stresses that are inadequately released and thus accumulate.

Stress not only has a negative effect on the mind, it also negatively influences posture and movement. The physical aspect of stress causes tension in the same muscles that have been affected and stiffened due to poor posture. In a habitual posture that constantly brings the body out of balance, some muscles are too short, and others are too long. This creates distortions in the skeleton. Stress, especially chronic stress, places these stiff muscles under even more pressure and causes the distortions to become permanent.

The distortions in the muscles and skeleton degenerate further and, in turn, affect other parts of the body. Because the pain threshold decreases, significant stress causes problems in the body to become agonizingly obvious. The body tries to avoid this pain by developing compensatory movements, and a downward spiral is created. Many people recognize this pattern in their own experience. High work pressure, for example, causes the body to become fragile, and problems are usually felt in weak areas. For some, it may be the lower back and for others, the neck or shoulders. It depends on the way we overload our body. The upper back, shoulders, and neck are well-known stress areas. The upper back often becomes stiff just under the shoulder blades and sometimes even develops an excessive kyphosis (rounding of the back). If stiffness increases in this area as a result of stress, the upper back just under the neck also tightens. The shoulders may stiffen and are pushed toward the neck. They also hang forward, limiting free movement of the ribs and chest and, as a result, breathing. If you sit a lot, the lack of mobility in your upper back will be compensated for in your neck. If you stand a lot, this immobility will occur in your lower back.

Physical problems related to stress have a mental component too; it is not really apparent where one ends and the other begins. The connection is complicated and usually has a long history that makes it difficult to determine the cause and see where changes should be made. The resulting feeling of powerlessness may be an additional stress factor.

A popular belief is that stress is necessary to perform effectively. This is true. A little stress increases concentration, motivation, and efficiency. But it is only harmless when it is minimal and temporary. Otherwise, the stresses multiply and become chronic. We are all confronted regularly with stress, in our relationships with partners, children, colleagues, and so on, and we must learn how to deal with it. A lot of attention is given in this book to a healthy alternative to stress—that is, alertness, based on the fundamental strength of relaxation.

Sports and Exercise
During the last century, Western culture has developed the belief that sports and exercise are the ultimate activities for positively influencing health. Indeed, for many people sporting activities are an important mode of movement and a superb way to balance a life that consists of long hours of inactivity or repetitive movements during work time.

Sports can be fun, but are they also healthy? Of course, vigorous play increases circulation, lung capacity, and body confidence, and it can also lower stress levels.

On the other hand, nearly all sports require strength that can only be developed by the constant contraction of muscles, which results in the systematic reduction of mobility. This applies to professional athletes as well as to amateurs who play competitive sports. Even though there is constant movement, certain parts of the body gradually become less flexible. The superficial movement muscles become so strong that the function of the postural muscles gradually diminishes. The long-term result is that the movement muscles become shorter and stiffer, and circulation to them decreases. These are clearly the first steps on the road to malformations of the skeleton. Over time, habitual postures and movements are formed that may ultimately not be healthy or beneficial

Stiffness is the first complaint that many athletes have. The areas of stiffness depend on the sport. Generally, football and soccer players have stiff legs and backs; tennis players develop stiffness in their backs and the shoulder and arm with which they hold their racket. Swimmers develop stiff upper and lower backs, and runners develop stiff lower backs, hips, legs, and knees. The common factor is that hardly any circulation is seen in the skin of the affected areas. Circulation is not even increased during yoga exercises that are meant to stimulate these areas.

3.3 Critical Alignment can stop the negative effects of habitual posture and movement patterns and restore the total experience of movement.

Movements and postures that are linked with ambitions, fears and other desire based complexes occur unconsciously. Critical Alignment offers a solution to stop these negative developments. It creates the space that is needed in order to recognize the unconscious negative process. This makes it possible to take action.

The goal of yoga practice is the conscious relaxation of the movement muscles. Then the postural muscles and related parts of the skeleton can stretch and pass movement along through the movement chains from one part of the body to the next (see chapter 2.4.1 for a detailed description of these processes). Yoga exercises force us into an intense confrontation with ourselves, because they are both difficult and painful, and above all, they are the total opposite of our normal (automatic) way of moving.

To practice yoga correctly, open awareness and attention are necessary. It is only through open and passive attention that we can see what our intention is during yoga practice. Otherwise, we remain in our automatic drives of ambition, fear, competitiveness, and so on, even when we practice. The danger then exists that yoga becomes yet another automatic, habitual movement.

When we perform the exercises correctly, we create space and energy in our body. This makes it possible to experience subtle qualities of movement and to be conscious of the time and space we are in. We experience the information that specific yoga exercises provide from the inside out—that is, from our body. Initially, we will not receive much more information than superficial feelings of pain or restriction. But as relaxation increases during the exercises, our body becomes more flexible, which then amplifies our physical sensitivity and ability to experience more subtle information.

As mentioned earlier, we can experience not only movement but also the time and space around us. This means that to have the total experience of movement, our awareness must be directed within and without. This consciousness is generally absent in habitual movements, but it is something we can cultivate. Only through this higher consciousness is it possible to become aware of the flow of information in our body together with our environment. If we do not have higher consciousness, we are either lost in the outside world or locked inside ourselves.

Experiencing both ourselves and our environment can be compared to driving a car. Our hands and feet are constantly busy controlling the speed and direction of the car. We are conscious of space and time (if we are not acting automatically). During the constant act of driving (acceleration, changing gears, steering, braking, and so on), we are continuously aware of the traffic situation—the space around us—and constantly react to changes in the situation. When we practice yoga, we are not driving from place A to destination B, but we are moving from pose A to pose B. During movement, we must apply the techniques in the correct way in order to achieve our final pose. Simultaneously, we are totally aware of the speed with which we move and the space around us, creating movement that has an open and free quality.

The following explanation will show the correct approach when practicing yoga and how the exercises can be used to develop higher consciousness.

Paschimottanasana: correct and incorrect ways to achieve open awareness

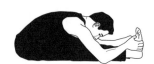

3.3-1

I have chosen Paschimottanasana (Seated Forward Bend; figure 3.3-1 and also chapter 10.5, number 6) because it is an exercise that most beginners cannot do correctly the first time, and it can be painful for both new and experienced students. This pose forces you to confront your abilities and limits and helps you see how you cope with the exercise. Do you avoid pain by doing the exercise poorly and incompletely? Or do you rely on willpower, again doing the exercise incorrectly? What is the correct mental attitude, and how can this be achieved?

The stomach and chest are pressed against the outstretched legs in Paschimottanasana. Because the back and leg muscles are usually too stiff to achieve such an extreme stretch, it is typically an extremely painful experience. This stiffness and pain are such great obstacles that almost everyone who does Paschimottanasana for the first time reacts emotionally. One reaction is that people are shocked and recoil back to the starting position. Another is that they stay in position but adopt a half-forward bend to avoid the pain; they are just waiting for the cue to come out of the pose. A third reaction is that they stay in the pose at whatever cost. They defy the pain and force their body into the pose—"no pain, no gain." A fourth option is to go into the pose, move no farther than the threshold of tolerable pain, and try to relax into this place. Then it becomes possible to see the nature of the reaction and what must be done, or not done, to develop the stretch.

These reactions reflect our motives and their attached habitual postures and movements, which can take over during yoga. In the first reaction, fear is the driving force; the second reaction reveals avoidance and pretense—for example, pretending to perform the pose by doing a half bend instead. The result of both of these reactions is that nothing develops that can dissipate the tension and pain in the long term.

In the third reaction, ambition and competitiveness are the driving force that leads to the application of brute force. The body is irritated rather than stimulated by this force. Too much effort leads to too much pain. You have to back off to avoid acute lower back pain or overstretched muscles. Working too hard is driven by willpower and has nothing to do with relaxation. Here, the art is to stand face-to-face with your ambition or competitiveness.

In the fourth reaction—the correct one—an open-minded, passive attention to the body is developed. You create an all-encompassing awareness where you can simultaneously observe yourself and your motives and consciously experience the qualities of the asana. Stretches such as Paschimottanasana are superb means for discovering how you cope with asanas. Too little effort, as seen in the first two reactions, leads to nothing. You have to go further, until you clearly feel the pain but it is still tolerable. Only then do you come face-to-face with fear, avoidance, or substituting easier poses. Without trying to push these reactions away or avoiding the pain, you stay in the asana with an open attention and as little pain as possible.

Even when you cannot fully complete the exercises, the right sort of exertion will always be rewarded. That is to say, you can consciously encounter your unconscious motivations and habitual movements. Relaxation is an important factor and has everything to do with balance, pressure, breathing, and attention. These are some of the building blocks from the protocol for practicing asanas (see chapter 2.4.1 for more details).

In Paschimottanasana, the lower back must be active. Proper use of the lower back ensures that the hips are used correctly, which in turn reduces the tension in the lower back, hips, and hamstrings. These dynamics ensure that the stomach, chest, shoulders, and neck can relax. Correct dynamics lead to creating space in the body, while the other "solutions" lead to contraction and restriction.

When practicing asanas, it is difficult to make a clear distinction between right exertion and overexertion. When we adopt a position, we exert our body by applying pressure to certain parts. In Paschimottanasana, we apply pressure to the hips (if we use the lower back correctly), thus creating more freedom of movement. This causes the pelvis to tilt, which creates more stretch in the leg muscles. The process is supported by breathing. The exhalation is directed toward the muscles that need to relax; it makes them soft so the dynamics of the body can steadily bring us deeper into the pose. Because it is directed to specific areas, our attention zooms in on them.

If your hips or legs are stiff, overload can easily occur in Paschimottanasana simply by pulling too hard on your legs. This causes not only pain but also an undesirable change in your breathing, and an important means for supporting relaxation is lost. Breathing becomes irregular and shallow. In addition, pulling too hard on your legs often leads to a lot of tension in your shoulders. This is the start of a battle with the exercise and carries with it a high risk of injury.

Relaxation is nonexistent in such an approach. Habits and ambitions, accompanied by willpower, want to dominate and control. So the will to achieve, competitiveness, and so on take over again.

As mentioned earlier, stress—especially chronic stress—is an important factor in promoting the development of habitual postures and movements. For this reason, I want to devote a separate section to the role that Critical Alignment can have in managing stress.

Stress management

Chronic stress negatively affects not only the psyche, as in depression and burnout, but also body posture and movement (see chapter 3.2). Stress management must occur at two levels: the psychological and the physical. However, hardly any therapies teach stress management techniques that direct attention to these two areas. Most therapies concentrate solely on one level.

Moreover, it is remarkable that the physical body gets so little attention in stress management systems. Psychotherapy is primarily focused on changing behavior, and the few methods that consider the body are focused on simple relaxation techniques, occasionally combined with easy breathing exercises. Only a handful of therapies prescribe vigorous physical activity to people with chronic stress. As mentioned earlier, vigorous physical activity lowers the concentration of stress hormones in the blood, allowing both the body and mind to relax. Whether or not these people learn how to actively manage their stress is questionable; exercise and activity may become a crutch.

Critical Alignment tackles chronic stress on both psychological and physical levels. The correct attitude when practicing asanas allows us to come face to face with our ambitions and stress, resulting in Critical Alignment also having a healing effect on the physical consequences of stress.

Practicing asanas is a totally different approach than that used during passive relaxation exercises. Admittedly, relaxation exercises can provide temporary respite for the body and mind, such as what is achieved with a good massage or a sauna. In these situations, relaxation is linked to a feeling of tiredness and sleep. But this kind of relaxation is generally not maintained in active situations. Passive relaxation exercises do not change flawed muscle patterns or get rid of stress, they just alleviate it temporarily.

In conclusion

Critical Alignment allows us to reawaken our awareness of the subtleties and qualities of movement and of the space and time in which they occur. This applies immediately to yoga movements, but we can strive to apply it to our everyday movements as well. (Higher consciousness is elaborated on in chapter 5.) Next, I would like to consider the logical outcome of habitual postures and movements, the physical malformations, and how Critical Alignment can rectify them.

4

MALFORMATIONS

4.1 Introduction

The word *malformations* obviously has a negative connotation, which is not intended here. The message of this book is not that you must learn to live with malformations but that body malformations are usually not permanent, which means that total or at least partial recovery is almost always possible. If, for example, you have had a bent upper back for many years, the constant pressure on the front of the vertebrae and the intervertebral discs would cause a wedge-shaped formation. These vertebrae and discs are not damaged and can return to their original shape once correct use of the spine is reestablished. That is, your bent back can become straight after pressure is applied to the rear of the vertebrae. The Critical Alignment method can play an important role in this recovery.

4.2 Natural predispositions, emotions, and lifestyle define the mobility and balance of the body.

Small children differ greatly from each other in their posture: the curve of the upper back, stiffness in the shoulders, a hollow lower back, and so on. Preferred postures are evident at an early age, as are personality traits. Children can naturally be quick-tempered, fearful, quiet, angry, sluggish, or mischievous. These emotional tendencies have an influence on the development of the muscular system and posture. Dreamy, relaxed children develop physically in a totally different manner than quick-tempered, energetic children. Open, enthusiastic children develop differently than timid ones. We all develop our dispositions partly because of genetic traits and partly because of the environment in which we grow up.

The family situation is crucial, and the characteristics of parents and siblings play an important role. The parents' own physical development has most likely followed a similar pattern. They pass this on partially through posture and partially through their behavior toward their children. This is why family members often have strong physical similarities. When physical problems develop, you often hear people say, "It runs in the family." Although this is true, there is often a tone of resignation in the statement, as if the problem is genetic. Actually, the problem is mostly the result of copying the posture and behavior of the parents, so change and recovery are possible. Different personality traits also cause certain abnormalities to develop in muscular patterns. Some children develop too much tension, others too little. This has consequences for the development and condition of the body in later years.

Muscle length and the suppleness of joints are important as well. Genetic predispositions and life circumstances play important roles here. Some adults can place their leg behind their neck without ever having done yoga. Some children have a natural aptitude for the Lotus Pose, while others experience extreme pain during even a modest attempt. Further individual differences can also arise following illness or accidents, and some people are more prone than others to develop physical problems.

These problems can take on serious forms, such as radiating nerve pain, impaired mobility, lack of circulation, ruptured discs, and repetitive strain injury. These are health threats and often lead to an inability to work. For this reason, they must be treated therapeutically.

A bent or hollow lower back, scoliosis (curvature of the spine), and rotations in the spine are some of the most frequent distortions that cause these problems. I define such health threatening distortions of the physical body as malformations. Sometimes no obvious abnormality is visible, but even then, the problem can give rise to a serious health risk. Because of the problems such a situation can cause, this is also a malformation.

4.3 Malformations often have a long and complicated history.

Malformations develop for a variety of reasons, but some causes are more prevalent than others. Most malformations are caused by habitual postures and movements; congenital malformations and those caused by accidents are much less common.

Those caused by habitual postures and movements have a long history in which physical, psychological, and social influences play important roles. Together with stress, they often cause stiffness to start developing in parts of the skeleton, often at an early age. This can lead to rotations and stiffness in the skeleton. Over time, these blockages can develop into malformations with their associated problems. They can initiate compensatory movements in other parts of the movement chains that then overload other areas of the body. (For a detailed description of the causes that lead to malformations, see chapters 2 and 3.)

Thus, compensatory movements and new blockages can develop far away from the malformations. For example, the pain and movement problems that develop in one of the legs as the result of a ruptured disc can ensure that the other (healthy) leg is overused and thus develops problems as well. Pain in the hands and arms that results from malformations in the upper back can easily lead to compensatory movements to relieve the pain. These compensatory movements, in turn, cause their own blockages in other areas of the movement chains and additional problems. For instance, when the upper back is stiff (first level) we need to release our core stability in order to stand up straight. This release produces tension in the lower back (second level), but further down, the hips can become painful and stiff (third level) because the lower back does not properly transport the movement or body weight toward the pelvis floor and hips.

4.4 The nervous system

A great deal of the complexity and diversity in malformations is due to the anatomical organization of the skeletal and nervous systems. Both the spine and the peripheral nervous system have a *segmented* organization that I want to consider in detail because it is important for understanding malformations and the problems arising from them.

Blockages in the spine can be found in single or multiple vertebrae. Reduced mobility in the spine hampers the function of the nervous system. There are thirty openings in the spinal column through which nerves exit: eight in the neck, twelve in the thoracic spine, five in the lumbar spine, and five in the sacrum. Nerves require space when exiting the spinal column, and this space is optimally maintained through movement. If the back stiffens, this can have serious consequences for the flexibility of the (muscle) tissue around the nerves and impinge on the free space the nerves need to function properly. Nerves can become partially or totally compressed, hampering their ability to pass along impulses.

Because there are so many nerve outlets and blockages can occur at different places, there is a wide diversity in the locations where and degree to which compressed nerves can develop. The extent of the stiffening of muscles and vertebrae determines the seriousness of the malformations and the resulting conditions.

Problems can develop in places that are far removed from the malformations. Abnormalities in the neck can affect the nerves that innervate* the arms. These nerves can become pinched or damaged where they exit the neck vertebrae, and pain and other problems can develop in the hands and arms. Problems can develop in the lungs as well because these nerves innervate the lungs.

Another (rare) source of complexity occurs when congenital deformities and traumas resulting from accidents combine with habitual postures and movements to create complex malformations.

The following is a short description of the organization and function of the skeletal and nervous systems to simplify understanding of malformations and the problems they cause. A lot of attention will be given to the spinal column, because the majority of the nerves that innervate the muscles originate there, as do the nerves that innervate the head, lungs, and other internal organs.

---

* During pregnancy, nerves grow from the central nervous system of the embryo to the muscles and other organs so that electrical currents originating from the central nervous system can reach the organs to control their activity. This contact between the nerves and organs is called *innervation*. It is because of the innervations of our muscles that we can move at will.

In a four-week-old embryo, the segmented organization of the body is already clear.

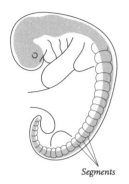

Segments

4.4.1 The spine and the nervous system are organized in segments.

During the early embryonic stage, a human being develops a segmented* body structure (figure 4.4.1-1). As the embryo grows, these segments partially disappear. The spinal column, however, remains segmented even in maturity. The ribs and their intercostal muscles reveal clear remnants of their segmented origin.

The spine consists of series of more or less identical vertebrae, all of which have a clear form and function. These are the cervical, thoracic, lumbar, and sacral vertebrae (figure 4.4.1-2).

All the vertebral bodies have a ringlike structure, and together they form the spinal column, which encompasses the spinal cord. One pair of nerves springs from the spinal cord at the level of each vertebra (figure 4.4.1-3).

After exiting the spinal column, these nerves proceed ventrally (along the front) and dorsally (along the back) within the body to innervate muscles and organs (figure 4.4.1-4). The nerves are named after the vertebrae from which they exit. There are eight pairs of

* During early development, the embryo consists largely of a series of almost uniform parts, or segments (figure 4.4.1-1). This is a way to create length in the body that is also seen in many other animals. Some, such as insects and crabs, remain clearly segmented even in maturity. In human beings, the segmented parts disappear at an early stage, and at birth, there is almost no trace left: ultimately, it is only a few structures, like the ribs and spinal column, that more or less retain their original segmentation.

4.4.1-2 Anterior, lateral, and posterior views of the spinal column showing the cervical, thoracic, lumbar, and sacral vertebrae.

4.4.1-3 Schematic view of different segments of the spinal column

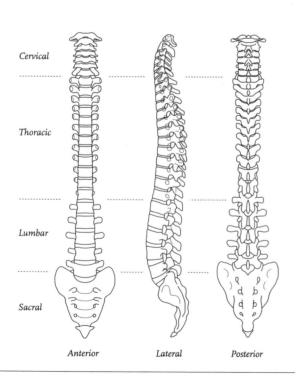

Cervical

Thoracic

Lumbar

Sacral

Anterior Lateral Posterior

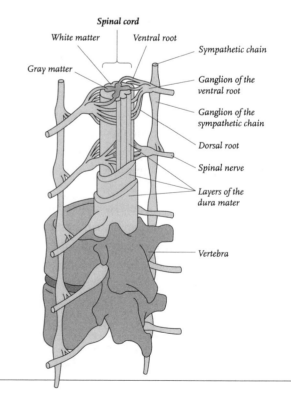

cervical nerves, twelve pairs of thoracic nerves, five pairs of lumbar nerves, and five pairs of sacral nerves.

The innervation pattern of the skin is noteworthy. The sensory nerves (those that give information about temperature, pressure, stretch, and so on to the brain) from the spinal column innervate the skin in striped formations called *dermatomes* (figure 4.4.1-5). When the limbs are fully grown, it looks as if these dermatomes are malformed. However, when viewed from the side, a person bending over shows that this is not the case (figure 4.4.1-6). The dermatomes are important for the diagnosis of functional impairments (discussed later in this chapter).

Besides skin, these nerves innervate muscles and connective tissue. This means that when nerves are pinched or damaged, the muscles they innervate can suffer a loss of strength. The skeleton and internal organs are also innervated in segments.

The body is divided into central and peripheral sections. The brain belongs to the central section, while all other organs and structures (skin, muscles, digestive system, limbs, and so on) belong to the peripheral section. Nerves that exit the spinal column belong to the peripheral section, as they innervate organs that are situated outside the brain. Therefore, the spinal nerves belong to the peripheral nervous system. In contrast, the nerves that function exclusively within the brain, such as the optic nerves, belong to the central nervous system.

Let's briefly discuss the organization and function of the peripheral nervous

4.4.1-4

Posterior view of the body showing the various sections of the spine and their nerves. C = cervical; T = thoracic; L = lumbar; S = sacral; Co = coccyx.

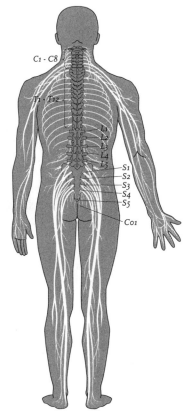

4.4.1-5 Illustration of the dermatomes. C = cervical; T = thoracic; L = lumbar; S = sacral.

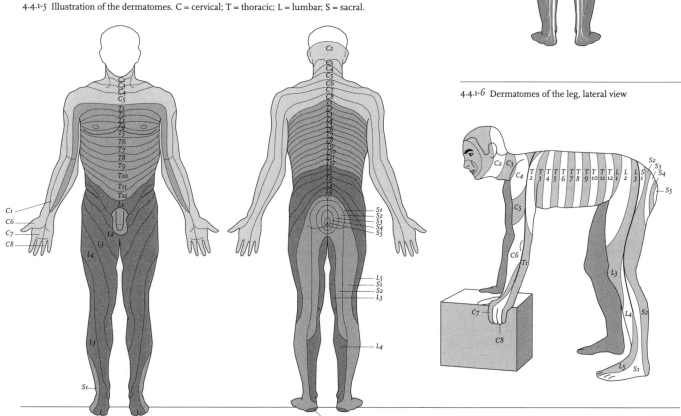

4.4.1-6 Dermatomes of the leg, lateral view

system, which consists of two parts: the *somatic* (physical; figure 4.4.1-7) and the *auto-nomic* (independent; figure 4.4.1-8).

The somatic peripheral nervous system

All spinal column nerves that innervate skin, joints, and muscles and are under our *voluntary* control belong to the somatic peripheral nervous system. This system consists of two parts—motor and sensor—and is sometimes called the somatosensory system.

The *motor component* provides contraction of the muscles and movement of the skeleton and is thus essential for the generation of movement. These motor nerves descend from the brain through the spinal column and exit via the ventral roots to innervate the muscles (see figure 4.4.1-7).

The *sensory component* innervates the skin, muscles, and joints and collects information about temperature, pressure, and so on from these structures. This information is then transported by the sensory nerves via the dorsal roots to the spinal column and farther up to the brain (see figure 4.4.1-8).

The *receptors* (the parts that receive the signals from the sensory system) are continuously giving information about the position of the body; pressure in the joints; and pressure, friction, temperature stimuli, and so on to the skin. Sensory information is then sent to the cortex of the brain where it is assembled in the sensory area. This area reflects the sensory body and is organized in the same way as the body itself, with the head, trunk, and limbs (figures 4.4.1-9a and b). However, the form of this sensory body is not in true proportion to the physical body. Some parts, such as the hands, fingers, and lips, are much larger. Other areas, such as the trunk, are relatively small. This reflects

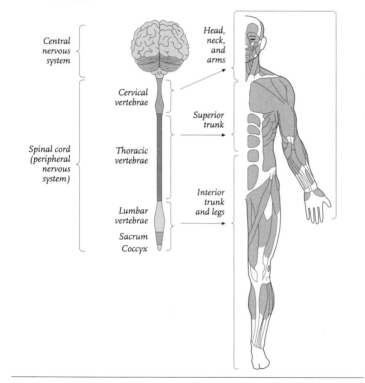

4.4.1-7 Overview of the somatic peripheral nervous system and the muscles that it innervates

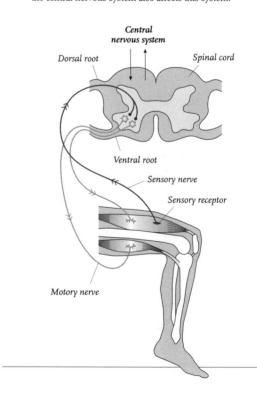

4.4.1-8 The peripheral nervous system of the somatosensory system has a sensory and motor nerve component. It has been shown that the central nervous system also affects this system.

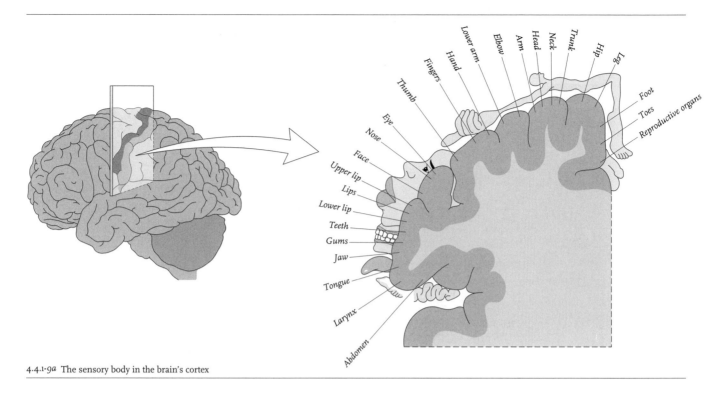

4.4.1-9a The sensory body in the brain's cortex

the density of the receptors in the different parts of the body. The fingers have an especially large number of receptors, which makes them very sensitive. As a result, they occupy a relatively large area of the brain. On the other hand, the receptor density in the trunk is small, making it somewhat insensitive. This is mirrored by a smaller representation in the brain.

The initial processing of sensory information is done in the sensory cortex. It is here that we become conscious of our posture and movement, physical contact, and so on. This information is then integrated with sensory information from other sources such as the eyes and ears. It can also be combined with information about possible danger, how we are moving, and the space around us.

Sensory information may be integrated within the motor system, making precise adjustments in our posture and movements possible. If we remain open to this information, we can use it constantly when practicing yoga.

We could say that that our body makes itself known to us in two ways: through visual observation from outside via the eyes, and from within via the sensory system and the brain. This stream of information becomes more conscious and increases proportionally as the body is better able to relax. In other words, when the body can perform yoga exercises through the postural muscles, thereby releasing compressed nerves and enabling information to flow freely, it leads to greater sensitivity, and we are able to observe more precisely.

4.4.1-9b

The sensory body is illustrated here in three dimensions to show how the receptor density varies in different organs.

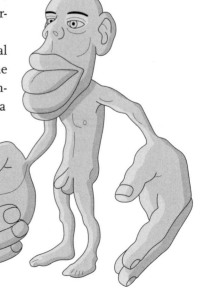

The autonomic (or visceral) peripheral nervous system

This system contains the nerves that innervate the internal organs, veins, and glands. Sensory nerves pass on information about the functioning of the organs, such as blood pressure and oxygen saturation of the blood, to the brain. The motor nerves from this system influence the contraction

The organization and functions of the sympathetic nervous system and the parasympathetic nervous system of the autonomic nervous system. It is important to recognize that these systems are opposite to each other and have opposite effects on the body.

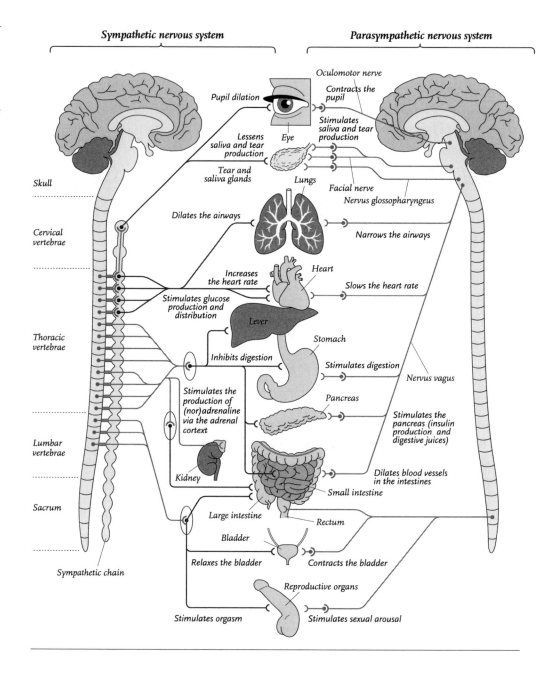

Sympathetic nervous system — Parasympathetic nervous system

Pupil dilation
Oculomotor nerve
Contracts the pupil
Stimulates saliva and tear production
Lessens saliva and tear production
Eye
Skull
Tear and saliva glands
Lungs
Facial nerve
Nervus glossopharyngeus
Cervical vertebrae
Dilates the airways
Narrows the airways
Increases the heart rate
Heart
Slows the heart rate
Stimulates glucose production and distribution
Lever
Thoracic vertebrae
Inhibits digestion
Stomach
Stimulates digestion
Nervus vagus
Stimulates the production of (nor)adrenaline via the adrenal cortex
Pancreas
Stimulates the pancreas (insulin production and digestive juices)
Lumbar vertebrae
Kidney
Dilates blood vessels in the intestines
Small intestine
Large intestine
Rectum
Sacrum
Bladder
Relaxes the bladder
Contracts the bladder
Sympathetic chain
Reproductive organs
Stimulates orgasm
Stimulates sexual arousal

and relaxation of muscles in the veins, intestines, heart, and so on. They influence secretions in both sweat and hormonal glands. This all occurs outside our control, or automatically.

The autonomic peripheral nervous system has two components: the *sympathetic system* and the *parasympathetic system*. These two systems are anatomically separate, as figure 4.4.1-10 clearly shows. They do, however, innervate the same organs. The sympathetic nerves exit the spinal column from the ventral roots of the vertebrae in pairs, and they branch out and innervate the organs via the sympathetic ganglia. They exit the thoracic and lumbar vertebrae of the spinal column. The parasympathetic (cranial) nerves exit the brain stem and the sacral segment of the spinal column (described later).

The two systems often act on the body in opposite ways; therefore, they must be coordinated precisely. A good example of this is the regulation of organs during times of stress. During stress, the sympathetic system regulates not only the secretion of stress hormones from the adrenal glands and the increase in heart rate and blood pressure but also the simultaneous decrease in the activity of the digestive system. When the stress situation has ended, the activity of the sympathetic system lessens, and the parasympathetic system becomes active. This leads to a reduction in the secretion of stress hormones, heart rate, and blood pressure, as well as a resumption of activity in the digestive system (compare this with chapter 3.2).

The peripheral autonomic nervous system is remarkable in that it regulates the activity of many organs simultaneously. Information about the condition of the internal organs is constantly passed on to the brain, which then regulates them as necessary.

The pain system
Pain receptors are located all over the body, except for the nerve tissue of the brain. Pain signals are transported via the dorsal nerve roots to the spinal column and on up to the brain, where the pain is recognized and processed as a feeling.

The cranial nerves
In addition to the nerves that exit the spinal column, there are also twelve pairs of cranial nerves. These spring from the brain stem and innervate mainly, but not only, the head. Some (such as the optic nerve) belong to the central nervous system, while others (such as the vagus nerve) are part of the somatic or autonomic peripheral nervous systems (see figure 4.4.1-10).

Two important conclusions can be taken from this short summary of the organization and function of the peripheral nervous system. One concerns the segmented character of functional impairments and their resulting complexity. The second concerns the physical (that is, material) basis of our consciousness.

Conclusion 1. Functional impairments have (secondary) segmented characteristics.
It is now obvious that malformations can simultaneously affect numerous functions in the peripheral nervous system. It will also be obvious that functional impairments (taking into account the organization of the peripheral nervous system) have segmented characteristics. Functional disturbances can affect one or more groups of nerves. The intensity and area of pain, loss of strength, and/or numbness all depend on where and how many nerves are compressed and the degree of compression. Problems can therefore have varying degrees of intensity and can occur in different areas of the body.

Functional disturbances have causes not only at the root level but also farther along the neural pathways, such as in the shoulder girdle, arms, or legs. Disturbances at the root level are mostly due to misalignment of the spine. For example, the nerve that springs out between the fifth and sixth cervical vertebrae controls, among other things, the strength of the biceps (the muscles located on the upper arm; figure 4.4.1-11). Root-level impairment to this nerve due to a misaligned spine can cause weakened biceps as well as other problems. However, functional disturbances in the periphery of the body (such as weakened biceps) are not necessarily caused by problems at the root level; they can also result from too much tension in the peripheral movement muscles that can, in turn, compress nerves.

Dermatomes are important for diagnosing functional disturbances in the peripheral nervous system (and damage to the spine). A loss of sensitivity in certain dermatomes

4.4.1-11

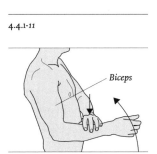

Biceps

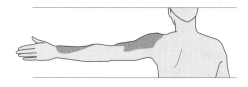

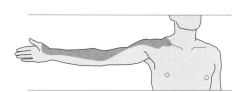

points to a functional disturbance in the nerves exiting the spine at the level of that dermatome. For instance, if the nerves in the shoulder girdle are pinched due to muscle tension, this can cause tingling and numbness to the skin in the fingers.

Some dermatomes extend over a significant length of skin; thus conditions can cause pain in areas remote from the inflammation. For example, during an acute phase of arthritis (inflammation) in the shoulder joint, movement of the shoulder can cause pain in the lower arm, wrist, and hand. This is explained by the fact that the fifth dermatome covers the capsule of the shoulder joint and the skin of the neck, lower arm, wrist, and hand (figure 4.4.1-12). Compression to the nerves at the level of the shoulder capsule caused by the arthritis results in a radiating pain to the arm and neck.

Conclusion 2: Our experiences are completely anchored in our body.
The second important conclusion elaborates further on chapter 3.1—that is, the total experience of movement within space and time. As shown earlier, our movements are constantly monitored by the peripheral nervous system and passed on to the central nervous system. This is also true for the autonomic nervous system and the pain system, which monitor and pass on information regarding the condition and health of the organs to the central nervous system. This information is continuously integrated within the sensory cortex, together with information from the senses and other areas of the brain. Hence, the experience of movement and information about the condition of the body unite with the experience of space and time. This gives us a total experience of our self that is strongly anchored in our body.

When seen in this way, there is no body-mind dualism in which the experience of space and time is attributed to the mind and the experience of movement is attributed to the body. Also, there is no mind-matter dualism, as all of our experiences are developed through physical (or material) processes. These are the processes that occur in the organs and in the peripheral, autonomic, and central nervous systems. Elaborating further on this important point, it is easy to see that malformations and their resulting blockages and functional impairments to the peripheral and autonomic nervous systems can have a negative effect on the total experience of our posture and movement and, more importantly, on our experience of our self.

The preceding has important consequences for the execution and experience of yoga asanas. An interesting sort of tension develops between the head (thinking and memory) and the body (feeling) during the execution of movement. I will discuss this later in detail when I explain the asanas. It is enough to state here that the balance between the three elements of thinking, memory, and feeling must be finely tuned during the execution of yoga poses:

· We acquire the necessary information and knowledge about the technical aspect of the exercise through thinking. This insight must be developed before we initiate movement, as it shows us the areas where we must "zoom in" before we move.
· Subsequently, we place this knowledge in the framework of our earlier experiences that have developed a physical feeling we try to recall. This, too, occurs prior to movement.

· Thereafter, we initiate the movement and let go of these aspects. They do not disappear, however; we keep them in the back of our mind in order to connect with the direct experience of our movement. Thus, we track (or monitor) the movement, directing our attention toward our body. The result is that we receive direct and clear information that can be adjusted according to the image, thought, idea, and memory of which we maintain awareness. The experience of movement is material, because the body itself, not thinking, is the source of this information. The stream of information from memories, feelings, and thinking often mix together; the art is to keep them separate and use them in the right order.

As a logical continuation to this sequence, the next section comprises a short discussion on malformations and their resulting ailments. Chapter 4.6 discusses the correction of malformations and the treatment of complaints.

4.5 Malformations can be divided into a small number of groups, each with a large number of ailments.

Considering the complexity of the malformations, it seems best to keep the descriptions straightforward by grouping them into three categories. The first comprises malformations in the frontal plane of the body (anterior/posterior abnormalities); the second comprises malformations in the sagittal, or vertical, plane (lateral abnormalities); and the third comprises malformations that are a combination of the two (rotations).

The following gives examples from each category. I have limited myself to malformations that occur frequently and that I regularly treat therapeutically. I have also given examples of common complaints caused by malformations.

The three categories of malformations

Anterior/posterior malformations
The stereotypical pattern of malformations in the upper back begins with the collapse of the lower part of the sternum: the heart region—the center of our emotions. It is not coincidence that the bending of the upper back begins at the same time that children change from feeling beings with free bodily movement and open posture whose hearts and stomachs dominate to children who are more cognitively orientated and whose heads start to dominate. The head literally moves forward; the sternum collapses and virtually pushes the heart deeper inside.

The bent upper back (figure 4.5-1) and the hollow (figure 4.5-2) and flat (figure 4.5-3) lower back all belong to the typical and frequent malformations that occur in the frontal plane. The events leading to these malformations have been discussed in previous chapters.

In the case of the bent upper back, the transfer of small movements is blocked at this level so that larger movements, like standing up, cannot be accomplished freely. To make these movements possible, the body often uses the lower back in a cramped manner, pulling it into a concave position or flattening it. The neck also becomes concave and excessively mobile.

4.5-1

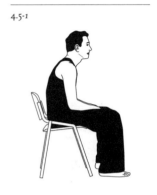

4.5-2

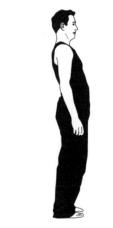

4.5-3

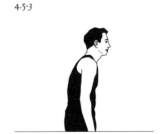

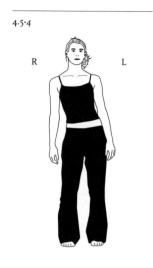

4.5-4

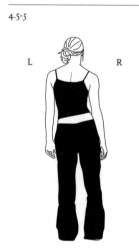

4.5-5

Lateral malformations

Lateral malformations often cause noticeable differences between the left and right sides of the body. Left- or right-handedness plays an important role here. In right-handed people, the right shoulder is often noticeably lower and more forward than the left (figure 4.5-4). In left-handed people, it is usually the opposite, although there are always exceptions.

The unevenness of the shoulders has a deeper cause that becomes clear when they are relaxed. The superficial tension in the shoulders disappears, but the underlying irregularity remains, showing that shoulder angle is just the tip of the iceberg. There is an underlying asymmetry in the position of the vertebrae, ribs, and/or pelvis. The lumbar vertebrae can often move more easily in one direction than the other. This is also the situation with the thoracic spine and ribs.

Similar mechanisms to those discussed in the anterior/posterior malformations (formation of local blockages and the onset of compensatory movements that in turn cause their own blockages) cause lateral malformations as well.

When standing, the legs also develop their own preferential posture. We often stand on one leg (usually the same one) when we have to wait, causing a lateral asymmetry in our pelvis and lower back (figure 4.5-5). This is frequently diagnosed as a "leg-length discrepancy." I have seen many a leg "grow" during my treatment of such complaints.

Rotations

Rotations are combinations of anterior/posterior and lateral asymmetries. The same physical mechanisms discussed in these categories of malformations play a role in the development of rotations.

Rotations predominantly affect the position of the ribs and vertebrae. They can have serious consequences for the costovertebral joints (the two joints which connect the rib with the vertebrae), which can become blocked from the asymmetry. This can have a negative impact on the free movement of the upper body and on the ability to breathe freely. This sort of blockage often makes people feel that, during a deep breath, they miss part of the movement and consequently part of their breath.

Common complaints caused by malformations

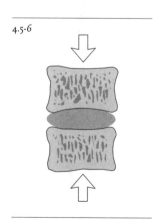

4.5-6

Most complaints related to these malformations are caused by functional disorders of the nerves and/or blood vessels, often at the root level. Such disorders are initially the result of malformations in the spine and subsequently due to tightness in the surrounding muscles. Typically, we feel these problems not only in the spine, but also in other areas of our body such as our arms and hands or our legs and feet. This is because the nerves and blood vessels, whose function is impaired at the spine, innervate these organs and supply them with blood. Thus, disturbances at the root level of nerves and/or blood vessels have logical negative effects in other, remote areas. We know this as referred pain (see chapter 2).

As we shall see, it is not that one type of malformation leads to a certain complaint but that many sorts of malformations can lead to the same complaint. The opposite is also true: different problems can originate from one sort of malformation.

Repetitive Strain Injuries

Problems that develop in the shoulders, neck, and arms are collectively known as repetitive strain injury (RSI), or complaints of the arm, neck, and/or shoulder (CANS). RSI is an older term that was originally used to describe an overload of certain body parts created by repetition of the same movement, which resulted in such things as tennis elbow or carpal tunnel syndrome. Lower back problems also belong to this category. They are not necessarily caused by excessive movement but rather by lack of movement. A good example is the "mouse arm" with radiating pain in the arm, neck, and shoulder. Loss of strength in the arm muscles and pain in the lower arm and wrist can be symptoms of this complaint, which is caused by a stiffening of the back combined with asymmetry in the vertebrae. This comes from continuously sitting in the same position. High work pressure, deadlines, and stress do the rest. RSI complaints are good examples of problems that originate from different types of malformations in the neck and the upper and/or lower back.

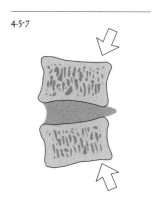

Spinal disc herniation

Our posture has an effect on the muscles of our back and the position and flexibility of our vertebrae and intervertebral discs. In a good posture, the thickness of the front of the intervertebral discs is equal to that of the back, as seen in figure 4.5-6. The outside of the intervertebral discs has a strength that can be compared to a car tire. The inside contains a jellylike ball called the *nucleus*.

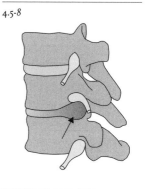

If the back is malformed, such as in a rounded lower back that cannot straighten properly anymore, the shape of the local intervertebral discs changes. In a rounded lower back, the front of the disc gets thinner and (together with the nucleus) gets pushed backward as the weight of the body rests on the front of the disc, as shown in figure 4.5-7. If this situation continues for years, the intervertebral discs will become chronically distorted. In the worst-case scenario, as the bulging increases, the intervertebral disc ruptures, allowing the nucleus to protrude (see the arrow in figure 4.5-8).

Spinal disc herniations are caused by ruptures in the intervertebral disc. A rupture can cause nerve compression that initially causes a radiating pain and, in later stages, can lead to a serious loss of strength and sometimes a total loss of control of one leg. Herniated discs mostly develop in the lower back, but they can also occur in the neck and upper back.

Obstructions to blood circulation

The changes that develop in the skeleton as a result of malformations in the upper back can have serious consequences for blood circulation (figure 4.5-9). The blood vessels that transport blood to the arms are a good example of this. They proceed from the heart upward to the space between the collarbones and the first ribs into the arms (see also figure 4.6-11). Malformations in the upper back always have consequences for the shoulders. In a bent upper back, the backs of the shoulders shift upward, causing the fronts of the shoulders to hang forward. This can make the collarbones drop and pinch the blood vessels, so circulation both to and from the arm is impeded. The tissue can become hard and painful as a result of the buildup of waste that leads to serious problems such as those discussed later in this chapter for the treatment of RSI and CANS.

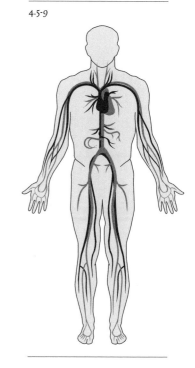

Problems with breathing

Nerves that innervate the upper part of the lungs spring from the upper section of the spine and the brain stem. The mobility of the spine influences the function of these nerves. Breathing problems develop partly due to malformations, such as a bent or twisted upper back, which leads to a lack of mobility in the affected areas and in turn causes a functional disturbance in the nerves that innervate the upper part of the lungs. Then the impulses to the top of the lungs are considerably reduced. This is one of the reasons why many older people mainly use the lower part of their lungs when breathing.

Other malformations of the spine can seriously obstruct free breathing: the collapsed lower back, for example, causes a person to breathe from the stomach, because there is not enough support to breathe open and freely in the chest. A chest that is too high pushes the diaphragm so far forward that a free and relaxed stomach breath is impossible; the breath remains "caught" and cramped in the chest. Tension in the midback causes the sternum to become fixed and seriously limits diaphragmatic breathing.

Peripheral loss of strength

Problems in the shoulder and neck that result from malformations and a bent upper back often lead to problems in the arms. These problems are not only related to radiating

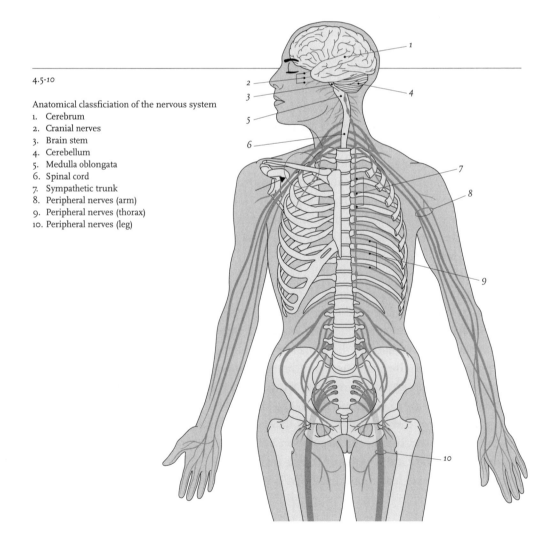

4.5-10

Anatomical classficiation of the nervous system
1. Cerebrum
2. Cranial nerves
3. Brain stem
4. Cerebellum
5. Medulla oblongata
6. Spinal cord
7. Sympathetic trunk
8. Peripheral nerves (arm)
9. Peripheral nerves (thorax)
10. Peripheral nerves (leg)

pain (see the earlier discussion of RSIs) but lead to reduced strength in the arm muscles caused by functional distortions to the nerves that innervate the arms. These nerves meet in a plexus (network) in the shoulders (see the arrow in figure 4.5-10), and this is the area where there is an enormous amount of muscle tension. Everyone wants a massage in this area. The tension in these muscles impairs the function of the nerves, lessening the impulse transfer and causing a loss of strength.

A similar story can be told in relation to a loss of strength in the leg muscles, caused by impairment to the nerves that originate in the lower back.

4.6 Critical Alignment is especially aimed at correcting malformations at the skeletal level to effectively address ailments.

Complaints that arise from malformations can only be eliminated by correcting those malformations at the skeletal level. Specific principles are must be followed to do this. First of all, a protocol defines the steps necessary for making corrections at the skeletal level. Second, the teacher's use of props and mobilization techniques is critical. Last, the mental attitude of the student is very important.

1. Principles for correcting malformations

Protocol
Critical Alignment endeavors to recover the alignment of the skeleton through the application of a specific protocol. As stated in chapter 2.4.1, the protocol consists of the following three steps:

1. Stiff muscles around the area of skeleton are corrected so they will relax.
2. This relaxation allows skeletal parts to move individually, thus activating the postural muscles.
3. The function of the postural muscles is optimized through regular practice.

The effect of successfully completing these three steps is that the weight of the body, which is necessary in order for the skeleton to move, can again be accepted by the stiffened areas of the skeleton by neighboring parts of the body: the vertebrae are able to pass the movement to their neighbors because they and the neighbors are mobile. Movement can again be passed on through the ideal power line from one part of the body to the next, making supple and open movement possible.

The role of the teacher, props, and mobilization techniques
If you have malformations with (serious) problems, it is impossible for you to complete the protocol independently, because your relationship with the malformed areas of your body is functionally lost. Therefore, your body does not feel like it is straight, even when it actually is. On the contrary, straight feels crooked, and crooked feels straight. It is precisely because the corrections run so contrary to the feeling experience that they are difficult to apply independently. This is why continuous work with a teacher is crucial.

During the treatment, the teacher will use the props and mobilization techniques that were introduced in chapter 2.5 and explained further there and in chapter 3. The tools and techniques can help to relax cramped movement muscles so that newly enhanced movement in the skeletal parts will stimulate the postural muscles in that area. You must actively participate with your teacher's mobilization, especially with respect to breathing, to learn the new way of movement.

The props are designed to support your body in areas where support is necessary. This initially feels uncomfortable, as pressure is applied exactly where movement restrictions are located. When you work with them, you should see these props as extensions of your body. Imagine your own hand pushing against your back when you lie on a roll or a strip.

The headstand bench is one of the most important tools. It supports the shoulders in such a way that the neck and head are free, and the correct connection between the neck and pelvis is maintained. The teacher can easily mobilize your spine, and you can incorporate the mobilizations directly and actively do them yourself.

The first objective in practicing with props and mobilization techniques is to free the nerves that exit the spinal column by eliminating blockages in the skeleton and the movement chains. The next phase, which you can complete independently, is concentrated on the practice of yoga asanas. This creates optimal circumstances for the unhindered transfer of information through the nervous system to the muscles so that open, free movement can occur.

Participation of the student

You must participate actively in correcting malformations; the teacher cannot do it alone. There are different phases to the process. First, you must learn to relax, making it possible for you to adopt the right attitude when dealing with pain and stiffness. It is about finding the right balance between too little and too much effort. (This was discussed in detail in chapter 3.3.)

Too little effort, often done to avoid pain, will not lead to tangible results. You must reach the point where the pain is experienced but is tolerable. If the pain becomes too acute, then the effort is too strong. Working too hard is based on willpower; relaxation has nothing to do with willpower. Too much effort can even lead to injury.

When the right balance is found and you can relax, the next phase can commence. This consists of observing your behavior during the exercises as objectively as possible. Here, you come face-to-face with your fears and avoidance tactics, ambitions, competitiveness, and so on. You do not need to analyze the history of this behavior or what led to its development. In carrying out such an analysis, it is easy to make things up. It also takes you out of the present moment and hinders you from determining the real nature of your mental and behavioral blockages. It is critical that you see your behavior clearly. Only then can you consciously understand it.

A good understanding of right effort is crucial. When we adopt a position, we challenge our body by putting pressure on certain joints and stretch on certain muscles. In the earlier example of Paschimottanasana (figure 4.6-1), this occurs by applying pressure to the hips, which allows them to move more freely, causing the pelvis to tilt and stretching the leg muscles more. The use of the breath is very important here; the exhalation is directed to the muscles that must relax, and the inhalation is used to increase relaxation and a feeling of lightness in the entire body. Open and passive attention is necessary for this development. The process of relaxation can easily be disturbed when we try to

4.6-1

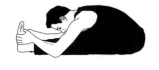

take control. We often pull too hard on our legs, causing more pain and irregular, inadequate breathing. Pulling too hard on our legs also causes excess tension in the shoulders. When we try to take control in this way, our habits, ambitions, and willpower begin to dominate, and there is no space for relaxation.

2. Treatment of malformations and complaints

The treatment of malformations and complaints is directed toward the parts of the skeleton where the free transfer of movement is blocked. Treatment is not initially meant to take away the complaints but to correct the parts of the skeleton that are causing the problems. The teacher has an important role here and will use props and mobilization techniques repeatedly.

Sirsasana in the headstand bench is of prime importance in treatment. Even though this has already been discussed in chapter 2, I want to emphasize it again here because it is so important for recovering the mobility of the spine.

A. Correcting Malformations

Anterior/posterior malformations

In the following description, I have assumed that the upper back is bent and very stiff (this is more or less the situation for most people). The tension that keeps the back in this shape must be dealt with according to the protocol described in chapter 2.4.1 (the three steps of relaxation, movement, and strength and coordination, in that order). When the student adopts Sirsasana, her back adopts its habitual curve, as this is the form it associates with strength. If she tries to relax her back in this position, she will probably fall over because the lower part of the curve (see the arrow in figure 4.6-2) is moving downward. To prevent this, the teacher must bear a large part of the student's weight and orient the lowest part of the curve upward (see the arrow in figure 4.6-3). Subsequently, the student must direct her exhalations toward the places where the teacher is applying pressure with the intention of relaxing those muscles. When the muscular tension lessens, the weight of her body slowly returns to her shoulders (figure 4.6-4). Through practice, her spine will become straighter and she will carry her body weight with increased relaxation (figure 4.6-5). Initially, this position will feel unstable as her deeper postural muscles

4.6-2

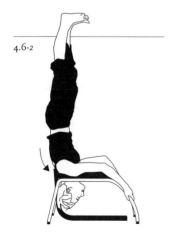

4.6-3

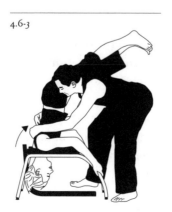

4.6-4

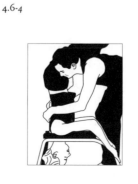

4.6-5

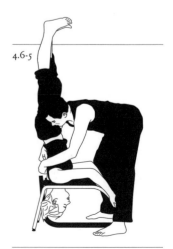

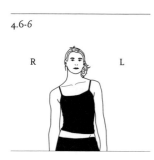

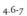

4.6-6

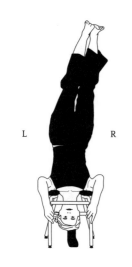

4.6-7

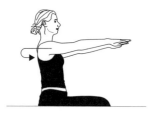

4.6-8

are suddenly activated and pressure is applied to the back of the vertebrae that are being mobilized. This will slowly improve as her postural muscles become stronger and her vertebrae become better aligned. Eventually, her spine will become stable and (almost) still and will remain in the midline.

This process can be applied to every vertebra in the spine that is stiff and out of alignment. Only one vertebra may cause a problem, but multiple vertebrae are usually bound together in an excessive concave or convex form.

Lateral malformations

When someone with asymmetrical shoulders gets on the headstand bench, the unevenness will be seen in the position of the head in relation to the pelvis and legs. If the right shoulder is lower and farther forward, and the left shoulder is higher and seems shorter (figure 4.6-6), then the legs will lean to the right (figure 4.6-7). Even though this is obviously unbalanced, the person experiences it as being straight!

To change this position, the teacher must be aware that the lumbar vertebrae on the left side are much stiffer than those on the right. Here, too, the tension that causes this must be dealt with according to the protocol of relaxation, movement, and strength and coordination. Subsequently, the teacher must examine the lumbar spine and ribs and place them in alignment.

At the end of this process, often in the first session, the student will probably say that she is standing on only one shoulder—in this case, the left. Even though her position is now straight, it will feel lopsided and strange, because her weight is now being carried correctly by the shoulder that was higher in the sitting or standing position. Subsequently, she has to release the tension in this shoulder without losing her balance. After some time, the feeling of being off-kilter will recede. After that (from a few days to a few months), the body itself will start to search for the correct posture.

Because these changes run so contrary to our feeling, it is difficult for us to develop and practice them alone. The new position of the body initially feels anything but straight. That is why it is important to follow lessons with a teacher who is experienced in the Critical Alignment (or a similar) method and can assess the situation correctly.

Rotations

Before discussing the treatment of rotations, I would like to note that they can cause the joints connecting the ribs and vertebrae (costovertebral joints) to become blocked. Treatment of these blockages requires considerable knowledge and experience, and learning the proper technique necessitates intensive personal guidance. It is for this reason that an explanation of the treatment of these joints is outside the scope of this book.

Here, I will only discuss the simpler malformations that exist as a result of rotations of the skeleton. In the earlier example of asymmetry, the right shoulder is rotated forward, which prevents a good connection between the arm and shoulder (figure 4.6-8). Traditional postural therapies emphasize the need to strengthen the muscles under the shoulder blade, pulling the arm back and the shoulder blade down. Obviously, such treatment has nothing to do with the misalignment of the spine.

Critical Alignment, on the other hand, endeavors to correct the underlying misalignment in the spine. The headstand bench is extremely effective for this. When the rotation is taken out of the shoulders by placing them exactly on the white lines (figure 4.6-9), the rotation will become evident in other places such as the chest, pelvis, and legs.

The exact location of the problem, which is probably between the shoulder blades, must be identified. Usually, large differences can be seen here between the left and right ribs.

The headstand bench makes it possible to compare the differences in mobility between the left and right sides through a special technique that is based on rotations. The protocol of relaxation, movement, and strength and coordination must again be used. In this way, it is often possible to place the spine and ribs in the correct position. Initially, the spine will keep falling back to its habitual posture, but it will gradually find its new balance. This is an important difference from traditional physical therapies, because no strength or tension is used to break through habitual postures. The changes are based on relaxation techniques that are applied to a body that actively carries its own weight. Thus, the body is not forced to change its posture by training the superficial movement muscles; on the contrary, it is the *ease* of movement that returns. This can best be explained by (once again) referring to the example of the bent upper back.

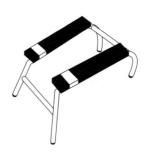

Regular physical therapies often prescribe an exercise program directed at strengthening the muscles between the shoulder blades. Such an exercise could specify that the client lie on her stomach, with her arms out to the sides, and lift weights toward the ceiling (figure 4.6-10). The back will certainly become straighter from such an exercise, but unfortunately it will also become stiffer. It feels awkward and unnatural to have to keep the body elevated with so much force. The tension built up by the muscles tightens and cannot be released. In fact, a new layer of tension is added. By correcting the position of the skeleton, as described earlier, the back will be able to use its new mobility and alignment to walk, sit, and stand with relaxed ease. Using the headstand bench, the vertebrae and intervertebral discs can return to their original alignment, and a coordination pattern based on breathing will develop.

4.6-10

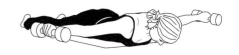

People who have experienced such changes usually say that their new posture feels normal. This is noteworthy, because that feeling couldn't have been anything but a distant memory. It would seem that with the return of correct alignment, the correct feeling also returns and is experienced as if it was always present and the problems never existed. This becomes obvious in the following example.

In my lessons, I had a student with very unpleasant shoulder problems. He had a lot of pain that kept him awake at night. It took a long time to release the tension in the shoulder area because his back was so stiff. Finally, after months of practice, a change took place. Such changes often occur suddenly rather than gradually; as if a button has been pushed. They can be extreme and occur during a lesson or during the night, as if the brain has to first process the information. Here, the change occurred suddenly; one day, during the lesson, his shoulder just aligned correctly. I was very enthusiastic and told him that his shoulder was finally straight. He replied, "Which shoulder?" Evidently the new posture felt so normal that he instantly forgot which shoulder had caused him so many problems.

B. The treatment of complaints caused by RSI or CANS

Obstructions in blood circulation

Complaints in the shoulders, neck, and arms that are collectively attributed to RSI and CANS are, according to Critical Alignment, caused by malformations in the spine.

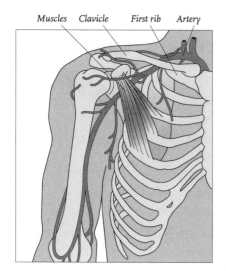

Muscles Clavicle First rib Artery

Backs often begin to bend and stiffen at an early age, causing elevated and stiff shoulders. This frequently compresses the nerves going to the muscles, skin, and bones of the arms and obstructs blood flow. Here, too, we have to change the structural alignment of the body so the tense areas can learn to relax, allowing the skeleton to return to its natural posture. This will free compressed nerves and obstructed blood vessels.

The following example shows problems that can be caused by obstructions to circulation. The large arteries that supply the arms with blood, run through the front of the body from the heart to the arms (figure 4.6-11). The most important artery has a difficult route between the collarbone and the first rib. When the upper back bends and stiffens, it can cause the shoulder girdle to drop forward, which in turn can depress this area and cause the collarbone and first rib to pinch the artery. Hands that suddenly or habitually become cold are an early symptom of this poor circulation. Western medicine sometimes advises enlarging the artery via angioplasty or enlarging the passageway by surgically removing the first rib.

Not so long ago a twenty-eight-year-old man came to me for a consultation. He informed me that the circulation to his arms had decreased to 35 percent. His specialist had advised him to have his first rib removed. Obviously, he was not enthusiastic about this prospect and had decided to give yoga a chance first. After seriously practicing yoga for a few months, he had learned to "open" the front of his shoulders so much that the circulation began to increase. He had eliminated the necessity of an operation.

Malformations in the skeleton also negatively affect the function of veins that return blood from the arms. This causes waste products to build up in the muscle tissue, which can lead to hard and painful tissue in the (lower) arms. Joint pain in the arms (wrists, elbows, and/or shoulders) often clears up when neurological control is recovered and blood flow is optimized. Even so-called trigger points, areas that are constantly sensitive and painful during use and rest, are the result of malformations of the skeleton.

Loss of strength in the biceps frequently occurs with CANS. This is caused by compressed nerves. Exercise programs are often prescribed to strengthen the upper arms. However, if the nerves remain compressed, this attempt to increase strength makes little sense. The remarkable effect of freeing impinged nerves by mobilizing the affected vertebrae can be seen in the following example.

One of my students regularly worked out at the gym. To increase his strength, one of his exercises was the bench press. The maximum weight he could press was 100 pounds. The week the vertebrae in his upper back mobilized and aligned during a session in the headstand bench, he was able to press 155 pounds.

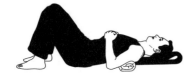

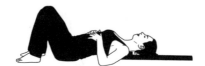

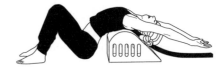

For the correction of CANS and RSI (which also includes lower back problems), Critical Alignment makes stretching and mobilization of the upper back central. Different types of exercises are used to achieve this.

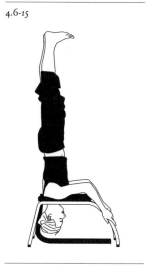

Passive Exercises
Examples of this type of exercise include lying with a roll under the midback (figure 4.6-12), lying on a rubber strip placed vertically along the spine (figure 4.6-13), and lying with the upper back on the backbender (figure 4.6-14). With these exercises, a lot of attention is given to free breathing and the free movement of the ribs. Shoulder exercises with the headstand bench are also included here.

Active Exercises
Examples include Sirsasana on the headstand bench (figure 4.6-15), sitting straight, twists while sitting (figure 4.6-16), supported Sarvangasana (figure 4.6-17), shoulder exercises (figure 4.6-18), and so on.

Coordination Exercises
Examples of these exercises include lying on the shoulderstand block (figure 4.6-19), sitting straight via the breath, and so on. Remedial exercises for the lower back are comparable to those for herniated discs (see the next section).

Spinal disc herniation
Lower back problems can develop independently from those of the upper back, but often there is a relationship. An examination of the spine will establish this. If there is a connection, then treatment of the upper back must also be initiated to prevent a recurrence of the problem.

4.6-16

4.6-17

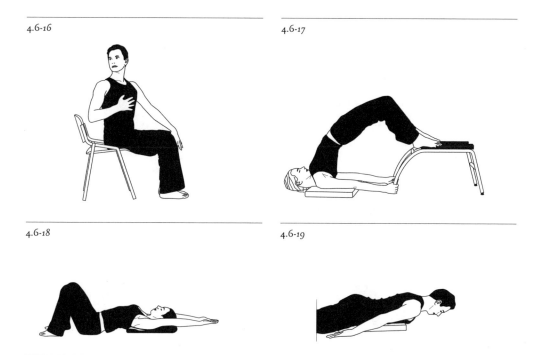

4.6-18

4.6-19

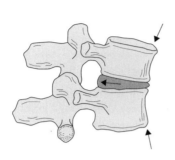

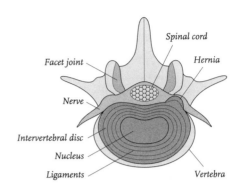

4.6-20   Lateral view of the vertebrae

4.6-21   Superior view of the vertebrae

Spinal disc hernias are ruptures in the intervertebral discs. The resulting bulge can compress the nerves that exit the vertebrae. This bulging often occurs following years of "hanging" in the lower back, causing too much pressure on the front of the vertebrae and intervertebral discs, which pushes the nucleus backward. Over time, the vertebrae and discs change shape (figure 4.6-20). These malformations alone can compress nerves, but a misstep, incorrect lifting technique, or other activity can cause the wall of the disc to rupture, pushing the nucleus outward. If a nerve is compressed (figure 4.6-21), which does not always happen, you will feel pain, numbness, a loss of strength, and finally, a loss of control of the leg and/or foot that the nerve innervates.

In such a situation, Critical Alignment (often together with other professional therapies) endeavors to free the compressed nerve through exercises that provide traction and space. Ultimately, pressure to the back of the vertebrae and discs is restored, and the (beginning) hernia can recede, relieving the compression. (If the exercises aggravate the vertebrae or cause pain you need to go to a doctor.) At the same time, the strength in the lower back must be increased substantially to ensure that the pressure remains on the back of the vertebrae. Here, too, we can divide the exercises into three groups.

Passive Exercises
Examples include lying on a lower back roll (see figure 4.6-22), lying with the tailbone on top of the backbender (figure 4.6-23), and so on. If the upper back is also involved, then the same exercises that were indicated for RSI and CANS are necessary.

Active Exercises
These exercises include Bhujangasana (Cobra Pose; figure 4.6-24), Urdhva Mukha Svanasana (Upward-Facing Dog Pose; figure 4.6-25), supported Sarvangasana with feet

4.6-22

4.6-23

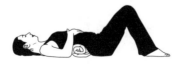

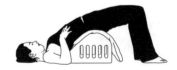

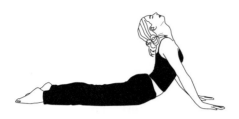

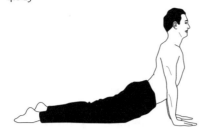

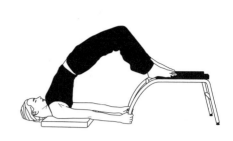

against the headstand bench (figure 4.6-26), supported Sarvangasana with feet against the wall (figure 4.6-27), and so on.

4.6-27

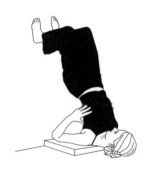

Coordination Exercises

Exercises in this group include placing the ribs with a hollow lower back (figure 4.6-28), lifting the legs with the lower abdomen pushed into the floor (figure 4.6-29), and so on.

Breathing restrictions

Most people who have a bent upper back do not use the upper part of their lungs. As soon as the back is mobilized, the necessary reflexes return, and the upper part of the lungs are reactivated. Again, exercises on the headstand bench give excellent results.

4.6-28

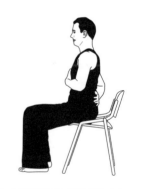

To learn the correct balance on the headstand bench, it is used with the backbender and the rubber strip (figure 4.6-30). When your pelvis is placed so your upper back can relax where it touches the rubber strip, the teacher can position your head to connect your neck with your mobilized upper back. This frees your cervical and thoracic vertebrae (figure 4.6-31). It mobilizes your entire spine, which often causes it to move in an uncoordinated manner. Over time, this agitation will subside, and you will experience a feeling of mobility. When your back is freed, there is an immediate change in the way you breathe. You suddenly start breathing much more deeply. Initially, this can be loud and extreme, but it will eventually stabilize into a fine, deep breath. This type of breathing is of enormous benefit in letting go of tension in your upper chest.

It is both interesting and satisfying to hear that a student experiences this process in a totally different way than an observer. The different parts of the student's body begin

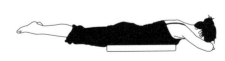

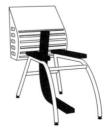

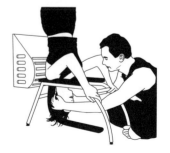

to work together, and this calms the mind. The tension that had taken over the body and afflicted behavior slowly begins to relax its grip.

Recovery of strength in the peripheral muscles

As mentioned in the RSI discussion, a medical diagnosis of RSI or CANS often includes reduced strength in the upper arms, leading to an exercise program to strengthen weak muscles. The same sort of pattern applies to weakness in the legs. From our point of view, this is about as intelligent as throwing buckets of water at a hurricane.

The first question that should be asked is, why has strength diminished? Most likely, this is caused by compression of the nerves that control the muscles. The earlier example of the nerves that join together at the front of the shoulder girdle (see the "Peripheral loss of strength" section on page 50 and figure 4.5-10) shows that the strength will return when the muscular tension lessens and the compression dissolves. Very soon, it is possible to maintain such exercises as Adho Mukha Vrksasana for longer periods.

A final comment

Traditional texts such as the Hathapradipika (written by Svatmarama in the fifteenth century) bestow strong therapeutic values to yoga asanas. From a modern scientific standpoint, these benefits are often described as unbelievably great. Possibly, in other times and cultures, they have had positive effects. For example, Mayurasana (Peacock Pose; figure 4.6-32) is described as follows: it "destroys all illnesses . . . stimulates the appetite . . . and allows the practitioner to swallow the most deadly of poisons without danger" (Hathapradipika, 1:3). I do not deny that the power of the asanas is probably greater than we think, but it is difficult to appreciate such statements or make them useful for our own purposes.

Critical Alignment draws support from the modern scientific tradition and does not claim to have any supernatural effects. Because of its close reliance on anatomical considerations for information and supervision, Critical Alignment can easily be combined with existing science-based therapies such as physiotherapy, massage therapy, and manual therapy on the condition that such treatments are given by a skilled therapist.

4.6-32

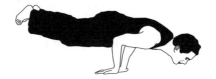

5

MEDITATION, PRANAYAMA, AND ASANAS

5.1   Introduction

Just about all of us have had the experience of going somewhere and being so lost in thought that we found ourselves in the wrong place. Without the cooperation of our conscious mind, our body continued on automatic pilot and ended up where we did not intend to be. The opposite is also possible: we can be so lost in our body and/or emotions that we lose the connection with conscious thought. This is typical of the disjointed lives that many of us lead. Our body, thoughts, and emotions become disconnected and, left to themselves, take over. When this occurs, we can barely cope with social and psychological stresses such as competition, relationship problems, and ambitions, let alone the more life-changing stresses of poverty, loneliness, unemployment, or the death of a loved one. We become victims of our circumstances.

Recovering wholeness
Critical Alignment helps to alleviate this loss of coherence by allowing us to recover a sense of wholeness when we practice yoga. Yoga exercises are totally different from normal movements. They are more complex, difficult, and above all, much slower. To practice in the correct way, we must first develop a total awareness. This can only occur when the fragmentation of our own selves ceases and our mind, body, and emotions start to cooperate and unite.

To this end, Critical Alignment is initially concerned with recovering the total experience of our selves. This can be achieved in various ways. When we practice yoga, a functional relationship develops between our thoughts, body, and emotions in which they are constantly exchanging information about various aspects of the asana. As part of this exchange of information, we consider elements of what we wish to accomplish before initiating a particular exercise. We recall these elements again during the exercise. Information about technique, earlier experiences, our feelings, and, of course, our direct experiences of movement are constantly exchanged between our mind, body, and emotions. These practical exchanges, which are always necessary when practicing yoga, generate an all-encompassing (total) attention; that is, an attention that is able to observe these interactions. (This was discussed in detail in chapter 3.)

Subsequently, this total attention, or absorption in the moment, can be intensified by directing it toward mental and physical tension. We are confronted with our own habitual postures and movements and with personal ambitions and mental tensions when we practice yoga. Total attention is necessary to become aware of this. This attention can only develop when we practice the exercises in a balanced way, allowing our body and mind to relax. Together with deep, slow breathing, this practice reveals areas of tension. The collaboration between our thoughts, emotions, and body creates a physical and mental openness that is maintained by a subtle circulation of energy. This energy is the carrier of a total (meditative) attention (see chapters 2 and 3).

Higher levels of consciousness (*manonmani*, literally "mind beyond mind"[1])
Next, we can access a higher level of consciousness from total attention. It is not so much about cooperation between mind and body, as a uniting of body consciousness with mental consciousness to form a higher consciousness that can eventually serve as a basis to access even higher levels. A necessary condition is that the "I" consciousness is surpassed. (Indian texts on the metaphysics of aesthetics refer to this as *sadharanikarana,* meaning "universalization," or a transcendence of the narrow, ego-constricted mind). Higher forms of consciousness are typically accompanied by feelings of deep relaxation, a radiating sense of wholeness encompassing the space around us, harmony and bliss, and a strong presence in the here and now. As such, they form a road to deep spiritual experiences, which is the subject of this chapter.

There is a clear difference between normal thinking and meditative attention, which I will try to clarify using the same example given in chapter 1. Imagine a street where three people are watching a girl walk down the opposite side. Each of these people—her mother, the boyfriend with whom she just broke up, and her best friend—have their own thoughts about the girl. In other words, they have all added their own "I" element to their observations. The girl is certainly not seen as she really is but through the tinted glasses of personal feelings, memories, and so on that color each person's observation.

The general sequence occurs as follows: we perceive a situation and fill it in with the residue of our own "I" element (personal interpretation); this gets stored in our memory. Every time a similar situation occurs, we use this distorted, or colored, memory and consistently strengthen it. (Indian philosophy calls this the wheel of samsara—the revolving wheel of perception, memory, and perception.) This clearly explains how much our thinking influences our direct perception. All of our learned "knowledge" is determined through this process.

Meditation is about breaking this cycle by excluding the "I" element, so we can remain present with our perceptions without interpreting them according to our ego-related predisposition; in other words, without thinking. This is the goal of pranayama, asanas, and meditation itself.

Higher consciousness is necessary for practicing yoga in a meditative, purely contemplative manner and can only develop when the following precise conditions have been achieved. First, the body must be in balance. It must be "stacked," enabling the muscles to support the free movement of joints and vertebrae and allowing relaxed and open breathing. Only then is the subtle transport of energy that can carry body consciousness possible. The body should not be lazy and soft nor tense and hard. Either condition reduces the subtle experience of body consciousness and the (later) access to higher levels of consciousness.

Second, the stream of thoughts and the senses must be quieted. This is necessary for accessing mental consciousness that is characterized by an intense, all-encompassing attention from the nonthinking part of our brain; the *bindu* (literally, "spot" or "drop") located at the back of our head. Body and mental consciousness then merge together into a higher level of consciousness.

To access this higher consciousness, it is important that we add compassion, love, or devotion to our practice and transcend the ego-hampered mind. Then we are able to find something that transcends our (automatic and often negative) emotional and cognitive reflections about the situation in which we find ourselves. Then we can perceive people, other creatures, objects, situations, and so on directly as they actually are.

Relaxation, openness, compassion, and space can dissolve tension and tightness and transform our ordinary experience of life into an experience where our inner self (soul) reflects the wholeness of life, an intense and warm experience of harmony. It is a spiritual experience. This transformation can be attained in phases using a meditative exercise, which makes it possible to experience directly the space and relaxation that develops in our body and mind—without the interference of "I" elements.

Once you are able to experience the transformation from ordinary awareness to an awareness that includes a sense of wholeness, you can also apply this method in the dynamic exercises and asanas where disquieting factors are more evident. It will also become clear that the manner in which you access higher levels of consciousness is different for every exercise. It depends on the sort of exercise you are doing and the disquieting factors involved. The sequence ends with a pranayama exercise.

5.2 Accessing higher levels of consciousness involves three phases: body consciousness, mental consciousness, and higher consciousness.

If we concentrate on only one part of our body, we quickly lose sight of the rest. For example, thinking about one arm is not difficult, but thinking about both arms simultaneously and remaining present is much harder. It is certainly impossible in Sirsasana to be present while keeping track (thinking) of all parts of your body from top to toe. But this *is* possible with an open consciousness.

This conclusion has important consequences for practicing asanas. Critical Alignment is based on the concept that asanas are realized via movement chains where different parts of the body must be connected correctly so that large, full movements can occur.

The same problem discussed earlier—of being present in all parts of your body—also occurs here. For example, when standing up straight, the head and neck must be connected with the lower part of the sternum (see chapter 6.3, connection 2). Subsequently, the sternum must be connected with the pubic bone (see chapter 6.3, connection 8). Finally, the pelvis must be connected with the legs (see chapter 6.3, connections 10 and 11).

Each connection has its own elements to be considered, and additionally, all four connections must work together in a fluid manner to achieve the relatively simple total movement of standing up straight. Our attention must constantly zoom in and out to realize a posture in which the participating parts of the body are vertically stacked and in balance. Higher forms of consciousness provide an open attention that encompasses the totality of body and mind, and this makes it possible to observe all the chains involved in the total movement.

This open and all-encompassing attention is the opposite of the concentrated attention that focuses on only one or two aspects of the movement chains. This does not mean that concentrated, specific attention and higher levels of consciousness cannot work well together. When, for example, relaxation or movement in only one or two parts of the body is necessary, this can be achieved by concentrating specifically on those parts (or zooming in). To achieve a higher level of consciousness after that, movement or relaxation of specific areas must be carried out with an open and positive total feeling that includes all of the movement chains.

Full consciousness is not only about an open, total attention to the body; it includes the space around us. This will be discussed in detail in this chapter.

Three phases for accessing higher consciousness

Phase one: body consciousness

The body has an important role as the vehicle of higher consciousness. It can complete this task fully if it is in balance, meaning relaxed and open. A body that is tense and tight is not a strong vehicle for reaching higher consciousness. We can achieve correct balance using the following steps.

First, our attention must be focused so that our thoughts, input from our senses, and so on do not take over. In Critical Alignment, our attention is mobilized by concentrating exclusively on the technical and physical aspects of the exercise. This attention does not intervene in an aggressive manner if something goes wrong; it carefully follows the movement, giving our body the chance to complete the exercise in the correct way, without tension.

During the second step (without losing the alert attention for the correct technical implementation), we relax and deepen respiration.

Finally, we can release tension from our body with exhalations. In this way, our entire body can slowly relax during the exercise without losing strength in the (postural) muscles.

These steps produce feelings of lightness and openness in the entire body. It is as if our breath unites every part of our body in an open connection. As a result, we can experience a tangible, subtle energy that carries our body consciousness; we become consciously present in our body. This body consciousness is characterized by a feeling of physical openness, or spaciousness. It covers all voluntary and involuntary processes in our body.

Phase two: mental consciousness

An observational, nonthinking consciousness is essential to maintaining body awareness when we hold a pose. This means we need to get rid of all our unconscious thoughts that distract us from the direct experience of openness. Unconscious negative thoughts are based on fear of change or on ambitious behavior that has traditionally dominated our actions. These thoughts do not stop instantaneously; we have to block them. That can be achieved by the following steps. First, we focus our attention on the feeling of spaciousness in our body, which we developed in the previous phase and is still present. Our attention follows the development of body consciousness with an involved but passive interest, supporting that consciousness.

At this point, we can release mental tension caused by unconscious thoughts through this constant attention. The moment we are no longer connected to our body consciousness, unconscious (negative) thoughts can start to take over. This takeover is not in terms of clear thoughts, but comprises noise, disturbance, and unease that can easily produce restless behavior. When we become aware of this, we need to restore the connection with our body consciousness immediately. When we are able to do so, our attention can gradually be directed to compassion and appreciation that come from understanding the position we are in. Instead of interpreting the situation as working against us (the confrontation with pain, effort, and/or strain), we should realize that our situation gives us a unique opportunity to release ourselves from (old) tension patterns. This lessens the stream of thoughts without diminishing body consciousness. The stream will most likely lessen in intensity, allowing a nonthinking, observational consciousness to develop. With the greater intensity of this observational consciousness, we are able to enter the next phase.

Phase three: accessing higher levels of consciousness

In the last phase, the open, observational, nonthinking mental consciousness unites with body consciousness to create an intense, higher level of consciousness. The uniting of mental and body consciousness is a critical event that can easily be disturbed by slackening attention and letting habitual desires, intentions, and negative thoughts take over. It is therefore important to observe this union closely with a passive yet acute attention, an attention that follows the actions of the body closely in a loving way. Breathing plays an important role in this process. It allows us to relax deeply and initiates movement when we practice asanas. The difficulties we encounter, such as pain, reverting back to habitual postures, and so on, start to lose their power. This allows us to release deeper layers of tension and distance ourselves from our ego. Then we can develop feelings of relaxation, lightness, and openness. When we successfully maintain this state, we can experience a heightened feeling of joy that starts to accompany us when we are fully engrossed in the here and now.

Once we have entered this initial higher consciousness, even deeper levels become possible. There are several points to consider here. First of all, we have to abandon all desire. This is a paradox because we first have to desire something (namely, the cessation of desire) to be able to abandon desire. But this paradoxical situation is the only road toward a completely empty mind (or heart or soul or self), a mind that is no longer engrossed in trivialities of any kind. Within this framework, here are a number of tips for dealing with common difficulties you may encounter when developing higher consciousness:

- Recognize that movement based on willpower prevents higher consciousness from developing.
- Exchange willpower for attention to your body.
- Approach your body gently and with compassion
- Be willing to investigate pain.
- Move slowly.
- Use your breath to initiate movement.
- Become sensitive to and absorbed by your breathing.
- Continue moving even when it becomes difficult.
- Do not allow yourself to develop habitual postures or other compensatory movements.
- Move from a feeling of relaxation.
- Move from a feeling of lightness.
- Move with awareness of the space around you.
- Allow your movements and concentration to grow from a feeling of joy.
- Regard your body as the best possible means for experiencing yourself.
- Recognize jealousy, competitiveness, and other emotions, and allow them to dissolve.
- Allow the connection with your ego to lessen continuously so you can experience deeper levels of consciousness.
- Investigate and appreciate overwhelming physical changes.
- During such overwhelming experiences, return your focus to the exercise and continue with the movement.
- Be prepared to extend the experience.

The discrepancy that existed in the perception of our inner and outer worlds is replaced by an intense, direct experience of ourselves in the here and now. This may be so acute that our perception of passing time dissolves into a direct experience of eternity.

We must stay alert and remain completely absorbed, because the development of bodily tensions, mental intentions, and so on will immediately break our newfound awareness. Only when we are fully absorbed, can the self (or heart or soul) become receptive to the eternal Self (or eternal Being) and be deeply immersed in it. We become overwhelmed by feelings of infinite harmony, joy, and bliss. This is beyond language—and very private.

The body, in a completely relaxed state, has an important function here. It is not only the receptacle of higher consciousness, it is the vehicle for the experience of that.

I call the experience of intense feelings of harmony, bliss, and joy at the start of a meditation the *lightbulb consciousness*. This experience is a gift. We do not have to do anything for it. More often than not, it does not transpire; we have to work conscientiously and continuously for long periods to achieve higher levels of consciousness. This can change from day to day. Following is a personal account of flashbulb consciousness.

Meditation through movement: a personal story

Initially, I used to move from willpower; I was concerned only with results. In retrospect, I realize that this created a sort of tunnel vision; my consciousness was debilitatingly limited. There was no way I could experience space or develop a meditative attitude that would allow me to attain higher levels of consciousness. I allowed myself to be driven by the wants and automatic patterns I had developed in normal activities like competitive sports. I call this the *functional power of the ego*: *functional*, because my actions were goal-oriented; *ego*, because my efforts came from my conscious and unconscious wants and desires. For example, I might have had any of the following thoughts:

- Next time, I want my Urdhva Dhanurasana to be better.
- Today I am going to stand in Sirsasana longer than yesterday.
- I want to show the group that I am not a beginner like the new people next to me.
- I want to show the teacher that I understand his instructions better than the rest.

It took a long time before I could admit that these thoughts defined my behavior. Finally I realized that it was exactly these thoughts that blocked the development of relaxation, and I become rather tired of them. I wanted to cultivate my practice and progress from feelings of relaxation. I wanted to enjoy my yoga and learn to change my behavior through yoga.

How did I achieve this? The most important realization for me was that willpower is directed through *thinking*, while relaxation can only be *felt*.

This realization and the experience of movement being initiated by relaxing certain muscles gave me enormous focus. However, I did not know exactly how to develop this focus: should I approach it through my ego-bound decisiveness or through something else, something in my body? I noticed that I could couple the feeling of letting go with my breathing. I felt how my breathing could promote relaxation in my muscles. I experimented with using my breath to maintain relaxation while moving into the end pose. That worked. I also tied the second point for attention—movement—to my breathing.

This created a shift in my behavior, a shift from an ego-bound, cognitive control (willpower) to an emotionally bound, physical control whereby the focus of the movement was maintained. I was able to visualize a rough image of the total picture of how the movement should be done and then accomplished it *without falling back into my habitual postures.*

I developed the routine of connecting myself with essential technical points of attention in every asana movement. Relaxation was always the central point within these directives. For example, when doing forward bends, I concentrated on relaxing the tension in my hamstrings and hips.

I felt that I had found the solution for a complicated problem: if I allowed myself to complete the asana purely from feeling, then there was a risk that my technique would suffer, but if I focused on technically correct movement, willpower would take over. As it turned out, neither happened: I was able to maintain the correct technique and remain relaxed. This also became *the* way for me to release my tunnel vision. My thoughts became quiet, and I was able to view the experiences of my body in an open, respectful manner. Through this experience with consciousness, and because I confronted my tension in an entirely new way, I was able to attain a new, higher level of consciousness. I was able to approach my tension from a feeling of relaxation together with a positive contact with my body. The "I"-focused, old manner, which was based on desires and driven by willpower, felt hard and aggressive when compared to this new experience.

I got the feeling that *I* was no longer the initiator of the movement; I felt how my body reacted to the focus of relaxation and movement initiated through my breath. I was able to observe this peacefully, without interfering, like an interested spectator.

The lightbulb

At a certain moment, I felt that my body itself started to organize the movement. It was an awe-inspiring and, above all, totally physical moment:

My body underwent a transformation, and I became very warm. I felt light and full of energy and sensed a transparent connection with the space around me. This new development in my consciousness felt like a lightbulb suddenly went off. I was so surprised by this that my thoughts immediately took over, causing the experience to end. Luckily, I found that by starting over at the beginning (body consciousness) and without longing for this particular end result, I could replicate the experience.

I was less surprised the second time and so was able to lengthen the experience. It felt like an unsteady (but not frightening) connection with myself. Slowly, I regained a clearer overview of the situation without losing the physical sensations. This "gathering" of myself felt complicated, because I was eager to return to my habitual manner of movement—namely, control. And control was the one factor that immediately stopped the experience. When I was able to continue moving without losing the sensations in my body, I once again experienced a large shift in consciousness. This could be described as higher consciousness.

As a disclaimer, I would like to say here that yoga is certainly not the only manner to experience this sort of change of consciousness. I would also like to add that I do not think that my experiences should become a model experience for anyone else. Everybody will have their own personal experience of such events. I do think it is important to write of my experiences as it gives an idea of what can happen.

Insights developed

- I learned to remain in this state for longer periods by not trying to control it, by simply remaining in the here and now. Strong feelings of joy started to develop: I was practicing intensely, even though it did not feel intense. The exertion was absent, and I felt at ease and full of self-confidence.
- Following this, I felt a strong connection with the space around me that transcended my normal experience of my surroundings. I felt connected to a sort of universal space, and it gave me a feeling of invulnerability.
- I felt that these strong feelings had their source deep within me, within my true nature. I realized that all these experiences came from my own actions.
- I felt connected to myself, and looking back, I realized that this transcended any feeling of suffering. It was as if I had risen above not only my own suffering (the pain in that moment) but the suffering of humanity. As if I understood (without expressing it through cognitive thought or speech) it was the *experience* of understanding, or compassion.
- The most striking aspect of this experience was that it brought me back to my true essence, my heart (or soul).
- A deep intuitive knowledge developed regarding this essence—namely, that it is good and radiates space.

Experiencing higher levels of consciousness on a regular basis may well change your point of view in life. You will become more compassionate toward other people and the world in general, and you will cease to feel that you are alone. Returning to your self is like coming home. There will be less room for doubt and mental distraction, and you will develop a constant positive and creative inner support toward your actions.

Some notes on the here and now experience in stillness, action, and the process of learning

I distinguish the experience of "here and now in action" from the experience of "here and now in complete stillness." Being here and now is often seen as a spot that resembles perfect balance: we are not in the future, not in the past, not at a high energy level or a low energy level; we are in the balanced space between the extremities. When we meditate or do passive exercises like lying on a rubber strip or roll, we can create that momentum and lengthen it by staying aware without any disturbances. But when we look at being here and now in action, it is a different matter.

When we act, it may be helpful to change our perspective from a dot to a circle. We have to plan our movements; we have to think about our previous experiences, and when we do so, we have to leave the dot—a fixed point. Sometimes we need to be active during the performance of an asana, but as long as we move within that circle with the fixed point as its center, we do not lose contact with the dot, which acts as a benchmark. In other words, it is possible to plan the next step in our development without being ambitious. It is also possible to work in certain asanas without building up strain. We calibrate our benchmark from the experience of higher consciousness in passive circumstances. When we lie down on a rubber strip or support our lower back with a roll, we become aware that we have built up tension through the years. We become aware that we have drifted away from our original circle (and benchmark dot) and built up another circle that is far from it.

Unconsciousness rules in that new circle. Most people are not aware of their stressed state. Those who fall victim to the slow buildup of structural stress also have moments when they experience total relaxation. We cannot deny them that. But they do not realize their reference for relaxation is completely different from their "original" feelings of relaxation. When exploring full body consciousness, the benchmark (the dot versus the circle) is different.

The practice of supported exercises, meditation, and pranayama brings us back to reality, back into the original circle with the original benchmark where we are able to experience real relaxation. We are safe here, because within that circle, we are no longer victims of mental or physical negativity (as mentioned in chapter 14). From that awareness, we are able to use relaxation in more difficult circumstances like asanas. Seen from this perspective, yoga practice prepares us to stay connected with our original benchmark in complex situations that can occur during stressful moments in daily life.

5.3 Applying these three phases to access a higher consciousness during meditation

The meditation exercise that is used to enter higher consciousness is tranquil; it does not contain the same dynamic characteristics that are found in asana and pranayama practice. It allows you to concentrate fully on accessing higher consciousness, using the preceding three phases. The exercise can be done in 20 to 60 minutes. Once you are successful in this meditation exercise, you can then attempt to access higher consciousness in the more dynamic asana and pranayama practices (to be described shortly).

First phase: realizing body consciousness

Sit on a shoulderstand block in Padmasana or with crossed legs; if this is not possible, sit on a chair. (For instructions on how to sit correctly, see chapter 7.2.) It is important that you establish your sitting posture with attention right from the beginning. The correct position keeps you focused and supports your body in its search for a posture that is correct and relaxed. Close your eyes and follow your body with a passive attention as it searches for an exact, erect, sitting balance. It is important that you do not actively interfere. Give your body the chance to find the correct posture, wherein you can sit straight for a certain length of time without tension.

Next, concentrate on breathing slowly and deeply, in and out. Breathing into your stomach gives a feeling of stability and increasing relaxation in the body's main center of gravity (*hara*). Sitting in a grounded manner is necessary to develop body consciousness and, later on, to enter higher consciousness. Continue to breathe into your stomach for a while to increase your physical stability and relaxation. Allow the relaxation to penetrate your entire being to the point where the need to maintain attentive control of your body and breath stops. It may feel as if your posture is collapsing; however, as long as your lower back remains straight and your head is in the same place, this will never happen. These two areas become the focus of attention for further relaxation.

After 5 to 10 minutes, begin observing your body in its entirety. It is essential that you sit absolutely still. Do not allow yourself even the smallest movements of your hands or shoulders, and keep your eyes closed.

Because your body and breathing are relaxed, you may start to perceive a subtle flow of energy in some areas. This process can be intensified by directing your breath to different areas of your body. Without breaking your passive attention, send your breath into one arm so that it can relax further, increasing the awareness of energy flow. An important aspect of this energy is that it gives a warm, agreeable feeling that moves through the arm, "carrying" the consciousness of the entire arm. Only total, deep relaxation can activate this flow of energy.

Without breaking the process in the first arm, direct your breath to the other arm and then your legs, trunk, and so on, until the flow of energy streams through your entire body. Then you can experience your body in its entirety. The flow of energy carries your entire body consciousness. You feel light, alert, open, and spacious. There are no areas of compression, tension, or hardness to block the flow of energy. You are totally present in your body.

Second phase: realizing mental consciousness

During the second phase, when mental consciousness can be realized, you must not forget the light and open body consciousness. It must remain intact; otherwise, you will find it impossible to achieve the third phase, higher consciousness.

If your neck is balanced, you may experience a lessening of tension in your face and a feeling of open awareness developing in the back of your head. This awareness allows you to distance yourself from external distractions and the stream of thoughts in your head. You will always hear noises, and your thoughts will continue to arise, but you will be able to observe them without getting involved. This is the beginning of the mental consciousness you can now develop further.

To make this possible, you must be careful not to take your body's relaxation for granted. This can cause you to *imagine* that you are relaxed, but in the meantime, tension starts to arise here and there in your body. You must consistently renew and deepen your physical relaxation with the help of your attention and breathing. You remain constantly, tangibly present in your body.

Nonthinking, mental, and observational consciousness occurs mainly in the back of the brain, whereas the assimilation of sensory input and the stream of thoughts occurs mainly in the front. In fact, thinking is continuously stimulated through sensory impressions. The senses: eyes (vision), tongue (taste), nose (smell), ears (hearing), and the skin (touch) continuously pass information on to the brain. The brain absorbs this information and colors our perceptions by adding our "I" element in the form of thoughts, fantasies, and so on. These thoughts continuously cause tension to build up in the forehead and especially in the eyes.

Therefore, by sitting tranquilly with your eyes closed, you lessen the dominance of sensory input. Contact with the outside world is largely blocked. The function of your eyes is reversed: when they are open, they stimulate the development of thoughts, but when they are shut, their movements can relax, allowing them to fall deeper into their sockets. This significantly reduces the stream of thoughts and develops a strong mental consciousness in the back of the head. The reverse is also true; your eyes will begin to move restlessly when you are taken over by your thoughts. The eyes, through their restless movements, give you an early warning sign that you are becoming lost in conscious or unconscious thinking. For this reason, it is important to observe attentively, from the consciousness at the back of your head, any changes in your eye activity.

Admittedly, the other senses cannot be shut off from the outside world as easily. But they can be calmed by passive mental attention and can contribute to the development of a positive physical feeling. For example, when your nose is not constantly trying to identify smells, it can relax and become tranquil. Inhalation can fill the nose with a pleasant sensation of space and relaxation and thus promote the subtle flow of energy throughout the body. This also applies to the other senses, such as hearing. You can actually listen to the sounds around or you can use the memory of the effect of beautiful music on your body contributing to the flow of energy. This process of stilling the senses is called *pratyahara,* and it is of great value when realizing mental consciousness.

Mental consciousness is characterized by the passive attention located in the back of your head. It makes it possible for you to hear sounds, smell odors, feel the surrounding temperature, and have mental images without getting involved in them. If you can sustain this for some time without disturbance, your mental relaxation will intensify.

Third phase: accessing higher consciousness
In the last phase, you are ready to access higher consciousness. This process is set in motion by allowing the passive, nonthinking observer at the back of your brain to move farther down your neck and spine into your heart region. Then you are able to "observe" your body from that region in a purely sensory way. The two aspects of

consciousness—body and mental consciousness—can meet and merge to become a single intense higher consciousness. You must remain completely aware, allowing the process to occur without trying to control it. Many students experience intense feelings of harmony.

Higher consciousness is now firmly anchored in your entire body and mind. You can experience yourself as open and spacious and experience the wholeness of life in a positive way. By feeling your breath—not only within your body, but also in the space around you—you can become aware of both areas, and they become a single continuum. Thus, you have the feeling, "I am conscious here and now."

Pain, the need to move, and so on lose their power, and you enter a state in which you develop a loving, interested connection with your body. After some time, it becomes possible to recognize other forms of ego objectives; desires and so on lose their power as well. Then the experience of being here and now becomes acute, as do feelings of harmony and bliss.

If you do not access higher consciousness continuously by allowing your mental consciousness to merge with your body consciousness, you will automatically return to your normal, distracted, and habitual condition. Thoughts, intentions, discomfort, or pain will easily claim your attention and take over when you lose focus. If you do lose focus, you have no option but to start the entire process over from the beginning. Instruct yourself in a pleasurable and friendly way by carefully observing your posture and correcting your breathing. (Again, follow the directions in chapter 7.2.) Afterward, you can concentrate on accessing higher consciousness.

In reality, the experience of higher consciousness alternates between being intense and somewhat relaxed. This natural rhythm is bound to the quality of movement that is natural for the mind. It is pointless to become frustrated if you do not access higher consciousness, and it is equally pointless to think you can remain in a state of higher consciousness for prolonged periods. If you feel you are there permanently, then it is merely your imagination. You only become aware of accessing higher consciousness afterward; when you realize that it has been lost.

5.4 Factors that can hinder accession to a higher consciousness

Because the preceding meditation exercise develops feelings of relaxed tranquillity, it is a relatively easy way to get to higher consciousness (an even simpler, supine variation is given in chapter 7.2). Higher levels of consciousness are more difficult to access during dynamic exercises, certainly in the beginning, because the problems you face tend to take over your attention. I will now discuss how you can neutralize such hindrances and continue the process of accessing higher consciousness.

First, I will identify the most important obstacles and follow with explanations of how these obstacles try to take over our attention, preventing us from achieving higher consciousness. I will use a moderately dynamic shoulder exercise while lying on a rubber strip as an example. (This exercise is described in detail in chapter 6.3, connection 4.)

The following obstacles can be encountered in every dynamic exercise, although not necessarily in the same order that they are given here.

Obstacles

1. Restlessness

Observing the slow rhythm of our breath often causes restlessness. This unease prevents us from relaxing fully and thus accessing higher levels of consciousness.

2. Discomfort

The pressure on muscles and joints that develops when the movement muscles relax can cause discomfort. This, in turn, can block our road to higher consciousness.

3. Movement

Normal movements are fast and unconscious. The tendency to move unconsciously and quickly is also present when practicing yoga. This presents a serious obstacle to higher consciousness.

4. Effort and strength

Effort and strength can quickly take over our attention and build up tension and compression in our body, thus blocking access to higher consciousness.

5. Pain

As yoga practitioners, we are often confronted with pain from mobilizing stiff joints and stretching stiff muscles. This pain can easily disrupt higher consciousness.

6. Incorrect balance

When our body loses its balance, we must use extra muscles to stay in position. This extra effort causes us to lose free movement in our body and breath, and it obstructs higher consciousness.

7. Uncertainty

Uncertainty about whether or not we are doing an exercise properly causes us to move hesitantly, restlessly, and vaguely. This too blocks higher consciousness.

5.5 How to cope with distraction during a simple, dynamic exercise: Shoulder Stretch

This exercise includes three parts. The first two are performed while lying on a rubber strip; the third is a seated twist. This sequence has been chosen for its simplicity and moderate activity level, making it possible to concentrate on accessing higher consciousness and the factors that can disrupt this process in a movement context. That is why I have placed this exercise directly after the meditation exercise.

The first part, lying on the rubber strip, is passive, with no active movement. The intention is to access higher consciousness. With respect to the three phases described earlier for this process, the first (body consciousness) will be described in more detail, as the use of the breath differs somewhat from that used in the meditation exercise. The following two phases are approximately the same as in the meditation exercises and are described only briefly. For a more detailed explanation, see the meditation exercise.

The effect of distraction or disquieting factors on higher consciousness will be discussed in the second part of the exercise, stretching while lying on the rubber strip. This exercise is especially suitable for stabilizing the shoulder joint. This is a good exercise for demonstrating disrupting factors, as it is easy to distinguish relaxation from activity. Because the upper back is supported by the strip, the back and shoulders can remain passive and relaxed and not be affected by the activity of the arms.

The seated twist is described in detail in chapter 12.3, number 1 (Parivrtta Siddhasana, or Revolved Perfect Pose). This exercise is especially good for demonstrating the effect of such disquieting factors as loss of balance.

As described in chapter 2, the body needs pressure to relax. Pressure can be applied by using the weight of the body or, in areas that are difficult to reach, props. This last factor certainly applies to the area between the shoulder blades. It is impossible for many people to place their head directly above the spine because their upper back is stiff and bent. The rubber strip, folded in two and placed under the head and between the shoulder blades (figure 5.5-1), solves this problem, allowing the upper back to relax and stretch.

I will now describe how we can access higher consciousness. As already stated, I will explain the first step, body consciousness, in more detail because of the role breathing has in it.

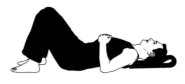

5.5-1

First step: realizing body consciousness

In a normal breath, most people regard their inhalation as the beginning of the cycle. In this exercise, the initial emphasis is placed on the *exhalation* and its relaxing effect; the inhalation is included at a later stage.

Place your hands on your lower ribs, near your abdomen. Next, bring your attention to the area of your back where the strip exerts the most pressure. It is here that stiff vertebrae are located, and they need this pressure the most. Direct your exhalations to this area so the muscles around the strip can relax, allowing the vertebrae and their discs to move slowly toward a straighter position. Use every exhalation to zoom in on this area with more precision, the goal being to release the stiff areas so they can become supple again. As you do this, your body will become heavier, which is a good indication of relaxation.

Next, include your chest in the feeling of relaxation, allowing the muscles around your ribs to become passive. This passive feeling initiates the inhalation. The movement of your ribs does not come from the ribs themselves, but from inside. The movement of air entering your body, together with the action of your diaphragm, causes your ribs to expand. The decreased tension you experience during inhalation will create more freedom of movement in the sternum and the ribs.

Free movement during inhalation does not occur by itself; you must consciously develop it. Thus, when you guide your breath from your stomach to the area of your chest where your hands are resting, your back should remain passive and heavy over the strip. Simultaneously, when the inhalation causes your ribs to spread, you should experience a feeling of lightness that starts where the air enters your body—in your nostrils. Feel the front of your chest become broad and spacious and the ribs in your back broaden in relation to the strip. This feeling in the ribs is important, because it shows that your back is relaxed. If your ribs cannot broaden, this indicates that your back is tense, probably because you are forcibly holding it straight.

Feel the breath gradually expand from the lower part of your chest to the upper areas. In front, it glides upward, past your sternum, to connect with your collarbones. In back, the movement follows the line of the strip, allowing you to experience a broadening of the ribs between your shoulder blades. Finally, when your lungs have reached their full capacity, your ribs will stop broadening, but the light feeling that came with the inhalation can develop even further, reaching your shoulders, arms, neck, head, pelvis, and legs. Try to observe yourself from a distance while still being conscious of your arms, legs, trunk, head, and so on. In this way, you achieve body consciousness carried by the flow of energy, and it becomes a tangible, physical experience. The feeling of lightness associated with the flow of energy will become more obvious as your relaxation deepens.

Second step: realizing mental consciousness

Next, feel the back of your head becoming heavy and the tension in your face easing, so a feeling of openness can develop in the back of your head. Take the time to passively observe fleeting thoughts from this place of deep relaxation. Consciously allow your sensory organs to relax, especially your eyes. The stream of thoughts will most likely lessen as time goes on, allowing you to achieve mental consciousness in the back of your head.

Third step: accessing higher consciousness

Remaining totally passive, observe how your body and mental consciousnesses merge together to form one intense, higher consciousness. This should be accompanied by a strong feeling of harmony and physical wellness. Higher consciousness is now firmly anchored in your body and mind. You may experience your body as being open or spacious. You become conscious of it and the space you are in not by breathing only into your body, but by including the space around you. The inhalation and exhalation become one continuum. You will feel, "I am conscious here and now."

Effects of disquieting factors and how to neutralize them

I will now discuss the effects of the above-mentioned factors on accessing higher forms of consciousness. This will be done using parts 2 (the shoulder stretch) and 3 (a seated twist) of the exercise. These are performed after accessing higher consciousness.

1. Restlessness

Directing your attention to the slow rhythm of your breath can initiate mental restlessness. This restlessness is caused by feelings of irritation or impatience or anger and its corresponding stream of thoughts. If you get caught up in this (unconscious) stream of thoughts, your attention—and, with it, higher consciousness—is immediately lost.

As soon as you realize that your attention to your breath is lessening, create a pause at the end of your exhalation. Allow your thoughts to calm down during this pause. Try to maintain the tranquillity in your head during your inhalation. This can best be achieved by once again directing your attention toward passive observation of the movement of your breath.

2. Discomfort

Relaxation achieved with exhalations makes your body feel heavy. This heaviness can cause discomfort, which in turn disturbs your feelings of relaxation and causes you to lose higher consciousness. Discomfort in this exercise is felt as a burning sensation in the skin, followed by a dull pain around the vertebrae. Your body will choose to move, but that instantly disturbs the depth of your relaxation. The strong desire to move causes restlessness, and that can become the first step in increasing tension. To cope with this, it is important that you deal with the restlessness caused by pain first by analyzing why the sensations are getting stronger and are causing your pain and aches. Understanding creates peace. Without going into detail about exactly what happens in your back, the rule of thumb is if the pain disappears, or diminishes substantially once the exercise is finished, you can regard it as a signal that something positive is taking place. That painful feeling, for example, can indicate that the vertebrae are becoming straighter and the structural tension in the muscles is starting to dissolve.

Your body will not immediately react in a positive way to discomfort and pain. If you do not respond to the desire to move, your body will look for another "solution" and react with tension. By directing your exhalations precisely to areas of tension, you can break this reaction, helping tight muscles around your vertebrae to relax so that movement can occur. If this does not work and the resistance remains, then the load is too large, and you must lessen the thickness of the strip so your body can accept the pressure. The free movement of inhalation will give a feeling of spaciousness to the areas of discomfort where the strip gives the most pressure. It is as if the inhalation washes away the tension in these areas. When you have acquired more experience in accessing higher consciousness, you will notice that being present in the here and now allows feelings of discomfort to remain increasingly in the background until they finally disappear.

The following three disturbances to relaxation and higher consciousness—movement, effort/strength, and pain—can be analyzed using the second part of the exercise, in which you move your arms over your head.

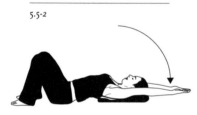
5.5-2

3. Movement
Slowly stretch your arms over your head until they can go no farther (figure 5.5-2; and chapter 6.3, connection 4). As soon as you initiate this stretch, you may be confronted with the third disturbance that can affect relaxation: movement. Normal daily movements are fast, direct, and automatic. They are dictated by the speed of thought, which is much faster than the movement of breath. With the initiation of movement, you often switch back to this fast, thought-controlled pattern, causing your body to tighten and you to immediate lose contact with your breath.

4. Effort/strength
The goal of the exercise is to allow your shoulders to move freely, so the movement of your arms can be passed on to your shoulder blades (there is a power line in your arms that leads to your shoulders). The shoulders themselves must remain relaxed. Because your back is on the rubber strip, it is straighter and your shoulders are relaxed. This allows your upper arms to develop strength, if you keep your elbows straight.

The increase of strength causes the fourth hindrance to higher consciousness: effort demands your attention. This is understandable because your daily efforts are also directed toward work, such as picking up (heavy) objects. This often occurs in a tense manner: your face tightens, your muscles tense, and your breathing becomes irregular or stops temporarily. Needless to say, if you do this during yoga, you immediately lose higher consciousness.

Although Critical Alignment does not make effort a high priority, the strength discussed in this exercise supports relaxation. There is a clear difference between tension and strength. Tension that develops when lifting a heavy object restricts and tightens the body. It occurs unconsciously and disturbs higher consciousness. The opposite is true for the strength that is developed in this exercise, which actually provides the possibility to deepen relaxation. If you release the tension in your shoulders, the strength in your upper arms will ensure that your chest receives more space and relaxation can deepen even further as a consequence. For this reason, during exertion, it is essential to direct your attention toward the area where the relaxation occurs as a result of strength (your chest) and to take advantage of the space created with the breath. Keeping your upper arms firm causes fatigue, but at the same time, it helps to create relaxation in your shoulders and chest. To cope with this fatigue, during exertion, you should remain connected with the positive feeling created by each inhalation. This is a conscious process that neutralizes your effort and makes it possible to maintain higher consciousness.

5. Pain

Practitioners of yoga are generally confronted with feelings of pain caused by stiff joints and muscles. An experienced teacher will explain that most of the pain is the "good" pain associated with change. However, sometimes the pain is inexplicable, and then it is up to the student to explore where it is coming from and what can be done about it. It is important to approach this pain with total attention. This is necessary because your body will react to the pain before it is actually felt. For example, if your shoulders are stiff, your elbows will start to bend during the shoulder exercise *before* you actually feel the pain. This "moving the pain around" is a common compensation. When it is corrected by keeping your elbows firmly straight, your body may harden and resist the movement. This resistance also occurs before you actually feel pain. Therefore, the question remains: does the pain exist because of a stereotypical reaction to pain, whereby the shoulders tighten even more and increase the pain, or is the pain caused by stiffness in the joint?

Only when your attention remains open and your respiration uninhibited, can this stereotypical resistance of the body be broken. When this occurs, you will often feel that the pain has gone, is greatly reduced, or has dissolved quickly. This principle also applies to stretching muscles, for example, the hamstrings in Uttanasana (Standing Forward Bend; see chapter 10.4, number 4).

6. Incorrect balance and uncertainty

A seated twist will now be used to study the effect of the last two disquieting factors on your experience and maintenance of higher consciousness. After you have completed the preceding exercise (lying on the folded strip and stretching your arms overhead), sit up straight on a chair as shown in figure 5.5-3. (For a detailed description of how to sit, see chapter 7.2.)

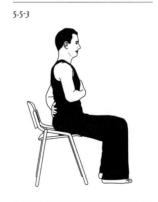

5.5-3

The previous exercises will make it easier to straighten your upper back, providing stability without tension in the movement muscles. Check the free position of your back by feeling if your back ribs are broadening with each inhalation (indicating that your back is relaxed) and narrowing with each exhalation (indicating that it is erect). You make the connection between your neck, upper back, and sternum with deep inhalations. This erect, free position of your upper body is the foundation for the twists you will perform and must be monitored via your breath.

Inhale, elevate your sternum, and pull your spine inward between your shoulder blades. This places your neck directly above your trunk. Maintain this connection during exhalations. Keep your shoulders relaxed. At the end of every inhalation, rotate to the

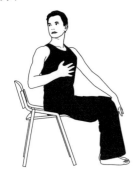

right by pushing your left hand against your left knee (figure 5.5-4). Relax your shoulders as you exhale. Retain the alignment of your head on top of your spine. Do this movement in small stages so you can learn it properly. After each stage, use an inhalation to check the proper alignment of your body. Inhalations keep your sternum and spine in correct balance.

A lot can go wrong during this exercise. You can lean too much to the left or right, your head can fall forward, your upper back may bend, you may lean too far back, and so on. Then you become stuck mentally and physically. When a vertebra or rib gets too much load, the free transfer of movement becomes impossible. This instability causes pressure and/or pain leading to tension, which directly disturbs your breathing and achievement of higher consciousness.

By continuously using your breath to monitor your posture, by staying present in the here and now, and by being conscious of the space around you, your body can maintain its balance. This allows you to perform the exercise accurately.

The feeling that you are on the right track helps to remove the last disruption to higher consciousness—uncertainty. When you are uncertain whether you are doing the exercise properly, your movements become vague and unsure. The dynamics of the exercise disappear, and your attention will dissipate. Obviously, you will lose higher consciousness.

You can remain unaffected by these obstacles by observing when they threaten to take over your behavior. Then you can neutralize them by focusing your attention on their opposites: space and relaxation. This gives you access to the deeper layers of mental stress that cause this tension, which is best described as an undercurrent of unease that may be related to the fear, anger, jealousy, uncertainty, envy, and so on that often control our actions.

5.6 Higher consciousness and disquieting factors during a complicated exercise: Paschimottanasana

It is more difficult to access higher consciousness in Paschimottanasana (see figure 5.6-1) than in the previous exercises, because it is a complex asana with many disquieting factors. Thus, I have placed it here in the order of exercises.

The technical description of Paschimottanasana can be found in chapter 10.5, number 6. This asana was also used to explain preferred poses (chapter 3), giving special attention to the right mental attitude needed to perform such a complex asana that can easily

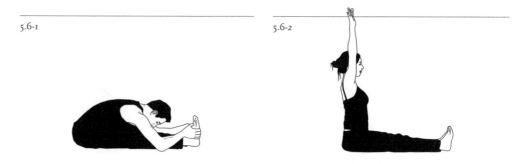

5.6-1

5.6-2

cause pain. This chapter uses Paschimottanasana as an example for accessing higher consciousness in a dynamic asana with complex movements. The degree of complexity is a source of many disquieting factors that make higher consciousness difficult to access in this and other complex asanas, so I will provide an extensive description of how these factors can be recognized and neutralized.

Paschimottanasana is initiated from seated Dandasana (see figure 5.6-2). Make sure your spine is stacked above your pelvis so that your lower back is solid and erect. You can align your body effortlessly above your diaphragm through your breath. (For a detailed description of Dandasana, see chapter 10.3, number 3.)

First, I will give a short description for accessing higher consciousness while performing the asana. For a more detailed description of consciousness, refer to the preceding meditation exercise.

Accessing higher consciousness

First phase: realizing body consciousness
You realize body consciousness in Dandasana, during which you calm your thinking in order to bring your spine into alignment. The correct positioning of your lower back gives it the strength needed to initiate movement. You consciously deepen and relax your breathing. You form an image of the movement and the final position together with one or two important points for attention.

Second phase: realizing mental consciousness
You use breathing to develop this step, creating an open, total awareness of your body without losing the points of attention for both sitting and movement. Your eyes have a soft focus, and you "look" from the back of your head, so you are not distracted by your surroundings. If restlessness begins to dominate, shut your eyes. Thus, without becoming distracted by external stimuli, you can perform the movement from Dandasana into Paschimottanasana with open attention and unrestricted breathing.

Third phase: accessing higher consciousness
In the final asana, body consciousness and mental consciousness merge into a full or higher consciousness, which includes consciousness of the space around you. This is the stage at which you are able to witness the positive intelligence of your body.

It may be compared with the moment when a child is learning to ride a bicycle, and the parent running alongside suddenly lets go. The child is free, and the parent witnesses how all the previous efforts instantaneously come together—at first there is an unbalanced, swaying movement, but within a few seconds the body starts to grasp the idea and balance itself. It starts to cooperate, and a badly coordinated movement becomes a well-balanced, completely new movement. Both the parent and the child experience this moment—the parent with a sense of relief and the child with a transformation from fear and stress to freedom, ease, and immense joy.

This transformation point where effort becomes freedom and strain becomes joy can also be experienced during this stage of yoga practice. Your body no longer resists and starts to cooperate. It begins to make decisions on its own to increase levels of relaxation, leading to a deepening of the asana.

Disquieting factors that disturb higher consciousness can develop in the following ways.

1. Restlessness

When you lose focus on your breath, willpower, enthusiasm, or ambition takes over, causing you to make hasty movements toward the end of Dandasana. Your attention to technique is lost, because you do not take time to form the correct image and the points for attention; you certainly do not take time to realize an open body consciousness. It is through body consciousness that you can observe the totality of your body and movement while maintaining the image and the points for attention. Instead of relaxing, you are taken over by haste and/or ambition.

2. Discomfort

An erect lower back transfers pressure to your hips, which can be unpleasant. This discomfort can disturb higher consciousness.

3. Movement

The movement from Dandasana to Paschimottanasana is complex. This complexity tends to disrupt higher consciousness. For example, if you lose the connection from your arms to your lower back, you will also lose higher consciousness. It is essential that your movements remain open, within the context of breathing and the space around you. If you become completely absorbed in movement, you will again lose higher consciousness.

4. Effort/strength

The effort of your lower back and the strength required from your legs and for lifting your arms can quickly demand all your attention, resulting in the opposite of higher consciousness: you hold your breath, your open attention narrows to a constricted concentration, and free movement becomes forced effort.

5. Pain

The more the movement develops, the greater the confrontation with pain in your hamstrings. This can hinder breathing and causes your body to develop compensatory movements to avoid the pain. Or your attitude may harden, and you see your legs as opponents that must be won over. All of this leads to a disturbance of higher consciousness, which must be present to oversee and guide the right dynamics, precise technique, and free breathing in the pose.

6. Incorrect balance

Incorrect balance causes you to lose attention. Your thinking becomes distracted and causes an immediate loss of higher consciousness. You do not know what you are doing anymore. For example, if your axis point moves from your lower back to your shoulders, your body will no longer be in a position to give you accurate feedback.

7. Uncertainty

Consequently, uncertainty will develop and lead to mental and physical restlessness.

5.7 Higher consciousness and disquieting factors during pranayama

The pranayama exercise is last in line, because pranayama is a formidable obstacle for many people due to a fear of suffocation. I will discuss this in detail and explain how to deal with it.

Slowing your respiration is an essential characteristic of pranayama. It helps you access higher consciousness by deepening relaxation and making it possible to connect your consciousness precisely with your breath. Also, your slowed beathing can help you access higher consciousness by "translating" important concepts such as space and relaxation into a physical experience (the subtle flow of energy). Then your mentally abstract understanding can be "transported" by your breath from your head into your body.

Furthermore, you hold your breath in some exercises, initiating a confrontation with the deeper layers of tension that determine your behavior. This confrontation gives you the opportunity to become acquainted with these deeper layers of tension and neutralize them. We will use the simple pranayama exercise Nadi Sodhana (Channel Cleaning Breath) to demonstrate higher consciousness and possible disquieting factors. To do this exercise, sit as shown in figures 5.7-1a and 5.7-1b and follow the instructions for breathing described in chapter 7.3, number 3.

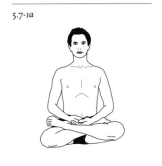

5.7-1a

First phase: realizing body consciousness
You can develop body consciousness when your body is both actively erect and in complete balance (and thus totally relaxed). To sit correctly, follow the instructions in chapters 5.3 and 7.2. This makes it possible to thoroughly work out the experience of the characteristics of the two gravity points (see chapter 6.3, connection 1).

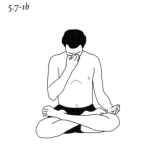

5.7-1b

The correct placement of your lower back provides space for your body's main (*hara*) gravity point. Inhalations subsequently fill this space with feelings of relaxation. Exhalations push the area below your navel forward, preventing the gradual buildup of tension.

The correct placement of your neck creates space around your heart gravity point. In this space, you develop a feeling of lightness through your breathing. This feeling is passed on to your entire body, allowing you to experience a subtle flow of energy. The open and transparent feeling that develops is supported by the solid foundation of your diaphragm, lower back, pelvis, legs, and contact with the floor. All of this leads to an open and positive body consciousness that is firmly anchored in the body.

Second phase: realizing mental consciousness
Before beginning the pranayama exercise, your thinking must be brought to a tranquil state by carefully releasing tension in your body and face and by relaxing your eyes (described in detail in the preceding meditation exercise). You achieve mental consciousness by calming your senses and thinking. As soon as you get caught up in a passing thought, an idea, an image, or a sound, this open mental consciousness will be lost. You can develop alertness within this mental consciousness by following the rhythm of your breath and the corresponding movement of your body.

Third phase: accessing higher consciousness

Before lowering your head and starting the actual exercise of Nadi Sodhana, allow your mental consciousness to descend through your neck and spine while noting these processes from your heart region. This way, you can observe the merging of body and mental consciousness into higher consciousness. The position of your head allows your neck to relax, which helps to calm your mind. Next, you direct awareness to the space around you. This does not mean only the physical space of the room or yoga studio; it also encompasses infinite space. When you achieve higher consciousness and continue the exercise with this higher consciousness, there is no more question of fear, suffocation, or reflexes of deep breathing. These disturbances can only exist when higher consciousness is broken by passing thoughts.

Disquieting factors can develop in the following ways during pranayama:

- Slowing your breath can cause strong reactions of *restlessness* or irritation. This can either be caused by a confrontation with stillness or be the result of a lack of stillness. Restlessness disturbs higher consciousness immediately.
- The unpleasant sensations of pins and needles and numbness that occur when your legs go to sleep often cause *discomfort*. These sensations are derive from the stretch on the nerve tracks or (temporary) compression to the blood vessels that supply these nerves. The discomfort is temporary; once your legs are stretched, the circulation will quickly return to normal. If you remain absorbed in higher consciousness, you register the numbness in your legs, but it does not cause even a hint of restlessness. Only when mental unease develops because you think, "My legs are asleep," can a new stream of thoughts be activated. If this occurs, the numbness in your legs will suddenly become annoying.
- *Movement* of the body — for example, the movement of your ribs during breathing — can demand so much attention that you become totally absorbed in it. This can be a good form of concentration, but if it interferes with higher consciousness, it becomes a disquieting factor.
- The strength (or *effort*) necessary to sit still for long periods can become a source of distraction. If your body is not stacked correctly, the movement muscles in your back will become tired.
- *Pain* can develop anywhere in your body and can be caused by the constant (unconscious) tightening of muscles. Tightness in the muscles around the middle of your back generally starts to dominate your attention. Inexperienced pranayama practitioners often develop a burning sensation in this area that disturbs higher consciousness. The cause of this enormous tension in the middle of the back is mostly caused by the gradual collapse of the lower back. The legs and hips can also become painful during long periods of sitting. If you sustain higher consciousness, this pain is nonexistent.
- *Incorrect balance* will block higher consciousness immediately, because it disrupts the free and regular rhythm of breathing. For example, if your lower back is not sufficiently extended, your exhalations become strained. Your stomach muscles tense at the end of each exhalation, pulling your stomach inward and causing deeper respiratory reflexes to occur. This, in turn, causes irregular breathing and disrupts higher consciousness.

· Deep respiratory reflexes are caused not only by physical instability but often by a purely physical reaction to the thought of breathlessness. As such, they become a source of *uncertainty*. Slowing your breathing may trigger the assumption that the supply of oxygen decreases. This activates a reflex center that initiates powerful deep breathing in order to bring the oxygen level back to normal. Everyone who has tried to hold their breath for as long as possible will have experienced this feeling of breathlessness and the ensuing deep respiratory reflexes. These strong physical reactions are also related to the profound (unconscious) uncertainty connected to a fear of suffocation, or a fear of death. This is purely a psychological phenomenon. Even a little breathlessness can be experienced as life-threatening, and nearly everyone panics in reaction to breathlessness. It is a confrontation that has a deep impact on our psyche—much deeper than confronting stiff muscles and joints when practicing asanas (see chapter 3.3 for a detailed discussion of this). The fact that pranayama exercises have a much more compelling structure than asanas also plays a large role: there is hardly any opportunity to compensate. The pranayama practitioner can easily become uncertain when confronted with such intense physical reactions and often begins to wonder if it is a good idea to carry on with this confrontation of tension.

The instigator of the respiratory reflexes is mental, not physical. There is enough oxygen in the body to stay alive. A good example of this is the Dutch free-diving champion who participated in my lessons. He could hold his breath for seven minutes. He also fought against his respiratory reflexes while underwater. He solved his uncertainty by continuously assuring himself that he had enough oxygen.

Relaxation and the associated experience of (infinite) space are the exact opposite of feelings of constriction and suffocation, so relaxation can help you to neutralize these reflexes, deeper layers of tension, and possibly unconscious patterns of fear. Thus, it is necessary to unite pranayama with the open experience of here and now, which is not marked by fear and worries. By observing the subtle forms of energy that circulate through your body, you can learn how to eliminate deeper layers of tension.

5.8   Conclusion

All-inclusive attention is the most important characteristic of higher consciousness and makes it possible to experience yourself and your surroundings in an objective way—that is, without your "I" element. While maintaining this consciousness, you can confront deep levels of tension and other problems in your body, as well as your ambitions and other motivations. When you see these issues as they are, without becoming involved or judging, they will slowly lose their power over you. Then it becomes increasingly possible to experience yourself here and now in asana.

Higher levels of consciousness promote intense feelings of harmony and freedom. These experiences form the basis of spiritual experience. They can be intensified through deeper relaxation and further withdrawal from the "to-do" mode. This intensive consciousness leads to an unprecedented direct experience of being in the here and now paired with a deep feeling of purpose and harmony. This experience is vital, because it is continuously renewed.

This is all we can do—or not do. Everything else, feelings of understanding, surrender, and so on, are given to us. We cannot strive for these goals; they come or they don't. We have no power over them.

In conclusion, accessing higher consciousness is obviously not limited to the yoga practices of pranayama and meditation. In spite of the many disrupting influences we encounter, we can attempt to realize this in our daily lives.

Part Three

Building Blocks of Movement Chains

In this section, I will explain important aspects of the function of movement chains, primarily through practical application—unlike Part Two, where I focused on the theory and context of the Critical Alignment method. Here I will discuss the building blocks of movement chains, or connections, with respect to yoga movements.

Connections are the links in the movement chains of asanas where movement is passed from one body part to the next. I will discuss this concept, which is new and has not previously been specifically considered within yoga, in detail in chapter 6.

6

UNDERSTANDING CONNECTIONS AND MOVEMENT CHAINS

6.1   Introduction

I introduced the concept of movement chains in chapter 2.1 and applied it to yoga exercises in chapter 2.4. Generally speaking, this concept explains how small movements are passed on through linked body parts and how series of small movements produce a final, larger, fluid movement.

Good communication must exist between the different body parts—such as the head, neck, upper and lower back, pelvis, and legs—to accomplish the full range of yoga movements. Connections between these different body parts allow smaller movements to be passed on like links in a chain, but a chain is only as strong as its weakest link. Similarly, connections that do not function adequately hinder small movements, preventing proper completion of a total movement.

First, I will discuss two important aspects concerning the function of connections: (1) the alignment of the body parts that form the connection, and (2) the sequence and momentum required to activate connections within a movement chain. Then I will talk about the different connections in detail.

6.2-1a–d

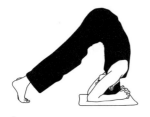

a

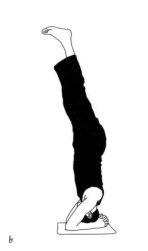

b

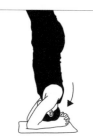

c

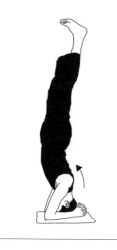

d

6.2 Optimal functioning of connections depends on precise alignment, correct sequence, and momentum when activating the skeleton.

The two most important aspects for the correct transfer of movement are establishing and maintaining good alignment and achieving the correct sequence and momentum when activating the skeleton.

Alignment of connections

It has been my experience that connections do not always function optimally. In chapter 2.3, I discussed the causes and processes that can lead to blockages in movement chains and cause physical problems. In chapters 2.5 and 2.6, I explained how Critical Alignment can eliminate these blockages by improving the alignment of the affected skeletal areas.

It is important to realize that movement chains can stretch in opposite directions. The spine is a good example. (Other examples are the connections of the arms with the hands and the lower back with the pelvis; see chapter 6.3, numbers 5 and 9, respectively.) The spine can stretch toward the head *and* toward the pelvis. Thus, small movements are passed on smoothly in opposite directions from vertebra to vertebra. The result is that small movements at the front (anterior) of the spine enable you to stretch toward the crown of your head (see chapter 6.3, connection 3), and small movements at the back (posterior) of the spine allow you to stretch toward your pelvis (see chapter 6.3, connection 10). The act of stretching in opposite directions strengthens the power line through the connections. The relevant body parts are placed in a better position where they can make optimal use of gravity and body weight.

The sequence and momentum for activating connections

As already discussed in chapter 2.2, the diversity of movement chains makes a large variety of asanas directly relevant to Critical Alignment. Differences in movement chains become evident when practicing asanas that use gravity and body weight differently.

Now I would like to detail the unique characteristics of movement chains, as well as how yoga movement is determined by the arrangement, sequence, and speed of the connections within the chains. In yoga practice, connections must be activated precisely by using the correct sequence and momentum. If done incorrectly, the weight of the body passes on from one body part to the next only partially (or not at all). This in turn hinders the larger, total movement, causing it to either falter or stop completely.

I will explain this using three asanas: Sirsasana (see chapter 8.2.1), Utthita Trikonasana (see chapter 9.3.8), and Viparita Chakrasana (see chapter 11.4.8). I discussed these asanas as they related to different movement chains and the use of body weight and gravity in chapter 2.4.2. Now I will focus on the differences in the arrangement of connections, their sequence, and their speed of activation. These descriptions are not complete, but they are an indication of the importance of understanding and using connections.

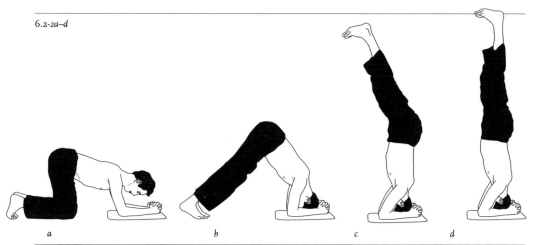

6.2-2a–d

a   b   c   d

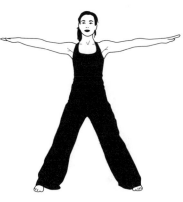

6.2-3a

6.2-3b

The muscles in the left side of the lower back have contracted.

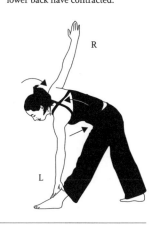

6.2-4a

Sirsasana

When moving into Sirsasana, the movements shown in figures 6.2-1a through 6.2-d often occur. In figure 6.2-1a, bringing the feet in toward the body causes the back to bend and tension to develop in the shoulders and neck. Pressure in the neck increases when the legs are lifted, as shown in figure 6.2-1b. Ultimately, the movement is obstructed in the neck and shoulders, increasing tension there even more (figure 6.2-1c) or causing tension in the middle and lower back, as shown in figure 6.2-1d. Tension develops in many areas of the body in the final pose because no attention was given to the right connections or the correct sequence of movement. This simply maintains and strengthens preferred postures.

Accurate connections, on the other hand, create space (all of the following connections are described in chapter 6.3). First, the shoulders are connected to the shoulder blades (connection 4), then the neck to the crown and upper back (connection 3). This can be seen in figure 6.2-2a. When you walk in to the pose, you use the connection between your lower back, pelvis, and legs (connection 7), as shown in figure 6.2-2b. Regarding momentum, when you lift your legs, you give connections 4 and 3 priority; your neck and shoulders move faster than your legs (figure 6.2-2c). This creates balance between the two gravity points (connection 1) in the final pose, illustrated in figure 6.2-2d.

Utthita Trikonasana

All of the following connections are described in chapter 6.3. Utthita Trikonasana is often initiated from a standing position (figure 6.2-3a). In a worst-case scenario, this causes tensions in the lower back, diaphragm, and neck (see the arrows in figure 6.2-3b).

The sequence of movement changes when the pose is initiated from Adho Mukha Svanasana. This allows you to develop the pose using connections. From Adho Mukha Svanasana, bring your right foot forward, connecting your lower back to that hip and leg (connection 7 and 10). Your neck can connect to your sternum and crown (connection 3), shown in figure 6.2-4a.

After stretching and straightening your right leg (connection 2), you stabilize your inner tube (connection 8) by arching your lower back. You can connect your head to your upper back (connection 2), creating balance and space between your two gravity points (connection 1). Your right arm connects to your shoulder

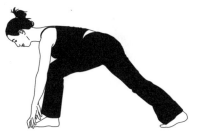

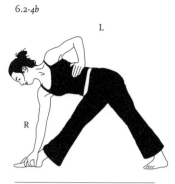

6.2-4b

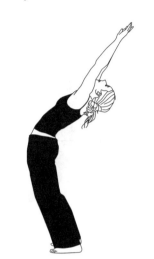

6.2-5a

blade (connection 4) and initiates the twist when you push with your right hand against the inside of your right ankle (figure 6.2-4b).

Viparita Chakrasana

This backbend is often done by "hanging" from the lower back and collapsing the chest (figure 6.2-5a). When this occurs, the arms cannot connect to the shoulder blades or the back, and the head cannot connect to the upper back. Support from the inner tube is lost. The movement hinges around the hips and lower back, making the transfer of movement through the spine impossible. Because the movement is initiated from the hips and not from the head, the result is an angular, jerky jump instead of an open, fluid movement.

From a Critical Alignment perspective, your arms must be connected to your shoulder blades and back (connection 4) first. Your head must be connected to your upper back (connection 2). (All of these connections are discussed in chapter 6.3.) Subsequently, the movement from your chest must be transferred via your inner tube (connection 8) to your pelvis and legs (connection 7), ending in your feet (connection 11). All of these connections remain intact during the dynamic phase (figures 6.2-5b and 6.2-5c). For an effortless jump, it is important for your head to initiate the movement and for your body to follow. The speed with which your head moves determines the progress of the jump. The result is an open, fluid movement; your two gravity points remain balanced, and you experience the movement as light and relaxed (figures 6.2-5d through 6.2-5j). Otherwise, this movement could never be repeated 108(!) times. (For more on this number, see page 298.)

6.3 Isolated connections within movement chains

I will now discuss two different connections, both of which are concerned with specific areas of the body that are easy to isolate. Most of the exercises make use of yoga movement components. As illustrated in the last section, asanas contain multiple connections that must be kept aligned and followed in sequence. The remainder of the exercises, described here, have the sole purpose of relaxing certain areas of the body; they are not asana movements.

6.2-5b–j

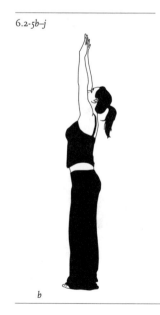

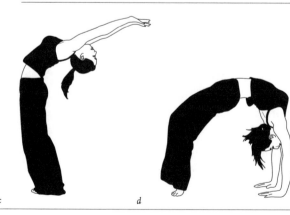

b   c   d

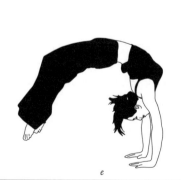

e

Yoga props allow you to become aware of the condition of your spine and locate potentially problematic areas. These props (discussed in chapter 2.5) include a felt mat, rubber strip, belt, shoulderstand block, and yoga mat.

The exercises described for connection 1 (the roll under the shoulder blades, the rubber strip between the shoulder blades, and the roll under the lower back) illustrate precisely how to develop diaphragmatic and chest breathing.

1. The connection between the two central gravity points: the lower abdomen and the heart region

When the spine is correctly balanced, movement is passed on, vertebra by vertebra, from the head through to the pelvis during such movements as standing, sitting, and walking. Movement that is correctly coordinated creates an upward movement from the lower abdomen toward the crown of the head. This maintains the space around both gravity points at all times.

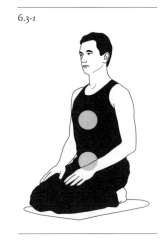

6.3-1

When this balance is disturbed, both centers of gravity become constricted, or one center of gravity dominates the other. In that case, it is difficult to experience a feeling of relaxation in the hara area in the lower abdomen or feelings of lightness in the heart center of gravity.

The first gravity point is located between the navel and pubic bone, and it is the main center of gravity in the body. As noted in chapter 2.2, it is called the *hara* in Japanese. The second point is located around the lower part of the sternum, near the solar plexus, in the region of the heart. It functions as the center of gravity for the spine (figure 6.3-1) and is independent of the hara.

When a gravity point feels spacious and relaxed, that indicates it is in balance. Movements that provide space to these areas can come from various parts of the body and from breathing. Feelings of spaciousness in the heart region come primarily from the neck, but the arms can also contribute. Similarly, space in the lower abdomen is principally provided through the dynamic use of the inner tube (this is the action of the lower back and the position of the pelvis and diaphragm). In some exercises, the legs can also provide extra support.

Of course, the two centers of gravity can be activated separately. However, in Critical Alignment, it is extremely important that they move simultaneously and with maximum ease, allowing an experience of the total movement as relaxed and free.

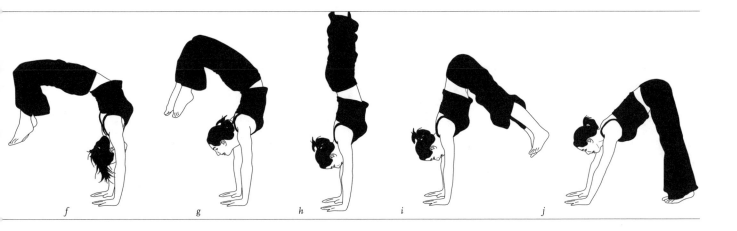

f   g   h   i   j

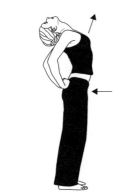

6.3-2a

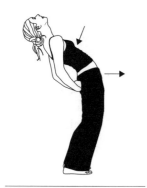

6.3-2b

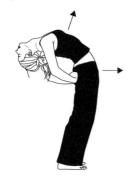

6.3-2c

Preferential postures that have developed as a result of normal everyday activities often cause one of the centers of gravity to dominate—always at the expense of the other. Or, even more detrimental, both centers of gravity can become inactive.

For a fluid, total movement in the spine, it is essential that the two gravity points maintain their equilibrium, so the continuity of the spine will remain undisturbed. Figures 6.3-2a and 6.3-2b illustrate the opposite situation, specifically, how the back can become strained when movements are done without balance between the two centers of gravity. The following example illustrates how this applies to a standing backbend.

When initiating the backbend, the following mistakes are common. The person in figure 6.3-2a has lifted her chest high to create space without allowing for space in her lower abdomen. The space in her chest is visible, but her lower abdomen is being pulled inward, because it has lost the support of her lower back. The strong chest movement "pulls" the support and strength out of her lower back (as indicated by the arrows). This immediately breaks the connection. The movement toward her pelvis cannot be completed properly and gets stuck in the middle of her back.

In the continuation of the backbend, the movement should be transferred to the pelvis. But the excessive lifting of her chest has removed the strength and stability from her lower back, which is no longer in a position to receive and assimilate the movement. This means the movement can continue to her lower abdomen, but when it reaches that point, her chest will collapse and become rigid. The open position of her chest needs the support of her lower back. The culmination of all this is that her body weight gets hung up in her lower back (see figure 6.3-2b).

Figure 6.3-2c illustrates how the movement appears when both gravity points are balanced. Both areas—the lower abdomen and the chest region—are supported and can move simultaneously with space and relaxation.

If we are not conscious of these two centers of gravity, their equilibrium will constantly be disturbed. This disruption can happen in various ways:

· The opening of one gravity point is done at the expense of the other, as described in the preceding example.
· Neither gravity point can be used because the back is excessively convex.
· Neither gravity point can be used because the back is overextended.

6.3-3a and b

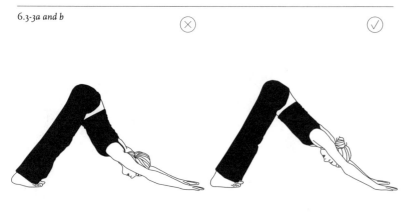

6.3-4a and b

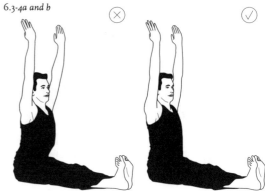

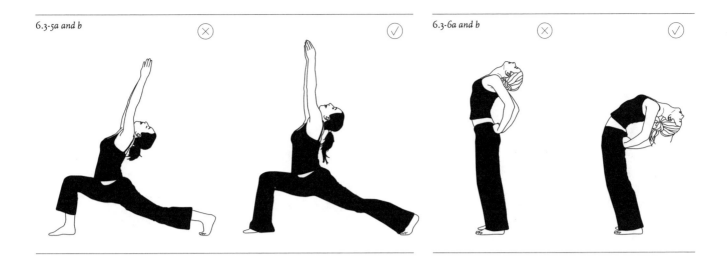

6.3-5a and b ⊗ ✓   6.3-6a and b ⊗ ✓

Incorrect movements belonging to these three categories, as well as the correct versions, are illustrated here

Opening the chest gravity point at the expense of the lower abdomen

1. Adho Mukha Svanasana I (see chapter 9.2, number 4); compare figures 6.3-3a and 6.3-3b.
2. Dandasana (see chapter 9.2, number 3); compare figures 6.3-4a and 6.3-4b.
3. Virabhadrasana I (see chapter 9.5, number 14); compare figures 6.3-5a and 6.3-5b.
4. Standing backbends (see chapter 11.4, number 9); compare figures 6.3-6a and 6.3-6b.
5. Tadasana (Mountain Pose; see chapter 9.2, number 1); compare figures 6.3-7a and 6.3-7b.

Opening the abdomen gravity point at the expense of the chest

1. Salamba Sarvangasana (Supported Shoulderstand; see chapter 8.3, number 13); compare figures 6.3-8a and 6.3-8b.
2. Standing backbends (see chapter 11.4, number 9); compare figures 6.3-9a and 6.3-9b.

6.3-7a and b ⊗ ✓   6.3-8a and b ⊗ ✓   6.3-9a and b ⊗ ✓

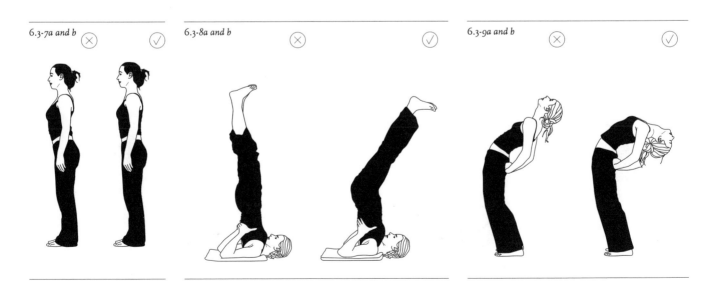

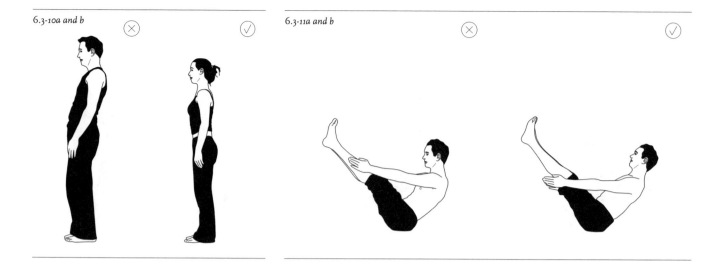

6.3-10a and b ⊗ ✓   6.3-11a and b ⊗ ✓

3. Tadasana (see chapter 9.2, number 1); compare figures 6.3-10a and 6.3-10b.
4. Navasana (Boat Pose; see chapter 10.3, number 1); compare figures 6.3-11a and 6.3-11b.

Lack of space in both gravity points due to an excessively convex back:

1. Paschimottanasana (see chapter 10.5, number 6); compare figures 6.3-12a and 6.3-12b.
2. Siddhasana (Accomplished Pose; see chapter 13.2, number 2); compare figures 6.3-13a and 6.3-13b.

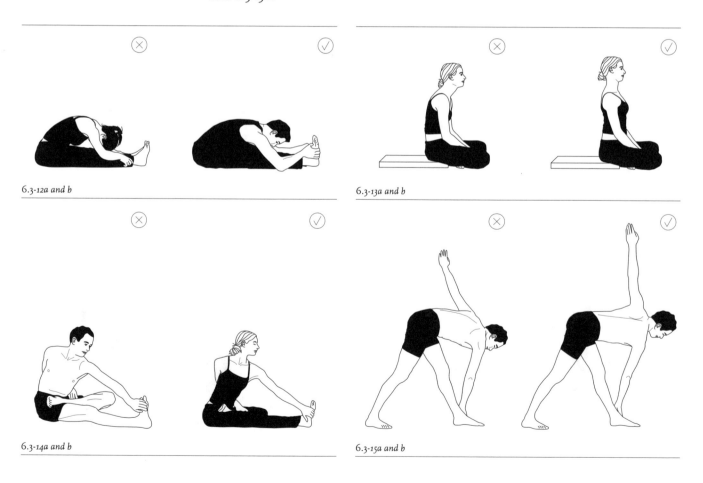

6.3-12a and b   6.3-13a and b

6.3-14a and b   6.3-15a and b

3. Ardha Matsyendrasana; see chapter 12.5, number 5); compare figures 6.3-14a and 6.3-14b.
4. Parivrtta Trikonasana (Revolved Triangle Pose; see chapter 9.3, number 9); compare figures 6.3-15a and 6.3-15b.

Lack of space in both gravity points due to overextension of the back:

1. Virabhadrasana III (see chapter 9.2, number 7); compare figures 6.3-16a and 6.3-16b.
2. Pincha Mayurasana (Feathered Peacock Pose; see chapter 8.4, number 19); compare figures 6.3-17a and 6.3-17b.
3. Utkatasana (see chapter 9.2, number 2); compare figures 6.3-18a and 6.3-18b.

If the two centers of gravity become constricted, they no longer feel free. It is precisely this feeling of freedom that determines whether or not we experience space and ease in our movements. Both of these gravity points are centers of feeling. Space in the lower abdomen gives a basic feeling of relaxation, whereas relaxation in the heart region gives a basic feeling of lightness and openness to our movements.

Relaxation can be experienced in these two gravity points when movement is correctly aligned. However, a conscious experience of lightness and relaxation can only be realized through correct breathing. By concentrating on our breath during movement or when standing tranquilly in an asana, we can observe (experience) relaxation and lightness in our body.

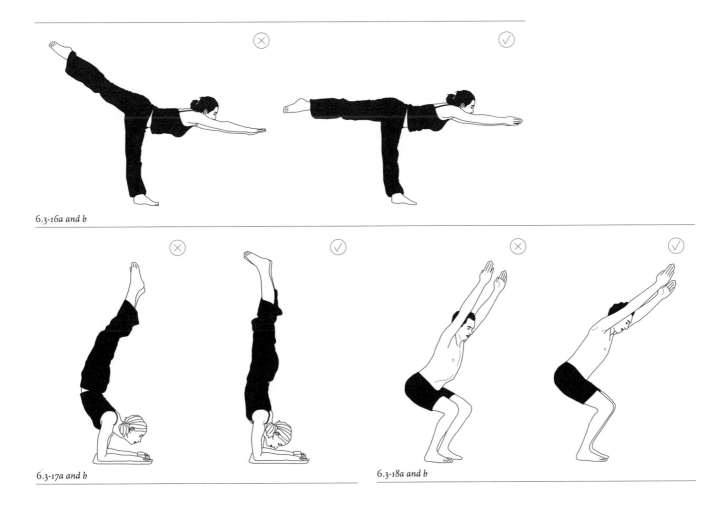

6.3-16a and b

6.3-17a and b   6.3-18a and b

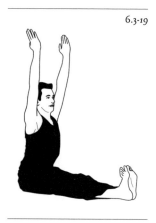

6.3-19

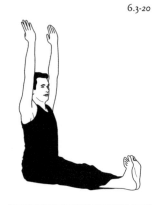

6.3-20

The most important component for achieving this equilibrium is the neutral position of the diaphragm, which is directly related to correct alignment of the lower ribs. The diaphragm is an important muscle for respiration. If one of the two gravity points is out of balance, the diaphragm also loses its balance. This causes the breath to "fall" back to one of these two areas, making it impossible to simultaneously feel, move, or relax both of them. The unity developed through open attention is also lost. When this occurs, at least one of the qualities related to the balance of the gravity points—either the feeling of relaxation or the feeling of lightness—is lost.

These disruptions are caused by the *intention* with which we direct our movement. Do we make a conscious attempt to complete the movement in a relaxed manner, or do we develop the movement from willpower, haste, or habit? If we are not conscious of these differences, we will again become prisoners of our habits, and the movement will be completed through effort. Such an attitude is clearly similar to that of many people when working out at the gym or playing sports. It aims at the automatic use of the movement muscles, which are controlled by willpower. To pursue relaxation in a dynamic situation, Critical Alignment focuses clearly on the postural muscles. Admittedly, the necessary movement muscles must also be engaged (as described in chapter 2.2). Priority, however, is given to an open attention that is carried by the breath and not to muscles directed by willpower. To be conscious of relaxation in the abdomen and chest simultaneously means that we have to be aware of two places at once. Such a complex attention can only develop when these areas become palpable through correct movement, breathing, and cultured tranquillity.

When we compare figure 6.3-19 (pose 1: Dandasana with the abdomen pulled in and the chest pushed forward) and figure 6.3-20 (pose 2: Dandasana with relaxation in the abdomen and chest), we can see alarming differences:

1. Pose 1 is created through tension; the muscles in the midback are contracted, pushing the chest forward. This causes the lower ribs to slide forward, disrupting the natural position of the lower back and creating more tension. In comparison, pose 2 makes use of two important connections that are brought into balance and linked; the inner tube is brought into balance with the neck–midback–heart region connection.
2. Pose 1 is based on the principle of "shoulders back, chest forward." This movement is directed by willpower and brought to completion by the superficial movement muscles. In comparison, the two connections in pose 2 are completed by engaging the postural muscles.
3. When the lower ribs shift forward, as shown in pose 1, the breath gets stuck in the chest, and the relaxing effect of abdominal breathing is lost. The space in the chest was not created by relaxed breathing and, as such, can only be enforced with strength. Thus, feelings of lightness and freedom in the chest are lost, and the pose feels strained: the body is working. In comparison, the breath in pose 2 is able to connect abdominal breathing with chest breathing, and the pose is created from feelings of relaxation and lightness.

When we consider the circulation of bodily energy, the disturbance between the two centers of gravity is interesting. When the awareness in the lower abdomen dominates because it feels relaxed, as most of us experience when we are sitting on the couch at the end of the day, we do experience relaxation. But it is the kind often connected with tiredness and sleep. In this state, we are inactive and not very interested in the space around us, but we are closely connected to ourselves. Because no action is involved, this kind of relaxation will not change our behavior during active (stressful) circumstances such as at work.

When the heart region dominates, as in the preceding example, we are connected with the space around us but in a hard, often insensitive way. It literally pushes the relaxation away. We are active but quite likely to build up strain, which can exhaust us. Our energy level is high.

When we are able to keep the centers of gravity balanced, we are able to connect our actions to relaxation. Even when the circumstances are stressful, we can learn how to behave without losing the connection with our own space and relaxation.

To clearly experience the feeling of these two centers of gravity being balanced, do the following exercise.

The balance between the two centers of gravity: prone

If you have a shoulderstand block, place it lengthwise on the floor. Otherwise, lie directly on your stomach.

Instructions

6.3-21

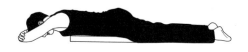

- Place the base of your sternum against the front edge of the shoulder-stand block; your abdomen and pelvis should be on the bottom of the block. Lengthen the back of your neck, and place your forehead on your forearms, as shown in figure 6.3-21.
- Relax your lower back, and press the area about 1 inch below your navel gently into the block. This will automatically pull the arch of your lower back into a neutral extension. Feel how every inhalation increases the space in your belly and adds more pressure on the block (or floor).
- During each exhalation, the space in your belly will diminish, but exhale in such a way that the spot below your navel keeps moving toward the block through the pressure of your breath. If you are able to coordinate your exhalation this way, it creates a perfectly relaxed base for the next inhalation, which can, very slowly, start from the same spot.
- When the spot below your navel starts to contract inward at the end of your exhalation, it will produce tension in your belly. Then the next inhalation will not start from the same area but a little higher, leaving some tension behind in your lower abdomen. When this happens again during the next exhalation, the tension will start to accumulate and push the inhalations farther up. This often happens when circumstances are stressful (due to a confrontation with discomfort or pain during the performance of asanas) or strenuous. After a while, breathing causes so much tension in your body that it will harden your shoulders, chest, and neck. When you are not able to change your breathing pattern through the proper support from your lower back, you are not able to neutralize this tension.
- Press the base of your sternum against the block and elevate your neck without losing its extension; your forehead lifts from your forearms. The weight of your head is now transferred to your heart region. Breathe into this area and feel how every inhalation intensifies the feeling of space there. Stretch your arms along your sides and let the back of your hands rest on the ground.

Note: You can actively press your sternum against the block, but the pressure against it can also arise through breathing. Inhalations press the base of your sternum against the block and pull your spine inward between your shoulder blades. As a result of this movement of the spine, your neck will move up and transport the weight of your head into the heart region (see also connection 3, the elevator (page 103).

If you elevate from your shoulders, you will reach beyond the bottom part of your sternum. You will be able to lift yourself higher and feel pressure in your stomach and abdominal areas. Your lower back will contract as your lower ribs shift forward—that is, away from the stomach. This is a wrong movement and to ensure that you avoid it, distribute the pressure equally between your lower abdomen and heart region, and intuitively connect these two areas with your breath.

The balance between the two centers of gravity: seated

Instructions

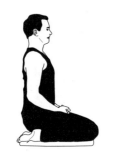

6.3-22

- While sitting on your feet (figure 6.3-22), first press one or two fingers against the spot 1 inch below your navel and send your exhalations toward your fingers. Feel the breath pushing against your fingers to avoid the tension accumulation already described.
- Breathe toward your sternum to feel relaxation in your heart region *without losing the pressure on your fingers*. The next inhalation will pull the area between your shoulder blades into extension. Use three or four breaths to develop this movement without losing the pressure on your fingers at the end of your exhalations.
- The movement of your spine will pull your neck into position on top of your trunk without strain. Breathe from your lower abdomen to your heart region as if you are still lying on the block.

By using your breath in this way, you can constantly scan your abdominal and heart regions. Pressing your fingers against the spot below your navel is a very effective method for verifying the relaxed use of your breath. It can be used in many ways during the practice of asanas. I will refer to this more often in the description of the asanas in the next part of this book. It can also be used in (stressful) daily circumstances, for instance sitting in your chair at your desk.

2 The connection between the head, the neck, and the upper back

The ability of the neck to transfer the weight of the head into the upper back depends on relaxing the upper back. Extension of the thoracic spine elevates the sternum and moves it forward. When this connection is disturbed, the postural muscles in the neck cannot transport the weight of the head toward the upper back, and the neck is no longer capable of extending fully. When this happens, the neck shortens, and the muscles of the neck and shoulders become structurally tensed.

The following exercises provide insight into how the connections between the head, neck, and upper back are developed.

The roll under the shoulder blades

The area directly distal to the shoulder blades is the middle of the back, and it corresponds with the base of the sternum. Ideally, when sitting or standing, the movement of the neck should continue right down to this part of the back. However, this area is often stiff, causing an increase in mobility in a lower part of the spine. The following exercise is designed to increase mobility to the area directly distal to the shoulder blades. It also demonstrates diaphragmatic breathing.

Instructions

- Sit on the floor with your knees bent and your feet flat on the floor. Place a roll (4 to 5 inches thick) horizontally on the floor behind you and lie on it so it is just under your shoulder blades (figures 6.3-23a and 6.3-23b). You can keep your knees bent or stretch your legs out, whichever feels best for your lower back. Your posterior ribs are supported by the roll just distal to the shoulder blades. The front of your body should feel as if the roll is supporting the base of your sternum.

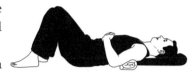

6.3-23a

- Place the rubber strip (or a book) under your head. This prevents your neck from becoming concave and tense.

6.3-23b

- Place your hands on the arch of your lower ribs to monitor movement there. Direct your breath toward your hands. Allow your ribs to move toward your abdomen, increasing the pressure of the roll on your back. Observe this area of extra pressure. Guide your exhalations there and relax your back. Inhalations remain in your abdomen because of your supine position. When the muscles in your back relax, the roll will stimulate your back to become straighter, allowing the intervertebral discs to change shape (see chapter 4.5). This can be painful, but it indicates that your back is moving.

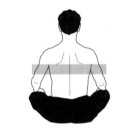

If you practice this exercise regularly, the vertebrae and their discs will be able to attain a natural alignment more quickly. The pain will also diminish faster. Within a few weeks, your back will most likely become more flexible, making the movement a lot less painful. (If you require additional relaxation in your spine, refer to the coordination exercise described in chapter 12.2.)

- The relaxation that develops with exhalations makes free and relaxed inhalations to your ribs possible. If you guide your inhalations from your abdomen to your ribs, you will feel the area under your hands begin to move. Your ribs must not move upward; they must remain low and become *broad.* The same occurs in your back where it makes contact with the roll. Feel how the ribs there broaden almost automatically, without effort. If you do not experience this immediately, keep the mental image of ribs that are relaxed and widening. You will eventually feel their actual movement.
- Try to allow the relaxed feeling from exhalations to encompass inhalations. Remember that the movement of inhaling begins inside the body: breath enters your nostrils, your lungs are filled, and they pass this movement on to your ribs. Your ribs will move with less effort if your muscles are relaxed. Allow your inhalations to become calm, so they feel like a soft breeze on the inside of your nostrils, as if you are inhaling a pleasant fragrance. This softness will be mirrored in the movement of your ribs.
- As soon as you feel your ribs broadening over the roll with a (relaxed) inhalation, guide your breath to the base of your sternum. The arch of your ribs will increase

with deeper inhalations. Your ribs can move in a relaxed way, even during exhalations, when there is no buildup of tension in your heart region. To feel this clearly, place a hand on the base of your sternum. When you exhale, feel your back narrowing. Admittedly, your sternum moves somewhat lower, but it remains free from tension. In this way, respiration massages tension out of your back muscles, intercostal ribs, and base of your sternum from the inside out. Continue this for 3 to 5 minutes. Repetition stimulates the effect and also influences your concentration. The speed of thought is normally much faster than the rhythm of breath. In this exercise, we try to join our attention to the slow rhythm of the breath. This can also cause unease, which makes breathing more rapid. Remain alert for such developments, and correct them as you become aware of them.

The rubber strip between the shoulder blades

This exercise increases mobility between the shoulder blades and demonstrates chest breathing.

Instructions

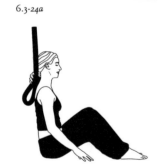

6.3-24a

- Fold one end of the rubber strip double; the folded part should be the length of your hand plus 1 inch.
- Place the edge of the double part against the seventh cervical vertebra (C7), as shown in figures 6.3-24a and 6.3-24b, and lie on the strip. You can locate C7, the last vertebra of the neck, as follows: bring your chin toward your chest and feel along the back of your neck toward your upper back. C7 is the protrusion you feel at the bottom of your neck.
- From this position, push your pelvis toward the ceiling until you are balancing on your feet and C7 (figure 6.3-25). Check with your hands that C7 is still resting on top

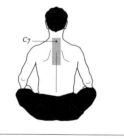

6.3-24b

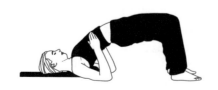

6.3-25

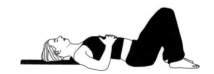

6.3-26

of the doubled-up strip. Push lightly with your feet toward C7. Your chest will move toward your chin, lessening the curve in your neck and developing length there. Your neck actually pushes the back of your head farther away.

- Place your hands on the arch of your lower ribs.

> **Note:** The neck can sometimes react in the opposite way, with the chin lifting and the back of the head moving toward the neck. If this happens, bring both of your hands to the back of your head and manually lengthen your neck.

☞ *Important Tip*

If your chest moves toward your chin and your neck muscles are relaxed, then your chin will also move toward your chest. *Do not* push your chin toward your chest; this will cause your neck muscles to contract and pressure will develop in your throat. When you relax your neck muscles, their places of attachment to the back of your skull will also soften. This allows the back of your head to stretch away from your neck.

- Try to keep your neck in this extended position by pushing lightly with your feet. This also increases the pressure to C7; use it to relax the surrounding muscles. Moving slowly, lower your chest and back toward the floor and feel the pressure of the rubber strip move from vertebra to vertebra. Guide your exhalations to these vertebrae.
- If your back moves sufficiently, then your neck will remain in the same position as seen in figure 6.3-26.
- When your pelvis touches the floor, your feet should still be pushing toward the areas of pressure on the rubber strip. Try to accept this pressure and relax your back with exhalations. This will allow your anterior (front) ribs to lower slowly without your neck lifting. When you have developed maximum relaxation with exhalations, you can use it to develop the inhalations. The rubber strip stretches across the entire area between your shoulder blades and provides enough support to prevent your sternum from collapsing.

> **Note:** If parts of your upper back do not move adequately with the pressure of the rubber strip, the back of your head will be pulled toward your neck, causing your neck to become more concave. This is not your neck's fault; the real cause is the inability of the vertebrae on the rubber strip to move. Slow the movement down and remain in that area. See if you can locate precisely which vertebrae are involved and allow the surrounding muscles to relax.

> **Note:** When your back stiffens, it becomes less sensitive, which means you do not experience feelings of inadequate movement there. The information will come from your neck, which will clearly show the lack of movement when it becomes more concave.

Note: Visualize the following: Your sternum, which is connected to your spine through your ribs, moves up during inhalation. Through this upward movement in front, your vertebrae, which are resting on the strip, can be pulled up a little. Thus, your spine can be stretched by the inhalation. To stabilize this straighter position of your upper back, press the back of your head gently against the strip. This will give a more active sense of support from your neck.

This coordination between the inhalation, the inward movement of your upper back and the position of your neck and head can be used in all exercises where your spine and neck are fully extended. Greater extension of the spine can be accomplished via the breath in backbends and forward bends as well.

Read the instructions regarding breathing from the previous exercise, as they also apply here. You can spend 3 to 5 minutes on this exercise.

In this exercise, the posterior ribs are suspended above the floor, which can make the broadening of the ribs feel freer. This differentiates it from the exercise with the roll. From the base of the sternum, the inhalation gradually develops in the chest and finally connects with the collarbones. In the back, the movement follows the rubber strip; the same broadening that occurs in the front ribs also occurs in those between the shoulder blades.

The following coordination exercise supports the correct position of the neck and upper back. It should be done immediately after the preceding exercise.

3. The connection between the neck and the sternum and between the neck and the crown

The neck will only be able to extend toward the crown if it can transfer the weight of the head into the upper back between the shoulder blades. This keeps the spine mobile and extended, supports space in the chest, and keeps the neck strong and free of tension.

When this connection is disturbed, it is impossible to use the weight of the head to extend the upper back. Therefore, the neck cannot support the space in the heart region. Then it is also impossible to lengthen the spine through the extension of the neck.

The neck has an important role in coordination; it must pass movement on in opposite directions: toward the head and the crown, and toward the upper back and the chest. For this reason, both of these connections will be discussed here.

6.3-27

6.3-28

6.3-29

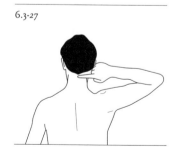
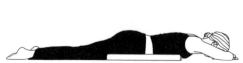
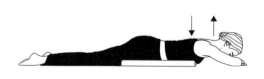

Preparation

In the following exercise, a specific part of the neck is involved in transferring movement in opposing directions. This part can be localized as follows: bend your head forward and feel with your hands where the muscles attach to your skull. Move your hands ½ to 1 inch inward, where your neck feels elastic and soft. Hereafter, this region will be referred to simply as the "neck" (figure 6.3-27).

The connection between the neck and the sternum (the elevator)

Instructions

- Lying on your stomach on the shoulderstand block, place the top of your forehead on your forearms. Allow your head to become heavy (figure 6.3-28). Place one hand on the upper part of your neck just under your skull. Check that your neck feels long and that the tissues feel elastic. If you move your chin forward, this point will collapse. When you move your chin back toward your chest, it will again become long. Do not pull your chin in too much, as this will develop tension in your throat.
- Place your hand back on the floor and inhale deeply. The inhalation will pull the vertebrae of your upper back inward, allowing you to lift your head from your forearms like an elevator (see the arrows in figure 6.3-29). Your neck remains extended, resembling the movement of an elevator rising, while the weight of your head sends pressure to the base of your sternum. Because the movement is directed through the midline of your spine, it is effected by using the postural muscles between your shoulder blades.

At this stage you can include your exhalations in the movement by exhaling toward your sternum and allowing your back to relax and deepen between your shoulder blades. This will cause more pressure to develop at the base of your sternum.

> **Note:** The connection between your neck and chest should also be active during normal activities, such as standing, sitting, and walking, and will even then be coordinated by your breathing.

The connections between the neck and the crown (exercise developed by one of my students)

The release of the atlas

Extending the neck can be difficult when the area around the atlas vertebra, right below the skull, is tense. To release this area, you can use the support of the rubber strip.

Preparation

Bring the tips of your fingers just below your skull and press firmly against the muscles and their attachments to find the exact spot to place the edge of the rubber strip. Slowly move your head up and down to feel the edge of your skull with your fingers.

Instructions

- Fold one end of the strip double; the folded part should be the length of your forearm from your wrist to your elbow measured on the back of your arm.
- Place the edge of the doubled-up part just underneath the edge of your skull and lie down on the strip. The edge of the strip will allow your skull to move away from your neck, and the back of your head will feel heavy on the single strip. Stay in this position for a few breaths and feel the heaviness between your shoulder blades on the strip and your shoulders at the sides.
- Very slowly roll your head to the right until you feel the pressure of the corner at the end the strip's edge. Remain aware of the strong pressure of the edge in your neck. The speed of your movement should be so slow that someone watching you can hardly see it happen.
- Remain here for a while, focusing on the release of your neck. The effect of this release often has a strong effect on other parts of the body. Many people experience relaxation in the shoulders, in the area between or underneath the shoulder blades, in the collarbones, and sometimes even in the lower back and legs. Just observe these areas in your body for 1 or 2 minutes. Then roll your head back to the center position equally slowly and repeat the movement on the other side.
- After doing both sides, roll your head to the right again, but this time, move as far as you can, passing the corner until your head hangs completely to the side. The corner of the strip's edge should still be pressing into the base of your skull. In this final position, the back of your head is still in contact with the edge of the single strip behind your head. Stay in this final position for 1 or 2 minutes.
- Repeat the head rotation on the left. After that, you can repeat rolling your head to the sides again, but do it faster and without a pause at the end of the movement.

Use this release of the atlas when you return to the prone position. Repeat the elevator exercise as explained earlier and allow your neck to push the back of your head forward. This will pull the tension out of your upper back. The back of your head transfers the movement to your crown, which will also move forward.

> **Note:** When you experience sensations indicating blockages in your neck, do not move any farther with force; wait until you start to relax. When your neck or the area below it starts to release its tension, your neck will start to lengthen, and the rotation will develop farther without strain.

6.3-30   6.3-31

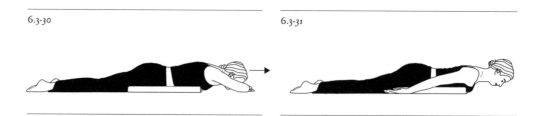

Note: If your back is straight, as shown in figure 6.3-29, then elevating your head in this manner will cause a burning sensation to develop in the postural muscles between your shoulder blades. This is a sign that they are working hard. By practicing this exercise regularly, your muscles will get stronger and your back will become straighter. This exercise trains the postural muscles, because you do not pull your shoulder blades together. If you do, you activate the movement muscles, which will harden your back and block the free, spreading movement of your ribs during inhalations. When you do this exercise correctly, you should always be able to move your shoulders freely.

If your back is bent similarly to that of the model in figure 6.3-30, then you will not feel your muscles contracting because your neck and upper back are not connecting. You desperately need to extend from your crown to pull the curve out of your upper back. Even though it may take a long time before you feel any change, it is very important to keep practicing. Only then will your upper back and neck be able to reconnect.

By repeating this exercise, you will be able to feel the pressure to the base of your sternum increase when you stretch your arms slowly along your sides. Allow the weight of your arms to rest on the back of your hands, as seen in figure 6.3-31.

Use of the neck when sitting
The previous exercises, in which you lie prone, are based on strength. When sitting, however, there is hardly any question of strength, because the spine, if correctly stacked, will be in balance. To sit upright without tension, the lower back must be erect (see connection 9).

When the pelvis and lower back have been positioned correctly, the shoulders and head are in a slightly forward position. The free connection between the neck, upper back, and chest is totally dependent on the mobility of the upper back. If the upper back is adequately mobile, the connection can be made through breathing, without using the back muscles.

Instructions

·   Sit with your lower back positioned as shown in figure 6.3-32, and feel the relaxation around the base of your sternum. Remain in this position, feeling the relaxation, for a while. Couple the feeling of relaxation to your exhalations. When breathing in, only fill your abdomen for the time being.

·   After you have done this for a while, with slow, deep inhalations, breathe in until you fill your lungs all the way to the top. Feel how this movement lifts your sternum and creates movement in your spine. The ribs that connect to your sternum also connect to your vertebrae, meaning the elevation of your sternum pulls your spine straighter. This movement automatically places your neck in the correct position.

·   After you have filled your lungs, hold your breath briefly to feel your posture accurately. When you exhale, your neck remains in the same position and pushes your crown up. Next, release the tension in your shoulders. Feel how this tension descends toward your lower back, where it is accepted and transferred to your pelvis.

6.3-32

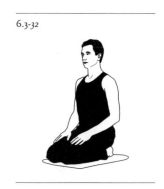

*☛ Important Tip

Observe your body carefully to ensure that it is responding to your breathing. Make sure your back muscles have not taken over the initiative to provide space to your chest. If your back does take over, it will block the broadening of your ribs, resulting in tension to your back and sternum.

You can complete the movement with one hand on the base of your sternum so you can feel whether it is in a free position and is sensitive to the movement of your inhalations.

In this connection, your head is virtually connected to your heart. Physically, there is space in both areas due to the fact that your neck and the base of your sternum are both in an open and free position. If you develop this connection further, the feeling center at the base of your sternum will occupy an increasingly prominent position in your movement and posture. But a lot of groundwork has to be done before you reach this stage. Your lower back must be positioned correctly to sustain the relaxation around the base of your sternum. Your neck must be able to connect freely with your upper back. And you need a good understanding of the correct use of breathing. This means your spine must be able to move freely and remain stable. It is not for nothing that the yoga tradition states that the practice of asanas is done simply to be able to sit steady and free.

When you practice these connections with increasing frequency, the results will be evident. You will be able to monitor yourself better. You will be able to observe and feel what happens in your body, allowing you to refine your posture in both asanas and everyday activities. More space will develop for breathing and the exercise of working out your posture will move from your head into your body.

4. The connection between the arms, the shoulders, and the back

When the upper back is extended, the arms can effortlessly connect with the shoulder blades. This allows the weight of the arms to transfer easily into the lower back and prevents overload to the shoulders. If this connection does not function properly, it will put too much strain not only on the shoulders but also on the upper back and chest.

Lifting the arms while lying on the strip
In the seated position described here, the back has to work harder to lift the arms than when lying supine, because this movement is not easy for the shoulders and back (figure 6.3-33). When the arms are hanging, the shoulders and back are reasonably relaxed, but when they are lifted, the back immediately assumes its habitual position (see chapter 3).

This action hardens the muscles in the shoulders. Additionally, the shoulders assume a position similar to the one they adopt when pushing the arms away. This reflex also happens when the head is raised. If this has become a habit, the head and arms will no longer be able to connect with the back. Over time, this causes a vicious circle of increasing tension to build up. For this reason, it is sensible, especially in the beginning, to do the seated exercise after doing the supine variation. This gives the body a chance to learn the correct movement without tension in the back and shoulders.

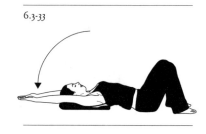

6.3-33

Preparation

This preliminary exercise localizes the transition area between the arms and back. The shoulder is important for transferring the movement of the arm to the back. You can find the necessary region as follows:

Sit on your feet and lift one arm up, as shown in figure 6.3-34; use your other hand to feel the area where the elevated arm meets your back. This is the deltoid—a strong, triangular muscle in the shoulder and upper arm. Immediately bordering this area, between your shoulder and back, is a hollow that transfers movement (as, for example, when lifting) from your arm to your shoulder blade without unduly taxing your shoulders.

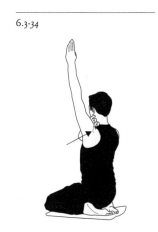

When your arms are raised, it is absolutely necessary to keeping them straight and parallel to each other. Then the upper arm is capable of transporting the movement to the shoulder blade, which causes a natural break in the movement of the arm. This is the stable position of the shoulder joint. When your arms bend, the upper arm moves around the bone of the shoulder blade without exerting any pressure; this makes the shoulder joint unstable. When the shoulder joint is stabilized, it allows your arm to support the extension of the midline of your upper back from the sides.

Fold the rubber strip in half so it is about 20 inches long and 2 inches thick, or make a roll out of a sheet with the same dimensions. You will also need a yoga strap.

Instructions

- Lie vertically on the double strip and feel how, when your back straightens, it gives your shoulder blades more room and they can descend toward the floor. Allow your back to become heavy over the end of the strip (middle of your back) and try to maintain this contact. Hold the belt or loop it around your wrists so your hands are shoulder-width apart, and lift your arms toward the ceiling.

- To experience the *incorrect* movement, push your arms as far as possible toward the ceiling. Your back will bend and start to resist the strip. Allow your arms to move back (correct movement), as shown by the arrow in figure 6.3-35. Your back will relax, allowing your shoulders to connect with your shoulder blades. Your shoulders should remain low in relation to your neck.

- Straighten your arms and pull lightly on the belt. Slowly bring your arms over your head, while keeping your back relaxed on the rubber strip. The final position of your arms is determined by the shape of your back. If your back is bent, your hands will end up higher above the floor than if your back were straight. If your back is straight, the connection of your upper arms with your shoulder blades will create an end to the movement. Keeping your arms straight, move up and down a little to feel this end position; it is a resilient sensation around your armpits, shoulder blades, and ribs. Do not move your arms past this point. If you do, the movement will become jammed in the hollow where your arms meet your back, breaking the connection with your back.

- The position of your arms supports the space in your chest. Take advantage of this space and breathe deeply for 30 to 60 seconds.

- Next, stretch your arms away from your back as far as you can. Your back lengthens over the strip, where the pressure is greatest. Your shoulders follow the arm movement, causing your neck to recede into your shoulders. Keep your hands at the same height above the floor during this movement. Then pull your arms back toward your

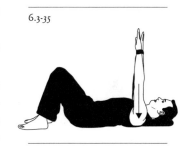

shoulder blades and raise them slowly toward the ceiling. Feel if the pressure at the end of the strip increases, and try not to lose this feeling when you repeat the exercise. If necessary, you can contract your stomach muscles slightly to maintain contact with the strip.

> **Note:** Pulling lightly on the belt helps to relax the muscles of the shoulder girdle. When these muscles relax, the muscles of the upper arms must activate to carry the weight of the arms. This can be hard work, but remember that it is a sign that tension is leaving your shoulders and strength is returning to your arms.

Lifting the arms when seated

When you practice the sitting variation after the supine exercise, end the supine variation by paying close attention to your breathing. Remain for a few minutes with your hands on your lower ribs and practice diaphragmatic chest breathing (see connections 2 and 3). Remember that the broadening of your posterior ribs indicates your back is relaxed and that narrowing indicates it is straight. This is easier to observe in the supine position than when seated. For this reason, try to imprint the feeling on your memory, so you can use it to help you to relax when seated.

Preparation

Sit on your feet or on a stool without a backrest, with a belt resting on your legs. Extend your lower back so the weight of your trunk is carried on the front of your sit bones (see connection 9). Breathe in the same manner as described for the previous exercise— broadening with inhalations and narrowing with exhalations. On a deep inhalation, position your neck as straight as possible above your back (see connection 3).

Instructions

- Holding the belt, bring your arms up until they are parallel with the floor (figure 6.3-36a). Allow your arms to move with the rhythm of your breathing. When you inhale, feel your ribs broadening your back and check to see whether your back is relaxed. When you exhale, your back narrows, indicating it is straight. Connect your arms with your shoulder blades. Keep your shoulders low while slowly raising

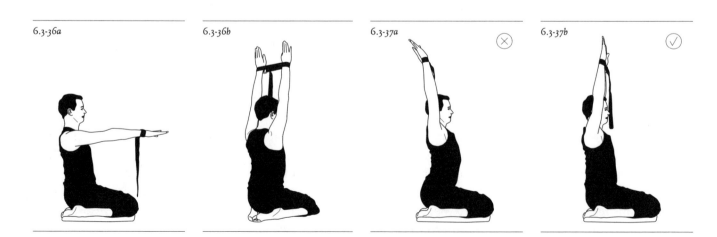

6.3-36a   6.3-36b   6.3-37a   6.3-37b

your arms with every exhalation (figure 6.3-36b). During inhalations, hold your arms at the same height and check that your back is relaxed. Your arms will finally be above your head, and you will feel the same end of the movement as you did in the supine variation. Move your arms back and forth slightly, and feel the elastic resistance of the end movement around your shoulders and ribs. Then lift your hands as high as possible away from your back. This is the same movement as in the preceding supine variation and will lengthen your upper back.

· Repeat this movement a few times.

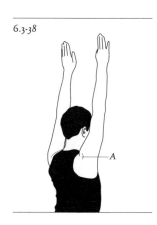

6.3-38

Note: Avoid lifting your chest. For clarification, see the differences between figures 6.3-37a and 6.3-37b. In figure 6.3-37a, the lower ribs are lifted together with the arms, compressing the back. In figure 6.3-37b, the back remains free and can extend out of the lower back. When your arms get tired, allow them to rest on your legs, keeping your head as straight as possible above your back and breathing deeply.

6.3-39a

✐ Important Tip

In both the passive, supine position and the active, seated position, your shoulders may be so mobile that they alone make the movement instead of passing it on to your shoulder blades. Then the movement is made through the hollow in the area between your arm and your back (point A in figure 6.3-38). This is a common compensation for a bent and stiff upper back. Your upper arms no longer end perpendicular with your back; instead, they and your hands move too far backward.

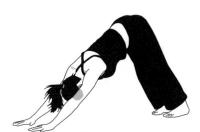

In forward bends, backbends, twists, and standing poses, an attempt is always made to connect the arms with the shoulder blades. In most of the exercises, the shoulders are kept low, but in, for example, Adho Mukha Svanasana (see chapter 9.2, numbers 4 and 5), both forms—pulling in or stretching out the arms and shoulders—can be applied.

6.3-39b

5. The connection between the arms and the hands

Correct coordinated use of the different parts of the arm creates a free passage of movement: the shoulder passing movement on to the upper arm, the upper arm to the elbow, the elbow to the underarm, the underarm to the wrist, and finally the wrist to the hand. This movement chain is always initiated from the spine, as it is the spine that determines the (free) position of the shoulder. Subsequently, the arm is able to reverse the path and connect the movement of the hand back to the shoulder and spine.

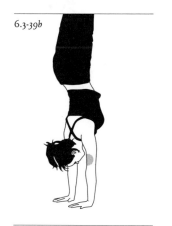

If the coordination between the different parts of the arm is disturbed, it can cause all sorts of complaints in the joints, circulation, and nerves of the arm.

The shaded areas of the upper arms in figures 6.3-39a through 6.3-39c, together with the act of actively stretching the elbows, create the connection with the shoulder blades. When the hands make contact with the floor or a wall—as seen in figures 6.3-39a (Adho Mukha Svanasana; see chapter 9.2.4), 6.3-39b (Adho Mukha Vrksasana; see chapter 8.4.18), and 6.3-39c (Setu Bandha Sarvangasana, or Bridge Pose; see chapter 11.4, number 8)—this same area of the upper arm creates the connection with the back of the hand. This can be seen in the following exercise.

6.3-39c

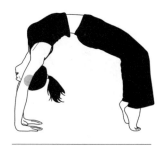

6.3-40

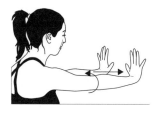

6.3-41

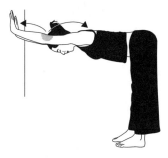

6.3-42

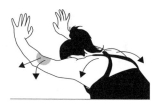

6.3-43

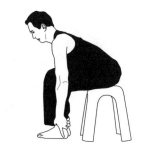

Instructions

- Stand facing a wall with a distance of about 40 inches between the wall and your feet. Place your hands against the wall at the level of your heart. Rotate your upper arms inward to increase the stretch to your thumb and index finger (see the arrows in figure 6.3-40), as well as the pressure to the palms of your hands. Your hands should be like two barnacles stuck to the wall.
- Slowly move your pelvis away from the wall to connect your arms with your shoulder blades (figure 6.3-41). Do this without releasing the pressure to your hands.

> **Note:** If your shoulders are stiff, your arms will end in the position shown in figure 6.3-42, bent with collapsed upper arms. The palms of your hands will have lost contact with the wall. To avoid this, you must move more slowly, allowing your shoulders and back to relax into the movement instead of fighting it.

6. The connection between the arms and the lower back

When your back is bent, as when you pick something up off the floor, your lower back can maintain its strength only as long as your arms remain connected to it. While this connection is maintained, the force of the movement (lifting, or pulling on your legs during an exercise) is passed on to your pelvis. If this connection is broken, it has a dramatic effect on your posture: your shoulders and neck become strained, your two centers of gravity are compressed, and your lower back is not able to transfer your body weight to your pelvis.

This connection is mainly used during forward bending and twisting, in which the lower back is slightly bent. When it is bent, as in Uttanasana (see chapter 10.4, number 4), the hands can pull lightly on the feet in such a way that the lower back can still extend. Even when the hamstrings and lower back relax in the end pose, the lower back can be supported effectively. This causes the pelvis to stretch farther back, creating space in the front of the body, shoulders, and neck.

The following two exercises isolate this connection—one in a seated position and one in an upright position.

Sitting on a stool

- Sit on a stool, with your back straight, and place your hands on your thighs. Lean forward until your upper body and legs come together. Keep your abdomen and chest as open as possible and grasp your ankles. Actively push your abdomen against your thighs while firmly holding your ankles. A tensile strength, which is powered by your lower back, develops in your hands (figure 6.3-43). Your head and neck should move upward. Do not allow them to move down when your hands start pulling on your ankles.
- Increase the pressure between your abdomen and legs, allowing you to shift the active strength from your lower back to your arms. The tensile strength is now activated by your hands. This pulls your lower back slightly inward and flattens it out a little, so your back can relax without losing the inward action of your lower back.

Standing from bent to extended legs

For a more detailed description of the coordination between the lower back, pelvis, and legs, see connection 7.

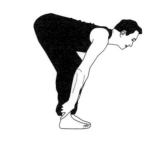

- Stand in Utkatasana (see chapter 10.4, number 4) with your hands resting on your thighs. Lean forward, keeping as much space as possible in your abdomen and chest, and take hold of your ankles. Push your abdomen actively against your thighs and feel the tensile strength in your hands (figure 6.3-44). Balance with your weight on the front part of your heels; this allows your hips to relax. By pulling on your ankles, increase the pressure of your abdomen against your thighs, giving support to your lower back by shifting the active strength from there to your hands. Relax your upper body over your legs without losing this connection.

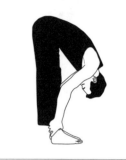

- Keep the connection to your lower back as you start to stretch your legs slowly. Whether you succeed in straightening them or not entirely depends on the length of the muscles at the backs of your legs. If they protest too much and the stretch becomes too painful, it is better to wait before deepening the pose.

☞ *Important Tip*

Often, stretching the legs gets priority, causing the connection between the arms and lower back to be lost (figure 6.3-45). The upper body then does not hang from the pelvis but from a spot in the spine. If you are a beginner and this movement makes you feel a stretch in the backs of your legs, this is sufficient initially. However, as soon as you can remain easily in the pose and can start to release the tension in your legs, it is advisable to initiate the correct structure.

- Allow your entire upper body, including your head, to hang forward. Use exhalations to dissolve the tension in your back and legs. In this vertical position, the muscles of your back are totally relaxed. At the moment of release, your arms are able to guide your lower back correctly to deepen your relaxation in the pose.

For this connection, it is essential to position your lower back dynamically. This occurs when the weight of your upper body is guided toward your lower back. When this has taken place, your arms can continuously stimulate the extension in your lower back. It is not about the strength you use when pulling on your ankles. If you pull too hard, your body will most likely harden and become insensitive to your exhalations. The relaxation you develop with exhalations is always the first step in such exercises. Your arms use this relaxation to create a good structure and deepen the asana.

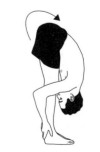

> **Note:** The traction developed with the hands is often used to tilt the pelvis farther rather than to flatten the arch of the lower back (figure 6.3-46). This movement can lead to too much of a stretch in the hamstrings. People who have practiced yoga for some time often complain about a feeling of irritation where the hamstrings attach to the sit bones. This tilting of the pelvis can also develop tension in the lower back. These problems can be avoided by keeping the critical connections in the lower back and allowing the stretch to develop in a balanced way.

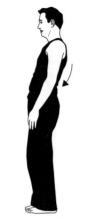

6.3-47

7. *The connection between the lower back, the pelvis, and the legs*

The distribution of body weight from the diaphragm downward should be passed through the midline of the lumbar spine. The transfer of weight is effortless when the lower back is in its natural, hollow curve.

When this connection is disturbed, it blocks the free passage of movement toward the pelvis. This can occur when the movement muscles of the lower back are so stiff that the vertebrae there cannot execute the hollow-shaped position anymore. But when the lower back is too hollow, it is also not able to transport the body's weight toward the pelvis properly. This will destabilize the lower back.

Critical Alignment divides the lower back into upper (the lumbar vertebrae L1, L2, and L3) and lower parts (the lumbar vertebrae L4 and L5, and the sacral vertebra S1). We will discuss the upper part of the lower back first. In some cases, this area can become stiff as a result of swaybacked posture (figure 6.3-47). The spine looks similar to the one shown in figure 6.3-48.

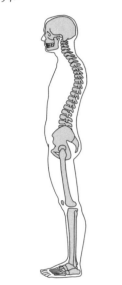

6.3-48

Stretching the upper part of the lower back (L1, L2, L3)

Preparation
Make a thin roll (approximately 4 to 5 inches thick) from the felt mat or from a sheet. You can also fold the rubber strip in two to serve this purpose.

Instructions

· Sit on the floor with your knees bent and place the roll horizontally on the floor behind you. Lie on the roll so it is exactly between your pelvis and rib cage, as seen in figure 6.3-49. Place your hands on the arch of your lower ribs. Try to accept the pressure of the roll while keeping your pelvis as heavy as possible. If this is painful, try to relax by directing your exhalations to the pain. When the stiffness decreases, increase your weight on the roll by allowing your ribs to lower with each exhalation.

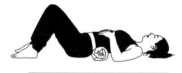

6.3-49

Note: The lying down movement is a fast one, and when it is done quickly, the muscles involved often start to harden. They actually resist relaxation. On many occasions, breathing helps neutralize this (unconscious) reflex once you have been lying down for some time. If the stiffness does not lessen within a couple of minutes and your back keeps resisting the roll, make the roll smaller. The pain may be caused by the muscles of your lower back or by deeper tissue structures.

It is a sign of improvement when your lower back starts to adapt to the pressure more quickly. You will experience this after (long) practice. When the negative response is broken, you can incorporate the movement into daily activities that are fast and unconscious, such as sitting, standing, or walking.

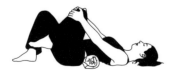

6.3-50

You can extend the stretch to include relaxation of the lower vertebrae and the muscles around the sacrum by pulling your knees toward your navel one at a time (figure 6.3-50). Your pelvis should remain on the ground during this movement. Try to visualize how this movement stretches your lower back. Sometimes you will feel the most resistance in your hip. When this dissolves by moving slowly, the pelvic part (L4, L5, SI) of your back and the sacroiliac (SI) joint—the joint between the sacrum and the hip bone (see figure 6.3-71)—will develop more freedom of movement.

Stretching the entire lower back (L1 to S1)

Preparation
Make a firm, thick roll (approximately 5 to 6 inches thick) from the felt mat.

Instructions

- Sit on the floor with your knees bent and hold the roll across your back at the same position as in the last exercise. Lift your pelvis as you lower yourself to the floor; this allows your lower ribs to move toward your stomach. Keep the connection between your lower back and roll light in the beginning. Then, as if you are going to lift your feet, increase the pressure on your vertebrae. Feel the contraction of your stomach muscles that results. The (upper) stomach muscles are important for keeping your ribs low during this exercise.

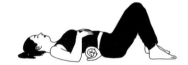

6.3-51

- Very slowly, paying attention to the relaxation that develops in your lower back, allow your pelvis to lower until your tailbone touches the floor (figure 6.3-51). If it cannot reach the floor, keep your pelvis as low as possible so you feel a firm pressure. This can be painful in the beginning, but the pain should lessen within 30 to 60 seconds.
- Lift your pelvis and repeat this downward movement slowly until the movement starts to feel more free, then repeat somewhat faster five more times. This way, you remain in the lower position for shorter periods of time, which can help you release tension. This is especially helpful if you experience a lot of pain and uncertainty during this exercise.
- Rotations can be very helpful to release the tightness in your muscles. Bring your ankles and knees together, and slowly rotate your legs to the right to bring your body weight onto the muscles in the right side of your spine. These muscles are responsible for the stiffness in your back. Exhale toward the spot and allow the muscles to become heavier with each exhalation. Repeat the same rotation on the left side.
- After becoming aware of your breathing, rotate as far as you can back to the right. Keep both feet on the floor. In the beginning, this exercise can be very intense.

> **Note:** When the rotation starts to develop, it will increase the pressure on the side you are moving toward with your legs and cause the spine on the other side to arch more and eventually come off the roll. It is important to keep both feet on the floor to enhance the arch.

- Repeat the rotation on the left. After doing both sides, you can repeat the movement on both sides again, moving a little faster after the initial tightness begins to disappear.
- Return to center and move your pelvis up and down from the floor a couple of times to find out whether the rotation has made the movement easier.

> **Note:** Don't worry if you are not able to touch the floor; just keep practicing. Do *not* change the thickness of the roll! You need that support to bring the movement into the bottom part of your lower back.

- When your tailbone finally reaches the floor, you can strengthen your lower back by pushing your tailbone into the floor. This causes your lower back to recoil slightly from the roll and activates its postural muscles because the strength is coordinated from the midline of your spine. Hold this position for a few breaths before you relax and then repeat the process. Breathe into your abdomen to release the feeling of resistance and spend 3 to 5 minutes on this exercise.

> **Note:** At this stage, you are allowed to raise your lower ribs so your tailbone can make contact with the floor. After pressing down with your tailbone, try to pull your lower ribs down gently with the help of your abdominal muscles. This will give you a strong sense of movement toward the roll (caused by your lower ribs) and increase the pressure on the roll. Make sure you combine the push of your tailbone with the downward movement of your ribs.
>
> This exercise is valuable for restoring the natural freedom of movement in your entire lower back. You can do the next exercise right after this one.

> **Note:** If your back is stiff in this area, the only solution is to do this exercise repeatedly. You can alternate lying passively on the roll with the more active variations described previously. It is definitely worth the effort to develop stability and mobility to this area of your back, as it can relieve a lot of lower back problems.

6.3-52

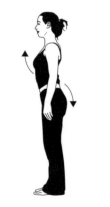

6.3-53a

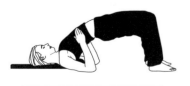

The lower lower back (L4, L5, S1)

Lower back problems affect the areas of the lumbar vertebrae L4 and L5 and the transition area to the pelvis (the sacral vertebra S1). For instance, people who hold their chest high with a backward pelvic tilt often have problems in this area (figure 6.3-52).

Preparation

Do the exercise with the rubber strip between your shoulder blades (see connection 2) first; it may be done right after the previous exercise. In this variation, the emphasis is on stabilizing the arch of your lower back with the use of its postural muscles.

Instructions

- Lie on the rubber strip—folded as in the connection 2 exercise—and lift your chest and pelvis high (figure 6.3-53a). Push your thighs and pelvis high with the medial arches of your feet and the insides of your legs. This forms an arch in your lower back.

- Feel where your back and the strip meet at C7, and keep pushing toward this area with your feet. This will keep your neck extended.
- Vertebra by vertebra, slowly lower your pelvis, keeping your lower back as arched as possible. During this movement, you can feel a strong contraction in the movement muscles of the lower back (the quadratus lumborum, or QL, muscles situated at the sides of the lower back; figure 6.3-53b). When your tailbone finally touches the floor, your lower back will have the same shape as it had on the lower back roll (see the previous exercise).
- The moment you actively push your tailbone into the floor (see figure 6.3-54), there will be an immediate change in the use of your muscles, because this movement organizes the strength from the center line. The strength at the sides will be released, and the deeper, postural muscles (the multifidus muscles, the smallest muscles connected to the vertebrae, on the left side of the spine in figure 6.3-53b) will take over. As figure 6.3-53b clearly shows, the muscles that are connected to the center line of the lower back move *into the pelvis* and support the stability of the vertebrae inside the pelvis (L4 and L5). This movement thus aligns the arch of the lower back using the deepest, smallest, and most powerful muscles of the spine—the multifidus muscles—rather than the movement muscles, which can only support the upper vertebrae of the lower back.

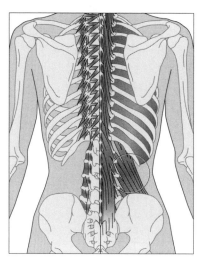

The quadratus lumborum is located on the lateral side of the spinal column (see circle). The small muscles on the left side are called the multifidus muscles.

Note: Remember that your lower back is excessively concave in these exercises. Normally, with your pelvis resting on the floor, the space between your lower back and the floor would be just big enough to insert your fingers.

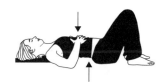

6.3-54

- To increase relaxation, direct your attention and breathing to the end of the strip where it meets your back just below the level of your shoulder blades. When you relax, the pressure of the strip increases. Then the increased mobility of your upper back allows your lower ribs to move toward the floor and makes it possible for your lower back to transfer the movement to your pelvis. The downward movement of your lower ribs is tranferred to the strong arch in your lower back.
- Practice this exercise for 3 to 5 minutes.

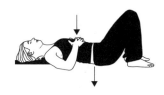

6.3-55

☞ *Take Note!*

The downward movement of your lower ribs activates the midline of your spine, since these ribs are connected to your spine at the back of your body. The movement directs your body weight toward your lower back and pelvis when your lower back is properly arched.

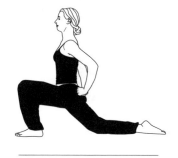

6.3-56

The most common mistake people make when doing this exercise is collapsing the lower back when the lower ribs descend. In our daily lives, this combination of movement often occurs when we sit. The lower ribs move toward the stomach, but the lower back nearly always collapses. This can be seen in a supine pose in figure 6.3-55. However, during the preparatory exercise for Virabhadrasana I (figure 6.3-56), this is prevented by the positioning of the back leg.

6.3-57a

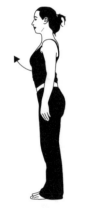

To learn how to apply this coordination when standing, arch your lower back well (figure 6.3-57a) before you bring your lower ribs down (figure 6.3-57b).

    The previous exercises break the collapsing lower back habit and teach your body how the relaxation of your lower ribs can be transferred to an alert and strong extension of your lower back.

    The exercise for the lower back is important because it illustrates the coordination of the lower back that should be used in almost all poses in which the lower back has a neutral arch, such as seated poses, inversions, and standing poses. Keep in mind that the pelvis never makes the movement itself ("tuck your tailbone in" or "rotate your pelvis"); it receives the movements from the lower back.

    During this exercise, the lower back can easily collapse. However, during the preparatory exercise for Virabhadrasana I (see figure 6.3-56), this is prevented by the positioning of the back leg. You can also complete this exercise while standing, with your fists pushing against your tailbone (see figure 6.3-56). Use your exhalations to find the connection between your ribs and tailbone.

6.3-57b

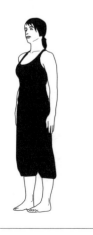

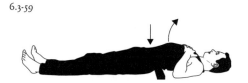

8. The connection between the sternum and the pubic bone: the inner tube

When the extension of the lower back coincides with the correct position of the lower ribs and the activation of the transverse abdominals, the abdomen is able to move with the breath, creating a natural feeling of relaxation in the abdomen and hara gravity point. When the abdominal muscles are too tight or too weak, they affect the shape of the lower back and prevent the breath from relaxing the lower abdomen.

The stomach muscles form the connection between the sternum and pubic bone. This connection should be firm but not hard as it is in people who do a lot of abdominal exercises. A stable connection depends on the ribs being able to move toward the pelvis and the area 1 inch below the navel being able to move toward the chest, *without* losing the arch in the lower back. To ensure that the lumbar curve remains intact during the following exercises, lie supine with the rubber strip (1 inch thick) under your lower back. The first exercise concentrates on the position of your lower ribs and the second on your pelvis.

The position of the chest

Instructions

- Lie on the floor with the rubber strip under your lower back (figure 6.3-58). Stretch your legs straight out and ensure that your lower back only touches the strip lightly. Place your hands on your lower ribs.
- Lift your lower ribs as high as possible and feel how your stomach falls inward toward your lower back (figure 6.3-59). Allow your ribs to come down and feel how your stomach rises. Feel the difference in your breathing. When your ribs are raised, your breath stalls in the lower part of your chest. As soon as your ribs are lowered, abdominal breathing can resume.

Good alignment between the position of your lower back and lower ribs results in a firm feeling in the column between your ribs and lower abdomen into which you can breathe easily. This connection provides extension to your lower back in all exercises where it should be neutral, such as inversions, standing poses, and seated poses.

> **Note:** Lifting your ribs too high causes your breath to remain restricted in your chest. Pulling your ribs too low makes chest breathing almost impossible. This occurs in exercises like Halasana (see chapter 8.3, number 14) and in daily activities such as sitting. The upper lower back (L1, L2, L3) loses its extension and collapses. It must be reactivated to support the space in the lower chest.

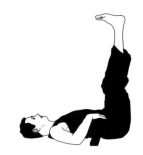

The position of the pelvis

Instructions

· Lie down with the rubber strip placed horizontally under your lower back and lift your legs to a 90-degree angle. Your lower back should touch the strip lightly.

· Place your hands on your pelvis and push your fingers into the fold where your legs end and your abdomen starts (figure 6.3-60) in the front of your hips.

· Slowly lower your legs to the floor without losing the contact between your lower back and the strip. If you feel this happening, stop lowering your legs. Use your lower stomach muscles to keep your pelvis in position. If you can lower your legs easily, you will feel (under your fingers) an increased extension in the front of your hips. Stop the movement when your heels are approximately ½ inch from the floor and remain in this position for 20 to 30 seconds. This will strengthen the movement muscles in your abdomen (the outer core) between your pubic bone and ribs. Keep breathing into your stomach despite the contraction in your stomach muscles.

6.3-60a

Anterior view of the transverse abdominals

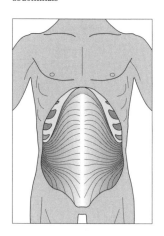

Note: When you bring your heels to the floor, you no longer need that "big" strength anymore, and the postural muscles will take over. When you do not re-lease the upward pull of the area below your navel, your transverse abdominals (see figure 6.3-60a) remain active; they are postural muscles. Your inner core, or inner tube, does not need much strength, and this makes breathing easier. The change from outer core to inner core happens during asanas when you jump up in Sirsasana or Adho Mukha Vrksasana.

If you tilt your pelvis backward (generally phrased as "tuck your tailbone in"), the lower two vertebrae (L4 and L5) will be pushed into the floor and the arch of your lower back will lose its neutral tension. You can easily test the ideal position of your pelvis by lying prone with your forehead resting on your forearms as described under connection 1. This activates the hara center of gravity. The base of your sternum should make an ef-fortless, relaxed contact with your stomach; your lower abdomen should touch the floor. If this is not the case, relax the muscles of your lower back so it can move inward and extend. Then push your lower abdomen toward the floor. This subtle movement will in-crease the strength of the neutral arch in your lower back. If you do not do this carefully, by pushing your pubic bone toward the block, your lower back will raise up. Stretch your knees and lift them off the ground to intensify the movement.

9. The connection between the lower back and the pelvis when sitting

Extension of the lumbar spine is organized through the correct positioning of the lower ribs. They ensure that the weight of the body is transferred through the lower back into the sacrum. This occurs effortlessly when the lumbar spine is in a neutral arch. If this connection is lost, the body weight never reaches the pelvis. Therefore, it also becomes impossible to stretch up from the pelvis.

When sitting, the correct position of the pelvis is where the neutral arch of the lower

6.3-61

Note: When your lower back becomes straighter, the strength of your stomach muscles increases automatically. Adversely, excessive and isolated training of the stomach muscles often leads to a bent upper back, as shown in figure 6.3-61. A lot of medical research has been done regarding the connection between the sternum and the pubic bone and the role of the more profound postural muscles in the lower back. The inner tube is formed by the following postural muscles: the diaphragm, the pelvic floor, the transverse abdominals, and the spinal muscles of the lower back (see chapter 2). Research has shown that training one part of the chain will trigger physical reflexes that automatically activate and thus positively influence the rest of the chain. For this reason, those who suffer from pelvic instability are advised to train the transverse abdominals (see chapter 13.4, number 7). In this way, strength in the deep postural muscles of the lower back, the diaphragm, and the pelvic floor — the entire inner tube — reflexively increases, allowing the lower back and pelvis to recover stability. When doing Sirsasana on the headstand bench (discussed in chapter 2.5; see also chapter 8.2, number 1), the spine is stacked vertically and carries the weight of the pelvis and legs. The latter can only take place if the lower back is in the correct position. Only then will the deeper postural muscles of the lower back be able to coordinate the correct strength for support. This activates the entire inner tube.

As discussed with the connection of the lower abdomen (the hara area) with the sternum, the connection between the ribs and lower abdomen must be kept stable. This means the lower ribs must be kept in place without losing the erect posture of the upper back. In addition, the pelvis must be positioned as in the foregoing exercise, where the lower abdomen is pushed into the floor.

These connections will be referred to in all exercises where the back is erect.

6.3-62

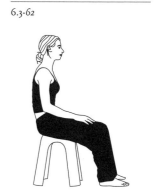

6.3-63

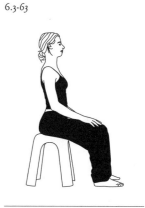

back transfers the movement to the hara center of gravity and where the lower abdomen, in turn, transfers movement to the crown. Whether or not the pelvis is able to achieve the correct position is largely determined by the structure of the lower back. For example, the pelvis can have an excessive backward tilt (figure 6.3-62) due to the habitual collapse of the lower back. A lot of physical therapies regard the tilting of the pelvis as central. But if the pelvis is tilted to make the lower back look straight (figure 6.3-63), it becomes frozen, because the lower back is kept straight by the quadratus lumborum muscles at the sides and not by the deeper postural muscles that activate all vertebrae in the lower back (see connection 7). The postural muscles are crucially important for movement in the lower back. Overly contracting the lower back with the quadratus lumborum muscles causes movement to occur exclusively in areas that are already mobile — usually the upper part of the lower back (L1, L2, L3).

Is it a good idea to use the pelvis to correct the posture of the lower back? Certainly. When moving from a forward leaning (figure 6.3-64) to an erect seated position, movement is passed from the head to the neck to the upper and lower back and finally to the pelvis. How the movement reaches the pelvis depends on the mobility of the spine.

Based on these considerations, the following question arises: how can you correct the position of your pelvis? The answer to this can be found in the following exercise.

6.3-64

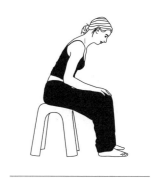

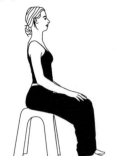
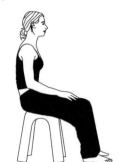
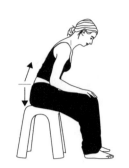

The correct position of the pelvis

If your lower back is not straight, its posture will either be cramped and excessively concave (figure 6.3-65) or collapsed. The cramped back must first relax, then it will probably look like the collapsed back (figure 6.3-66). When you have this collapsed back, your quadratus lumborum muscles will not interfere with the coming action. This makes it possible to guide the movement through your center line to realize a new posture.

Instructions

- Sit on a stool with your lower back slightly bent. Lean forward without changing your posture, so that your pelvis follows your trunk (figure 6.3-67).

6.3-68a

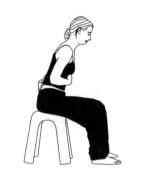

> **Note:** The pelvis follows the movement of the trunk because the muscles at the back of the legs (the hamstrings) relax. Therefore, the pelvis does not tilt because of the *contraction* of the quadratus lumborum muscles; it turns toward the legs because of the *release* of the hamstrings, which are attached to the sit bones of the pelvis.

6.3-68b

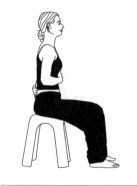

- The movement stops as soon as the gravity point in your lower abdomen moves past your sit bones. The weight of your body creates pressure in your thighs and hip joints.
- Relax the area where your quadratus lumborum muscles attach to your pelvis. This lets your pelvis move away from your lower back (see the descending arrow in figure 6.3-67).
- Your pelvis is now in the correct position. The arch of your lower back has changed from collapsed to an ascending position (see the ascending arrow in figure 6.3-67) and can now accept the following movement.
- Place one hand on the base of your sternum and the other on your lower back. With your upper hand, push on the lower part of your chest directly above your pelvis as if your diaphragm were a drawer that you are sliding shut. *Do not* contract your hamstrings; it will change the position of your pelvis. Ensure that your gravity point remains at the front of your sit bones (figures 6.3-68a and 6.3-68b). If you do this movement correctly, you will feel the vertebrae of your lower back moving into the correct position under your lower hand. Thus, your lower ribs, lower back, abdomen, and pelvis are in the correct position.

6.3-69a

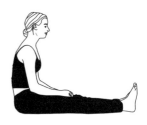

The position of your lower back virtually pushes your pelvis away from your back. The posture of your pelvis therefore feels grounded. However, this can feel strange in your upper back. The movement of your diaphragm causes your upper back to bend a little. Do not worry about this now. You need a good foundation to create a correct total posture. You achieve that by placing your lower ribs, lower back, and pelvis correctly.

The connections between the upper back, neck, and head were discussed earlier (see connection 2). The instructions for making those connections can now be followed.

6.3-69b

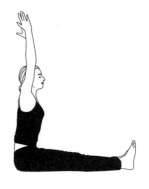

The connection between the lower back and pelvis in a seated position is important in many asanas, such as Utkatasana (see chapter 9.2, number 2). The connection should also be strengthened for forward bends with the pelvis on the floor, because if the legs are stiff, it can be difficult to position the lower back and pelvis correctly (figures 6.3-69a and 6.3-69b). Such stiffness can easily be released in standing forward bends, including Uttanasana (see chapter 10.4, number 4) and Prasarita Padottanasana (see chapter 10.4, number 5).

There are also exercises, such as Adho Mukha Svanasana (see chapter 8.4, number 18) in which the pelvis does not touch the ground, but the same connection applies. If the lower back is concave enough, the movement is transferred to the pelvis (figure 6.3-70a) and does not remain fixed in the lower back (figure 6.3-70b).

Whether or not an interaction occurs between the deeper postural muscles and the superficial back muscles depends on the position of the body. This interplay occurs during poses such as Utkatasana. But when seated, as already described, the weight of the body is carried entirely by the deeper postural muscles of the lower back.

6.3-70a

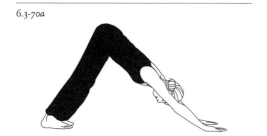

6.3-70b

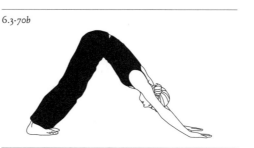

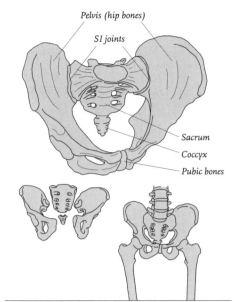

Pelvis (hip bones)

SI joints

Sacrum

Coccyx

Pubic bones

10. *The connection between the pelvis and the legs: the hips*

When the lower back has successfully passed the weight of the body on to the sacrum, the movement splits through the sacroiliac joints to both hips. Then the hips are included in the chain of movement. If this connection cannot be performed properly, the hips become stiff.

The pelvis

The body's center of gravity is situated in the lower abdomen, in front of the pelvis. The pelvis has three parts, the left and right hip bones (iliac bones) and the sacrum (figure 6.3-71). These are bound together in back by the sacroiliac (SI) joints and in front by the pubic bone. Because your hip joints are located at the bottom sides of the pelvis, you can easily feel your sit bones when sitting on a hard surface. The joints that form the pelvis have very little movement. Therefore, the feeling of movement experienced in this area is mainly due to the release of muscle tension. The mobility of the hips plays an important role in this connection. The following exercises are done with bent knees to prevent tight hamstrings from interfering with the correct movement, as would happen with extended legs.

Exercises with bent knees

The muscles around your hips can relax when your knees are bent. This relaxation is used in many asanas, especially standing poses, and the following exercise is a good example.

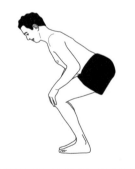

Instructions

- Stand in Utkatasana (see chapter 9.2, number 2) and rest your hands lightly on your knees, as shown in figure 6.3-72. Your lower back and legs carry the weight of your body. Make sure your lower back is straight. There is a crease where your thighs meet your abdomen. The mobility in your hips is largely dependent on whether or not the muscles in this crease can relax. When you carry your weight and balance on the front part of your heels, you will feel these muscles relax and your pelvis will be able to move.

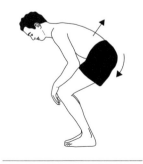

In this exercise, the lower back transfers the movement to the pelvis, but it is the hips that determine whether or not the movement can be accepted. The hamstrings are also important for the position of the pelvis and the lower back as well. When the hamstrings are tight, they can block movement by pulling on the sit bones (figure 6.3-73). This is sometimes a coordination problem: as soon as you become aware of the proper position—for example, when you see someone else do the movement and copy it— you can do it correctly.

But it can also be a matter of strain versus strength. If you commonly use the strength in your legs by straining your hamstrings, you will probably find it difficult to change this habit. The release of your hamstrings will activate your quadriceps (the muscles at the front of the thighs). It is very important to be aware of this change and do exercises such as standing poses that develop strength in these muscles. When your legs are not used

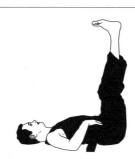

to coordinate the movement from these muscles, your body will never choose this option during daily, automatic movements, and your lower back will remain unstable.

Only when the muscles around your hips are relaxed will your pelvis be able to move.

☛ *Important Tip*

Two movements are actually made in this exercise. The posterior part of the lower back pushes the pelvis backward, but the front part of the lower back—the part of the abdomen that lies against the sacrum—moves forward and, together with the crown, upward.

Exercises with stretched legs

The following exercise shows how straight legs move in relation to your pelvis, without using your back. It can be disturbing to realize that your legs are stiffer than you think. This movement plays an important part in many asanas.

Instructions

·   Lie supine, with your legs stretched out and the rubber strip placed horizontally under your lower back, as shown in figure 6.3-74a. The strip should just touch the edge of your pelvis. If you allow your midback to relax, your lower back should touch the strip lightly. Push the inside of your ankles and knees together, and stretch your legs.

·   Lift your legs to a 90-degree angle without increasing the pressure to the strip. The weight of your legs should fall into your pelvis, not your lower back. With your fingers, feel the crease where your thighs meet your pelvis. See whether the muscles in this crease are relaxed and soft, or tense and hard (figure 6.3-74b).

> **Note:** The muscles in the crease are responsible for lifting your legs. In the first part of the movement, they may feel hard. However, once your legs have reached 90 degrees, the muscles should be able to relax and soften.
>
> If they are still hard when your legs are in the 90-degree position, you have either tension in your lower back (the area between the strip and your tailbone) or tight hamstrings or stiff muscles around your hips. This reaction of the hip muscles greatly affects the way your legs are involved. This also depends on the position of your lower back, which you can test in the following way.

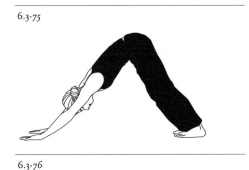

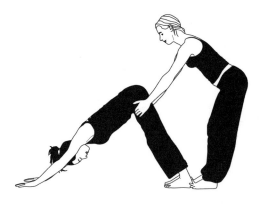

Instructions

- Stand in Adho Mukha Svanasana with a bent lower back (figure 6.3-75). Contract your quadriceps to stretch your legs; the muscles that produce the stretch are located just above the knee.
- Bend your knees and allow your sit bones to move up by releasing your hamstrings. This will straighten your back and cause your lower back to push your pelvis and thighs farther back and up. Stretch your legs as if someone were pulling on your upper thighs (figure 6.3-76). Your lower back makes this movement.

By using combinations of the preceding exercises, you can analyze the effect they have on the right and left sides of your body. To perform this analysis, do the following exercise.

Instructions

- Stand in Adho Mukha Svanasana again, and bring your right foot forward approximately three feet. Place your fingers on the floor directly under your shoulders and on both sides of your foot. Carry your body weight on the front part of your right heel. Simultaneously push your lower abdomen against your upper thigh and use your lower back to lift your upper body and head. Keep your fingers in contact with the floor and your arms stretched. Your lower back, which is not yet straight, pushes your right hip back. While this is happening, relax the area around your SI joints and your lower lower back (L4, L5). Your upper lower back (L1–L3) carries your weight. Although your fingers touch the floor, they do not support you. Your lower abdomen moves forward, together with your crown (compare figures 6.3-77 and 6.3-78).
- Remain in this position for 20 to 30 seconds, allowing relaxation to develop around your right hip.
- With your right hand, hold your right ankle or lower leg. This allows you to lift your upper body more so your lower back feels overly arched. Bring your lower ribs toward your belly until you feel the break in the movement of your lower ribs (also see connection 7, the lower lower back). This will bring the extension and strength to the center line of your entire lower back.
- Keeping your lower back active, stretch your right leg. Your right hip keeps moving back, but your abdomen, neck, and crown move forward. Slowly transfer your body weight to your back heel, pushing it into the floor.

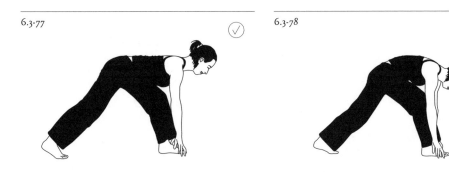

- Remain in this position so the movement in your hamstrings, lower back, and right hip can develop fully. Do not resist the movement, as that will cause it to remain in your hip, and the muscles there will harden immediately.
- Step back with your right foot and position your lower back so your head and chest can lower into Adho Mukha Svanasana. It should feel as if your lower back is pushing your upper thighs backward. Your right leg should now feel as if it is farther back than the left. The right side of your abdomen will also feel longer, creating more space between your right thigh and abdomen. You should also feel more relaxed around your sacrum and lower back.

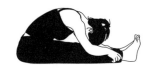

6.3-79

Note: If the muscles around your hips are stiff, the contrast between left and right will be much more obvious than if you have supple hips.

The preceding exercise clearly illustrates how the transfer of movement (with the help of body weight) is strongly improved when specific parts of the body can relax. Unfortunately, this seldom occurs in these types of exercises, because the movement is often impeded in the lower back, especially in seated forward bends, such as Paschimottanasana (see chapter 10.5, number 6). The back often looks like that of the model in figure 6.3-79 (collapsed lower back and chest) or figure 6.3-80 (collapsed lower back with the ribs, shoulders, and neck too high). In such circumstances, no movement can develop in the hips or the muscles in the backs of the legs.

6.3-80

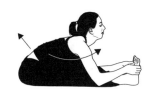

One solution is to work out the movement thoroughly in standing forward bends and standing poses so that, over time, it becomes easier to initiate the correct pelvic movement during seated forward bends. A variety of tips for the correct use of the back during these complex asanas is given in the introduction to forward bend (chapter 10.1). Read the information about connection 6 (chapter 6.3) carefully. Progress in forward bends is often very slow. It is easy to fall back into habitual postures (see chapter 3). Indeed, we often bend our backs all day long and nearly always at one particular point.

For this reason, it is worthwhile to take the time to analyze your forward bends. Start slowly, beginning with 5 minutes on a thin lower back roll (see connection 7). The following exercise is a good preparation, because it focuses specifically on freeing the pelvic part of your lower back.

Instructions

- Lean backward from Tadasana (see chapter 9.2, number 1) by pushing your fists against your tailbone and moving the top part of your body backward with space in your chest (figure 6.3-81). To return, pull the area below your navel up and move your lower ribs toward your stomach. When you can perform this movement well, it produces a break in the movement of your lower ribs that indicates your lower back is in a neutral extension and all parts of your core are connected. Repeat this exercise a few times, until your lower back starts to feel free.
- From Tadasana, bend your legs to allow your hamstrings to relax in Utkatasana, and rest your hands lightly on your thighs. Bend deeper until your lower abdomen

6.3-81

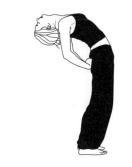

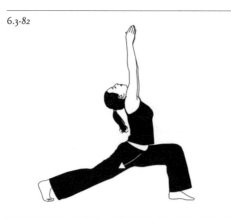

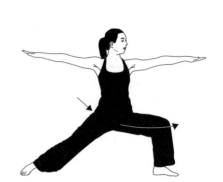

touches your upper thighs. Keep your lower back constantly active to stabilize the bend. Keep your chest and head high. Under your shoulder blades (midback), your back should feel shortened and engaged. Release the tension from the quadratus lumborum muscles and feel how your pelvis moves farther back, away from your spine. Do not lean on your hands or allow your chest and head to lower. Keep the center line of your lower back active; the sides of your lower back, SI joints, and hips can relax.

The hips and their free movement will be discussed with the standing poses. You can release the tension in your hips in a variety of ways: in Virabhadrasana I, the front part of the hip is freed; in Virabhadrasana II, the medial and side areas are stretched (see the arrows in figures 6.3-82 and 6.3-83).

It is important that your inner tube remain free and stable while you release the tension in your hips.

11. The connection between the legs and the feet

The (im)mobility of the hips determines the position of the thighs; this (in)flexibility is determined by the shape of the lower back. The transfer of movement through the legs is thus initiated through the spine. If the transfer of movement is correct, the thighs transfer the movement to the knees, which in turn pass it on to the lower legs, ankles, and feet. When the movement is correctly coordinated, the feet return the movement in the reverse order back toward the pelvis and spine.

If the coordination between the different parts of the leg is disturbed, it can cause all sorts of complaints in the leg joints, muscles, circulation, and nerves.

As well as the lower back, the knees also have an important role in transferring movement to the hips and feet. Stand with bent knees (figure 6.3-84) and the back of your pelvis against the wall. Make sure your knees are directly over your feet. In this position, your knees transfer the movement to the inside and outside of the crease between your upper thighs and abdomen. This creates space around your sacrum. You can experience the connection of your knees with your feet as a strength that moves from the inside of your knees to the top of your feet. From there, the movement spreads entirely over each foot. Your toes stretch, and your arches extend. The pressure to your heels is always evenly divided back to front and side to side.

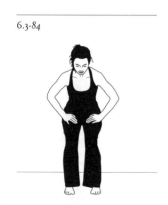

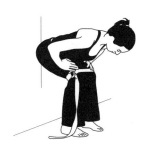

Note: When your hips relax, your knees often move sideways, causing tension to remain around your sacrum. Correct this movement by using your hands to lift the outsides of your knees slightly. Turn your feet in a little.

Note: In this exercise, the correct position of your feet and legs is crucial. Whether or not you can achieve this position is dictated by the amount of tension in your hips and lower back. You can relax these areas through a combination of pressure and balance, as in the preceding exercises.

6.3-85b

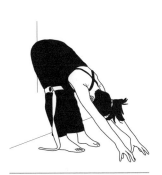

When you can realize this connection with bent knees, try it with your legs straight. Seek the same connection between the tops of your thighs and your pelvis as in Adho Mukha Svanasana (see chapter 9.2, number 4).

Instructions

- Stand with your hands resting lightly on your bent knees and the back of your pelvis against a wall. Without leaning on your hands, bring your lower abdomen against your upper thighs. Maintain your balance while your lower back moves toward your hips, and use the increase in pressure to relax your hips. Keep your knees directly over your feet, so the pressure remains even on the insides and outsides of your feet.
- Slowly stretch your legs from your midline, allowing your hips and SI joints to relax. If you are stiff, you will not be able to straighten your legs completely. As relaxation increases, this will become possible. A belt looped just above your knees makes it easier to align your legs (figures 6.3-85a and 6.3-85b).

PART FOUR

LEARNING THE
EXERCISES

The description of asanas, meditation, and pranayama should logically follow the preceding material. However, I have placed it in a separate section for the following reasons:

1. Asanas are the hands-on exercises that are ideally suited for realizing the essential characteristics of Critical Alignment; namely, how precise alignment of the body leads to feelings of lightness, relaxation, and strength. They also make the body fit and create a perfect working relationship between the parts, such as muscles, bones, joints, organs, the nervous system, and circulation. Thus, it is logical that practicing asanas can rigorously counteract physical stiffness and malformations.

2. I have divided each group of asanas into subgroups of similar exercises. I have done this to better isolate different parts of the body and to work more deeply with specific parts of the body. This allows deep layers of tension in the movement muscles to dissolve, providing better access to the postural muscles.

3. Asanas provide us with an extra challenge when we try to realize higher consciousness, because the body is in action. Because asanas are so diverse, there is always another approach through which to reach higher consciousness. Asanas truly are "meditation in action." Within this context, they give our physical activity structure; they channel our energy and thought processes. Balance is returned to the midline of the body. Asanas teach us how to remain relaxed in complicated situations and how to apply this relaxation in daily life.

4. Asanas have a strong meditative component, which is necessary both to handle the confrontations with physical and mental tension and for spiritual growth. For this reason, I have placed the technical description of meditation and pranayama exercises before the chapters on asanas.

7

MEDITATION AND
PRANAYAMA EXERCISES

7.1   Introduction

What is meditation?

To do meditation, the mind requires something on which to focus its attention. Some traditions use colors, sounds, mantras, pictures, or objects for this purpose. In Critical Alignment, the concepts of relaxation and space are essential, and they are the core elements on which to meditate. The purpose of this kind of meditation is to transfer the abstract (or cognitive) meaning of these concepts into the actual *experience* of relaxation and space.

We cannot develop meditative knowledge of these words intellectually; we have to enter our body to create a unique experience of them. Mental activity (thoughts) and physical tension block this experience. If we experience pain or discomfort when we are connected to our body in a negative way, it produces (unconscious) negative thoughts that usually lead to restlessness and discomfort. Further, the mind is restless by nature.

Observing relaxation and space from the unthinking part of our mind in a well-balanced body is the first step in Critical Alignment meditation. It produces an experience that can be described as, "I am space," rather than, "I am in this space." Some people have an immediate physical connection with space. Others do not, and they need the support of an image to keep their focus. Visualizations help us to remain in the process.

Many people do experience relaxation and space after a while but find it difficult to remain in that condition for long periods, because thinking pulls them out of the experience. This happens all the time in meditation practice. Developing the right attitude toward the confrontation of disturbance is part of learning in meditation and life. At its worst, disturbance can dominate a whole meditation session. But even then, our session is of great value if we use the experience of constant disturbance to correct ourselves in a calm, understanding way. To neutralize this tension, Critical Alignment advocates a return to body awareness, asking ourselves questions like, "Is my lower abdomen well supported by the arch of my lower back in order to produce relaxation in the lower abdomen?" or "Is tension in my heart region blocking my experience of space?"

Restlessness in our unconscious thinking patterns causes doubt. People often approach me after a class to ask what they are doing wrong. But it is inadvisable to interpret a situation from the perspective of right or wrong. It creates an attitude in which we are battling our own "wrong" nature. The mind is restless and moves around; that is natural, and there is nothing wrong with it.

Gaining confidence in what we are doing is the way to neutralize restlessness and feelings of uncertainty and doubt. We need to understand the posture we are sitting in to create a stable attitude. Instead of asking ourselves, "Am I sitting the right way?", we need to know exactly what we are doing when we assume a well-balanced position.

We can experience exercises performed on a rubber strip or a roll as meditative, because we feel a mental stability in these poses that leads to a feeling of openness. This is why Critical Alignment does not always place meditation on a higher level than asanas and pranayama like traditional texts often do. Through these exercises, we can develop meditation at an early stage of practice. They give passive support to the essential parts of our body, allowing us to experience lightness and space. This is why higher consciousness can be developed faster under Critical Alignment.

Patanjali states,[1]

> When there is activity carried out that is free from sorrow and radiant, then the mind becomes steady.

Once we can meditate for longer periods without interruption, we are able to transcend the meditation and experience our own nature. Then we enter the unknown in which teachers can no longer give guidance. It can lead us to moments of spiritual enlightenment. Vyasa, in the commentary on the *Yoga Sutra*, says the nature of mind is radiant and like space. We cannot enter this stage by willpower; it only comes to us like a gift.

The essence of all object-oriented meditation is the pure observation of the object without coloring it with personal thoughts, theories, feelings, fantasies, and so on—without adding the "I" component. This is difficult enough when sitting in a calm, meditative pose, let alone during such dynamic exercises as pranayama and asanas. Disrupting factors are more prevalent during dynamic exercises than during seated meditation. This makes pure observation without the "I" element especially difficult (see chapter 5 for a detailed description of this).

To understand what meditation is about, we should adopt a tranquil, meditative pose. This makes it possible to develop space and relaxation in our body. We can then successfully use the direct experience of relaxation, openness, and space that occurs during meditation to counter the tension and stiffness that constantly confronts us when practicing asanas and pranayama. A tranquil, meditative pose also allows us to become acquainted with the spiritual aspects of meditation. We can take that experience into the more dynamic exercises.

What is pranayama?

Prana means "breath, or life force" and can be compared with *chi* (energy flow) from the Chinese system; *ayama* means "lengthening, or stretching."

Pranayama is the lengthening, or stretching, of the vital life force. This life force is transported through a network of *nadis* (channels), which is comparable to the Chinese meridian system. *Granthas* (knots or blockages) can be found within this network of circulating energy. Acupuncture uses needles to release blocked energy from the outside in. Yoga, however, releases these blockages from the inside out through pranayama and asanas.

Ida and *pingala* are two of the most important nadis, but *susumna* is the most important. Pingala (the active, extroverted, solar nadi) is connected to the right nostril and stimulates the left side of the brain (this is a general principle—stimulation to one side of the body is processed through the opposite side of the brain). Ida (the passive, introverted, lunar nadi) is connected to the left nostril and stimulates the right side of the brain. It is for this reason that some pranayama exercises alternate breathing between the left and right nostrils. As well as clearing the nadis, pranayama has a significant effect on the deeper levels of tension stored in the body (see chapter 5.1). Pranayama and meditation have an obvious spiritual component, as discussed in chapter 5. It is this spiritual aspect that gives meditation a higher place than pranayama in the yoga tradition, and both stand above asanas. For this reason meditation, pranayama, and asanas have always been considered separate categories, described and practiced independently.

I am going to differ from this tradition and combine meditation and pranayama in the following technical description. I will also discuss them before asanas. There are two reasons for this:

1. A knowledge of meditation and correct breathing is essential for realizing higher consciousness during the practice of asanas. This is why this book combines the technical description of meditation and pranayama exercises and places them together before asanas. The exercises in this category, such as lying on a midback roll or a rubber strip, are simple and can be done easily at the beginning of an asana lesson.

2. Meditation and pranayama can both be practiced separately. Even then, however, they have obvious shared goals. One of these is to penetrate and ease the deeper levels of tension in the body and mind. Another is the achievement of spiritual enlightenment as mentioned earlier. From the point of view of technique, the exercises for this purpose are more complex. They will also be discussed in this chapter.

7.2   Meditation exercises

Meditation exercises have two purposes. They provide insight into the strategies we have developed over the years that have caused us to contract mentally and physically. We must identify and eliminate these strategies before we can experience genuine relaxation.

Then meditation exercises can support a spiritual experience. The concepts of relaxation and space play a central part in these exercises, as discussed in detail in chapter 5.

Meditation exercises to prepare for pranayama

In the first phase, the body is passive, and preparatory exercises are done using yoga props (a roll or rubber strip). During the second phase, a seated position is adopted wherein higher consciousness can be realized. In the third phase, the pranayama exercises are carried out.

Meditation exercises to prepare for asanas

Here too, the first phase consists of preparatory exercises (the strip and/or roll) to develop correct breathing techniques. From this foundation, the second phase of higher consciousness can be developed and maintained in slow movements. This is carried through to the third phase, in which movement becomes more fluid and asanas are combined. In practitioners with general restlessness, this gradual preparation is recommended.

1. Exercises to prepare for meditation

Do the roll under the shoulder blades and/or the rubber strip between the shoulder blades exercises, as described in chapter 6.3, connection 2. You can decide for yourself whether to do one or both.

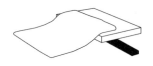

7.2-1a

Instructions: Meditation lying on the roll or rubber strip

In both of these exercises, you can develop higher consciousness through your breathing (see chapter 6.3, connection 2).

2. Sitting meditation practices

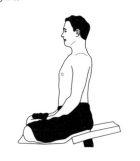

7.2-1b

Instructions

- When you have finished the preparatory exercise(s), arrange a shoulderstand block with a rubber strip underneath and a felt mat on top (figure 7.2-1a). Sit on the edge of the block and cross your legs in a comfortable, stable position such as Siddhasana (figure 7.2-1b; see also chapter 13.2, number 1, variation 2) or Padmasana (see chapter 13.2, number 1).
- Follow the instructions for sitting and stacking your spine from chapter 6.3, connection 9. Briefly, this should be done as follows: First, shift your pelvis into an erect position, then get your lower back and diaphragm into the correct position. Finally, with a deep inhalation, stack your chest, neck, and head on top. Shut your eyes and rest your hands, with palms facing up, on your feet (figure 7.2-2).
- When your back is stacked correctly, your head and neck are balanced effortlessly on top of your spine. Because your head is carried by the postural muscles, your neck will be able to relax. This can give your head a feeling of weightlessness. Your face can also relax, and you can begin to concentrate. Initially, this concentration is situated in the back of your head.
- Slowly develop higher consciousness (see chapter 5.2 for instructions on this).
- Take 5 to 10 minutes to deepen this consciousness. Remain aware of the space around you. Allow the openness in your body to communicate freely with this space.

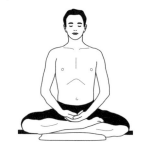

7.2-2

- As soon as you follow your thoughts, your attention will be lost. When you notice this has happened, correct yourself by carefully observing your pose and direct your attention to reestablishing higher consciousness.
- At this stage, your focus shifts more to breathing, which is essential to meditation. Guide your breath toward your lower abdomen, filling it until you feel your lower ribs move. Your ribs broaden during inhalation, then narrow and push the movement back toward your lower abdomen during exhalation. Your abdomen is not pulled inward when you exhale, because it is supported by your erect lower back, which also narrows during exhalation. This keeps your inner tube intact and allows your abdomen to remain relaxed and forward even at the end of the exhalation (see also chapter 6.3, connections 1 and 2).

> **Note:** This coordination of the abdomen, remaining forward and relaxed during exhalations, is difficult for many people and often ends in the opposite movement of the abdomen being pulled inward at the end of exhalations. This problem can arise when the lower back gives poor support to the abdomen. If your lower back cannot extend sufficiently when you are sitting on the shoulderstand block, try sitting higher. Experiment with different heights to find the best extension in your lower back. If you practice the lower back exercises in chapter 6.3, connection 7, the extension in your lower back will slowly improve.

- Breathing into your abdomen can give a feeling of stability, of being firmly connected to the floor. This feeling increases the experience of relaxation in the hara gravity point. Being "well grounded" while sitting is a necessity for higher consciousness. Your body functions as an anchor, providing the concrete experience of being here and now and preventing you from becoming lost in vague feelings and fantasies. To increase your feelings of stability and relaxation, keep breathing into your abdomen and allow the relaxation to encompass your entire body. This generally starts with the relaxation of your shoulders. The feeling of relaxation here can become so strong that you may feel like your pose is collapsing. However, as long as your lower back remains erect and the crown of your head extended, this will not happen. You must remain aware of these two areas as you continue to relax.
- Next, become more conscious of the movement of your breath above your diaphragm, and allow your rib cage to move in the same manner as when you are lying on the roll and the rubber strip (see page 134). Observe how the extension in your upper back allows your ribs to move freely. This movement gives important information about your pose. If your ribs broaden, then your back is relaxed. In a forced military posture, the ribs cannot broaden. Narrowing ribs in your back indicate that it is straight; a collapsed and bent back cannot narrow.
- Retain the extension of both your lower back and the crown of your head. This is not an exercise in strength but in a form of alertness and should be conducted as such.
- Breathe into the area above your diaphragm and allow your breath to circulate freely through your entire body.
- Sit completely still for 5 to 20 minutes, and observe your breathing. Every time you realize that your higher consciousness has diminished or been totally lost, start again with the three phases for realizing higher consciousness (see chapter 5).

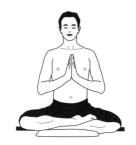

Note: There is another point in the body that symbolizes alertness. It is the area where the thumbs and the base of your sternum touch in the Indian manner of greeting called *namaskar*. Place your hands in a "prayer position" with your thumbs against the base of your sternum (heart gravity point), as seen in figure 7.2-3. Press your thumbs very lightly against your sternum, so lightly that the contact is established through the movement of your breath. You "push" your sternum toward your thumbs with inhalations. Breathing provides an ideal connection that is characterized by relaxation and space.

If your pose begins to collapse, your thumbs will push against your sternum. If you become overactive, your chest will take over the initiative from the rest of your body and push against your thumbs causing your body to tense. In both cases, you will lose higher consciousness instantaneously.

It is important to observe this point vigilantly, as the regular rhythm of breathing developed from open attention can easily be broken by the stream of your thoughts. These thoughts are often just below the surface of your conscious attention, meaning they slowly well up from your unconscious and, unnoticed, take over your attention. Generally, attention can be disturbed in two ways: it weakens (or wanders), or it hardens (because of a struggle with the breath). This is when the vigilant observation of the contact with your thumbs becomes valuable. It gives an early warning that things are starting to go wrong. When your attention begins to wander, your palms will lose contact and the extension to your crown will be lost. (See chapter 7.3 for more examples of this.)

- Finish your meditation by opening your eyes slowly without focusing on the area you are looking at directly. Do not become active right away. Observe from the back of your head, completely relaxed. Do not color your observations by adding something personal to what you see. (See note on page 137.)
- Move your arms and shoulders a little, unfold your legs, and lie down for two or three minutes before standing up.

7.3 Pranayama exercises

The instructions above said to build up your posture slowly after doing the preparatory exercises. Then there is another 10 minutes to build up the stage of higher consciousness and then we sit still for another 5 to 20 minutes. In total this exercise sometimes takes an hour. To prepare ourselves for pranayama we only need to do the meditation for 10 to 15 minutes.

Breathing is structured during pranayama exercises: it is lengthened and brought into a certain rhythm for a determined length of time. Some exercises use breath retention.

To lengthen respiration, position the fingers of your right hand as shown in figure 7.3-1; you will use this hand to close your nostrils partially or totally, as necessary. If the narrowing of your nostril(s) remains constant, you cannot possibly speed up your breathing. The positioning of the fingers also allows you to neutralize deep respiration reflexes.

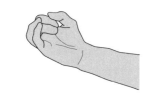

Note: Instead of narrowing your horizon to the spot you are gazing at, notice that your horizon is wide when looking from the back of your head. From this open, relaxed perspective, become aware of the space around you without letting your thinking distract you. Feel your connection with this space in the way that people become aware of their surroundings when they are in nature. Walking through a forest, being in the mountains, or looking at the ocean often gives us that same physical connection. That same space is around you in your room or at your office, even though the circumstances are different.

Instead of thinking that the exercise is over, it is more interesting to find out if the openness and relaxation you have experienced in your body and awareness are a meaningful foundation for your everyday actions out in the world. This awareness is the opposite of a narrow concentration and tense body where you lose contact with everything you have built up in the exercise. Remember that practicing Critical Alignment means that you learn not only how to balance your body and organize your movements without strain during practice but also how to connect this experience to (stressful) daily activities.

You need to accept your "new" posture in connection with feelings of relaxation and space. When you are straighter in your body and less tense at the end of an exercise or a class, you need to transfer that awareness to everyday circumstances. This is the moment to make the change because the experience is still fresh.

Visualize yourself in normal situations, and see yourself acting from this cultivated awareness of openness, relaxation, and sharp attention. Do it initially with simple circumstances like walking in your house or on the street, then when you are at work or in other more complex and stressful circumstances. When you become accustomed to ending your meditation (or yoga class) this way, you may remember cultivated awareness of openness, relaxation, and sharp attention when the imagined circumstances occur in daily life.

When you finish your practice this way, it is not the end of the exercise or the class but the beginning of a new awareness.

Pranayama exercises are initiated by developing higher consciousness. You practice the exercises with the open consciousness of being here and now.

You can do preparatory exercises aimed at quickly developing this consciousness. Follow the preliminary meditation exercises described earlier in this chapter.

As stated in chapter 7.2, we use the body to alert us to rising, unconscious thoughts during pranayama and to neutralize them. The positions of the fingers of your right hand against your nose play an important role here, as does the contact of your left thumb with your left index finger (figure 7.3-2). The fingers give more subtle indications of tension than the rest of the body. Being so sensitive, they are excellent and immediate "sensors." When the contact of your fingers lessens or breaks completely, it is a clear signal of diminishing attention. Conversely, too much pressure from your fingers results in the loss of relaxation and open attention. By maintaining an awareness of the signals from your fingers, you establish a working relationship with mental stress reactions. Other parts of the body also play a role in signaling the buildup of tension.

7.3-2

For example, raising your right elbow or one or both of your shoulders are clear signals of increasing tension.

Before you start your pranayama practice, it is useful to become aware of the possible tension at the end of your exhalations by pushing your fingers against the spot below your navel as described in chapter 6.3, connections 1 and 2.

3. Nadi Sodhana Pranayama (Channel Cleaning Breath)

Nadi means "channel"; sodhana means cleansing.
Nadi Sodhana clears blockages out of the nadis.

Instructions

- After spending 5 to 20 minutes on the preceding meditation exercise and developing higher consciousness, lower your chin to your chest at the end of an inhalation. This movement keeps your neck in a constant, open extension. Your neck is another area that warns you when thoughts are about to take over; it will immediately contract and lift your chin from your chest.

> **Note:** The extension of your crown provided an upward strength to the top of your sternum that is directly connected to the extension in your lower back. If your lower back collapses, this point under your chin will most certainly also collapse. The connection between the chin and chest is called *jalandhara bandha*. It produces the combination of mental relaxation and physical alertness that should also be present during Sarvangasana.

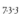

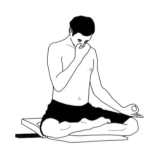

- Place your left hand on your left thigh so that your upper arm is relaxed and next to your trunk. Bring your right hand to your nose, placing the pads of your ring and little fingers just above the septum on the left side (the little finger supplies the pressure) and the pad of your thumb on the right nostril (figure 7.3-3).
- Connect your right arm with your right shoulder blade. Do not allow your upper arm to put pressure on your ribs.
- All of these actions take place within higher consciousness (see chapter 5 where the factors that can hinder the realization of higher consciousness are discussed).
- Gently close your left nostril with your ring and little fingers. Exhale through the right and then partially block the right nostril and inhale for 15 seconds. Close the right nostril, partially block the left, and repeat; exhale for 15 seconds, then inhale for 15 seconds. This is one cycle.
- Repeat this cycle ten times. End by stopping halfway through the exhalation from the right nostril. Allow your right hand to rest on your thigh and remain sitting totally motionless.

> **Note:** The 15 seconds mentioned here is an average. You should discover your own capacity; 10 to 12 seconds or less may be enough in the beginning. Ultimately, the timing should increase to 18 to 20 seconds or more depending on your ability.

General instructions regarding this exercise

1. You must use equal measures of time for all inhalations and exhalations during pranayama. This is often a problem when you use some mental method of timing, such as counting in your mind or using a mantra or a movement of your hand, rather than a clock. As the breaths become faster because of the surfacing reflexes, your counting will speed up also. For this reason, I prefer to count the ticks of a clock or a metronome.
2. Remain continuously aware of maintaining higher consciousness. That is the key to pranayama. If you lose it, use the steps described in chapter 6 to start again.
3. When deep breathing reflexes arise, you will immediately be inclined to enlarge the nostril to allow more air in. Try not to give in to this inclination. Allow the reflex to surface, and observe it with open attention. Try to neutralize the reflex by keeping the nostril partially closed and breathing slowly. Observe the end of your exhalations to find out whether the tension is originating there. Do not lose your posture when confronted with this tension. (Chapter 5.7 gives more instructions for dealing with these reflexes.)
4. If your nose is blocked, you can open the nostril by pushing the skin toward your cheekbone, raising the finger slightly higher on your nose. This will allow you to regulate the size of the opening.
5. You can also choose to do the following simpler version of this pranayama exercise.

4. Surya Bhedana Pranayama (Sun Piercing Breath)

Surya means "sun"; *bhedana* means "breaking (open)."
Exhale through your left nostril for 15 seconds, then inhale through the right for 15 seconds. Repeat this for 5 to 10 minutes.

5. Chandra Bhedana Pranayama (Moon Piercing Breath)

Chandra means "moon"; *bhedana* means "breaking."
Exhale through your right nostril for 15 seconds, then inhale through the left for 15 seconds. Repeat for 5 to 10 minutes.

A sound will arise inside your nostrils from the pressure of your fingertips against your nose. Observe the sound from higher consciousness, but do not engage with it or let it disturb that consciousness. When you maintain your attention correctly, the noise will be open and regular. When your thoughts begin to take over, the noise will become irregular or loud. This is a signal to retrieve your attention and higher consciousness.

6. Bhramara Pranayama (Bee Breath)

Bhramara means "bee."
Every pranayama session closes with this exercise. During the exhalations, you make a humming noise that resembles the sound of a bee.

Instructions

·   After completing the pranayama exercises, lift your head on an inhalation and position it directly above your spine.

- Breathing slowly and deeply, make a soft humming noise with every exhalation. This noise resonates and circulates through your mouth, into your entire body, and out into the space around you. Make the noise as if your entire body is producing it, not only your mouth or throat.
- Repeat this five times and end by sitting totally motionless for 1 minute. After this, stretch your legs and relax in Savasana (Corpse Pose).

8

INVERSIONS

8.1   Introduction

The achievement of free, total movements during inversions is not initiated from the lower back, as with standing poses and forward bends, but originates from stacking the vertebrae of the neck and upper back. Sometimes this occurs directly from the spine (Sarvangasana), sometimes from the extension of the neck (Sirsasana), and sometimes from the shoulders (Sirsasana on the headstand bench, Adho Mukha Vrksasana, and Pincha Mayurasana). Then the lower back can stabilize and pass movement on to the pelvis and legs.

Inversions can be divided into subgroups, each of which has unique characteristics. There are clear differences in their paths to the end pose based on their individual characteristics. The end pose offers the possibility of reaching deeper muscles, of achieving a level of tranquillity in body and mind, of finding and maintaining balance in the body, and so on. The following is an overview of the main characteristics of inversions.

1. Main characteristics of inversions

- The shoulders, arms, neck, and spine, together with the pelvis, legs, and feet, form the basic structure of the body. Inversions develop good structure and enhance significant function to the parts of the body located above the inner tube (chest, shoulders, arms, neck, and upper back).
- Pressure generated from body weight is used to strengthen the following connections: shoulder–back, neck–back, head–back, and arms–back.
- The subtle balance created through aligning the various parts of the body is unique to inversions.
- Inversions complement each other, allowing deeper penetration into muscles and bones. For example, Sarvangasana and Halasana stimulate and strengthen an extended upper back, while the position of the head allows the large back muscles to relax and stretch. This is a good preparation for learning how to extend the neck during Sirsasana. Adho Mukha Vrksasana and Pincha Mayurasana stimulate the extension of the back through the arms–shoulder blades–ribs–spine connection. This prepares the arms for the support they must provide to the shoulders and back in Sirsasana.

2. Developmental processes of inversions

Every asana takes a unique route to its end position. Once in the end position, all of these asanas increase the body's mobility and strength in their own way. The position of the neck is the most important characteristic for dividing inversions into the following three subgroups.

Inversions with an extended neck

On the headstand bench, the neck gradually comes into alignment with the back. This is due to the straightening of the upper back and occurs without the neck being encumbered with the weight of the body. The pressure necessary for this movement accumulates from the sides (the shoulders), creating a safe situation in which the extended neck can stabilize in relation to the continuously changing upper back. The constant extension of the crown, together with a light pressure from the back of the head against the rubber strip, develops strength in the neck.

This connection can be worked on during Sirsasana. In this pose, the neck must receive the body's weight and transform it into an extension of the upper back in the area between the shoulder blades. This allows the deep postural muscles to stabilize the neck and back.

Sirsasana on the headstand bench and Salamba Sirsasana with associated variations belong to this subgroup.

Inversions with a flexed neck

During Sarvangasana and Halasana, the neck is bent forward and relaxed. In this position, it has absolutely no weight-bearing function. This job is given directly to C7 (the last vertebra of the neck), to the thoracic vertebrae, and to the shoulders.

Because of this, these asanas provide relaxation to the movement muscles of the back and strength to the postural muscles around the spine simultaneously. Salamba Sarvangasana with its associated variations and Halasana belong to this subgroup.

Inversions with an arched (concave) neck

Adho Mukha Vrksasana and Pincha Mayurasana strengthen the arm muscles and the deep postural muscles of the shoulders. They work directly and dynamically into the midline of the body, which requires a concave neck that extends the upper back, as in a backbend. The support in these asanas comes from the sides, from the strength of the arms. This strength supports the spine as it stretches (indirectly) via the shoulder blades and is valuable for learning how to use the arms correctly in Salamba Sirsasana.

Adho Mukha Vrksasana and Pincha Mayurasana belong to this subgroup.

3. Meditative aspect of inversions

The delicate balance of an aligned body makes Sirsasana an alert meditative pose. Balance is provided mainly by the deep postural muscles of the spine and neck. The constant adjustments that are necessary to maintain balance develop an open attention that guards against overload or strain on any one muscle group. The extension of the neck is an important source of alertness. Through the mental stillness, open attention, and alertness that come with this asana, a spacious quality arises that allows optimal breathing. These qualities provide the open, meditative character that can be experienced during Sirsasana. This encompasses both the space in the body and the space outside it.

Sarvangasana has a meditative quality as well. But it is more tranquil than Sirsasana. The body is practically still in Sarvangasana; the constant adjustments necessary for balance characteristic for Sirsasana are totally absent here. Sarvangasana creates a more inward, passive stillness because of the lengthening of the neck.

Because Adho Mukha Vrksasana cannot be maintained as long as Sarvangasana or Sirsasana, meditation during this pose is much shorter but no less present. There is a direct and focused physical presence to it that has no peer and can only be achieved through the correct awareness. It is a mental warmup.

8.2   Inversions with an extended neck

Sirsasana on the headstand bench and Salamba Sirsasana with its associated variations belong to this subgroup. Both poses work primarily on the extension of the upper back in the area between the shoulder blades.

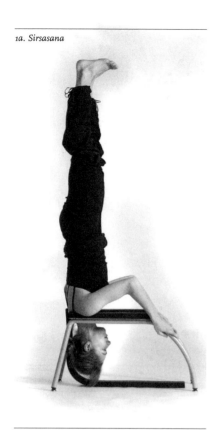

1a. Sirsasana

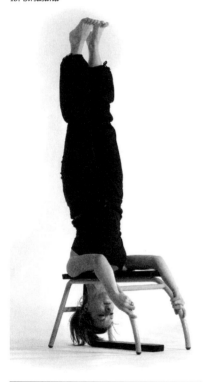

1b. Sirsasana

1. Sirsasana on the headstand bench

Sirsa means "head."

There are two ways to learn this asana. The first method provides extra support for your upper back, which prevents it from adopting its habitual position. In the second method, your body must learn to provide its own support to your back.

Method 1

Set up the headstand bench, backbender, and rubber strip as shown in figure 8.2-1.

Instructions

- Position your shoulders so that you feel the rubber strip pushing firmly against your back. Your head should hang free and *not* touch the strip. This allows your neck to extend and relax (figure 8.2-2).
- Holding the legs of the headstand bench, bring your feet closer in while lifting your pelvis as high as possible above your shoulders (see figure 8.2-2). This is called Ostrich Pose. Consider the following points before jumping up:
  1. Allow your shoulders to become heavy and relaxed and visualize how your upper back (between your shoulder blades) can move with the pressure of the strip during your jump. In other words, let go of the tension in your upper back while you exhale.
  2. At the same time, contract your stomach muscles. They must be in the correct position before you jump: your stomach muscles form the inner tube between your pubic bone and sternum, and you can feel them easily in this position. Breathe into your abdomen without relaxing these muscles, and do not lose this contact during your jump.
  3. Remember that the strength for the jump, and subsequently that for positioning your legs and pelvis on top of your upper back and shoulders, comes primarily from your lower back.
- When you are conscious of these points, jump up on an exhalation, and position your core above the area where the strip touches your back. Bend your knees and place your feet against the wall. Immediately after you jump, check that your neck is still relaxed and extended and that the breath in your abdomen is still under control.
- Without disturbing the inner tube, remove your feet from the wall, one at a time, and stretch your legs. Balance your weight on the back of your shoulders and not on your hands. Imagine driving a car with power steering — this is the same action your hands have on the legs of the headstand bench. If you start to lose your balance, all you have to do is adjust your hands slightly to find it again.
- Remain standing for as long as you like without timing yourself. Initially, a lot of blood will flow to your head creating a feeling of pressure. Do not be alarmed; this will lessen with practice. Do not cause extra pressure by holding your breath and/or tensing your shoulders and neck muscles. This can rupture the capillaries around your eyes. If this happens, gradually build up

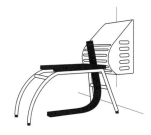

Note: If you cannot jump up on your own, lift one leg and ask for assistance in bringing it farther toward the wall. Your pelvis should be involved in the movement. See the difference between figures 8.2-3a, in which the pelvis follows the movement, and figure 8.2-3b, in which the pelvis is actively and correctly engaged in the movement.

Check your posture immediately after jumping, and try to determine whether your pelvis is stacked over your chest. When they are correctly aligned, the inner tube will provide stability between your chest and pubic bone. However, if your lower ribs have shifted forward and your abdomen has fallen inward, then you lost control of your abdominal muscles during the jump. If that is the case, jump up again. This will probably result in excessive tension in your stomach muscles, causing your hands to bear your weight and making it necessary to lean on your collarbones. This is not important; it only means that your upper back needs more time to relax around the rubber strip. Push downward on the legs of the headstand bench so your lower ribs can shift back gradually. As soon as your upper back becomes more mobile, your diaphragm will move into its correct position, your weight will shift to the back of your shoulder blades, and your inner tube remains active.

8.2-2

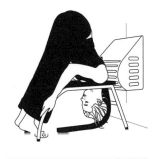

Note: This movement will make your back straighter, increasing the pressure to your shoulders and your back's contact with the strip. Admittedly, this can feel uncomfortable, but try to remember that the pressure is a good sign. This pose can actually be compared to lying on the rubber strip (see chapter 6.3, connection 3), only here you are in a vertical position. Try to relax into the pressure, allowing your upper back and shoulders to soften when you exhale.

8.2-3a ⊗

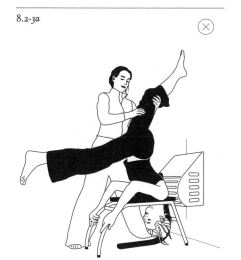

8.2-3b ✓

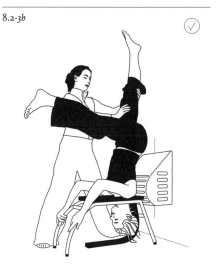

8.2-4

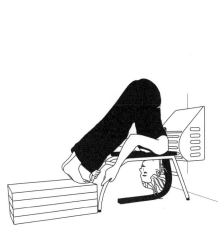

the exercise by beginning with Ostrich Pose minus the jumping up. You can also gradually raise your feet (figure 8.2-4). Remain relaxed; keep breathing; and soften your shoulders, upper back, and neck during exhalations. After holding this position for two or three minutes you can jump up again as calmly as possible during an exhalation, allowing it to soften your upper back.

☞ *Key points*

If your upper back is bent and stiff (this can encompass your entire upper back or just a few vertebrae that are not moving adequately), compensatory movements will cause problems.

The first series of compensations involves your neck and the position of your head and can arise in two ways:

1. If your shoulders shift forward (away from the backbender) on the headstand bench during the jump, your head will shift too far forward (figure 8.2-5).
2. If your neck has shortened and your head touches the strip after the jump (meaning your head has moved backward), then the movement has occurred in your neck and not your upper back.

The solution lies in keeping your neck, shoulders, and head stable. If you can do this during the jump, then your upper back must make the right movement. If you can't, then your lower back and pelvis will compensate. Your lower back will become excessively concave, and your pelvis and legs will then take one of two positions: a hollow lower back with your legs in a forward angle (figure 8.2-6) or a hollow lower back with your legs moving backward (figure 8.2-7). In both cases, contact with your inner tube has been lost, disturbing the alignment of your lower back. If your body looks like the illustration in figure 8.2-8, with a hollow lower back and your legs moving backward, your hands will bear the weight of your body. Allow your lower ribs to move back gradually, shifting your weight from your hands to the back of your shoulders. If this does not work because your upper back cannot relax, then you must move your shoulders a little farther forward on the headstand bench, away from the backbender, as indicated by the arrows in figure 8.2-9. Do not move too far, as that will allow your back to bend too much, and it will lose the stimulus to straighten supplied by the strip.

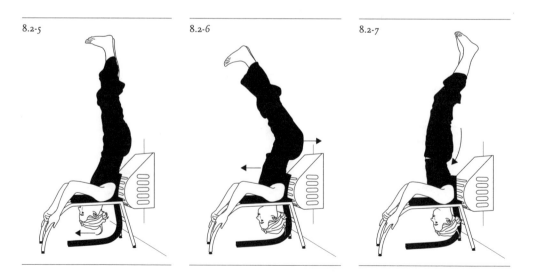

8.2-5   8.2-6   8.2-7

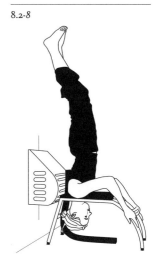

8.2-9 Superior view

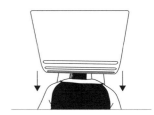

Note: Keep in mind that adjusting your lower back is not the starting point in Sirsasana. First you need to straighten your upper back by releasing the tension there. However, you do need to transfer your body weight to your upper back in order to direct pressure to the area between your shoulder blades and shoulders (as explained in chapter 2.4.1). The strength to do this comes initially from the movement muscles in your abdomen. You do not need that strength when your upper back becomes straight. Then you are able to transfer your body weight from your inner core muscles, like the transverse abdominals. When your upper back starts to straighten out, it affects the balance of your lower back. Initially the weight of your pelvis and legs is carried by a compressed arch in your lumbar spine (also see figure 8.2-8). Once you can lengthen the lumbar arch by extending your upper back, the weight of your legs will balance on a properly aligned lower back, which will make you feel that your legs are balancing on L5, the last vertebra in your lower back. This produces an unstable "wiggling" movement in your lower back. It will feel as if all the vertebrae can move separately and are controlled by the postural muscles in your lower back. Your transverse abdominals, activated by the upward pull toward your navel from the area 1 inch below it, supports this balance. Because your position is supported by your inner core muscles now, balance feels effortless.

☞ *Warnings*

1. If you experience a lot of pressure or pain in your upper arms, or if your fingers begin to tingle, come back down and wait until these sensations disappear. Observe whether these sensations lessen or take longer to appear in the following weeks. When that happens it is a good sign. If they do not diminish, seek advice from a qualified teacher who has experience making corrections on the headstand bench. The feeling of too much pressure or tingling is often caused by a misaligned upper back. In such cases, body weight is pushed to the front of the shoulders near the collarbones where all the nerves from the neck come together before they enter the arms. Pressure on the nerves may cause numbness or tingling in the arms or hands.

It is very difficult for the body to relax when movement is fast. Jumping up is fast, so the body sometimes unconsciously resists the pressure this causes and starts to contract muscles instead of relaxing them. This contraction can put pressure on nerves or the blood vessels that supply the nerves, which may cause the arms to become numb.

2. Large, heavy people who can easily let go of the tension in their shoulders must be careful not to lose the feeling in their arms. The rule of thumb is that if you are heavier than 220 pounds, it is best to build up your time in the pose gradually. Do not remain on the headstand bench if your hands or fingers become numb; instead, come back down and try again once feeling has returned. Do not squeeze the legs of the headstand bench with your hands, because you will not be able to tell if they start to tingle. After a while, the numbness will take longer to develop until it finally disappears altogether.

8.2-10

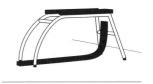

Method 2
Set up the headstand bench and rubber strip as shown in figure 8.2-10. Chapter 4.6.1 discussed how you can learn the three steps of relaxation, movement, and strength and

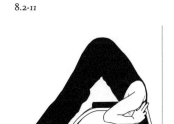

8.2-11

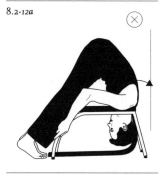

8.2-12a ⊗

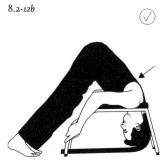

8.2-12b ✓

coordination from a teacher. That relaxation is directed primarily toward the stiffness in your upper back. The following description shows how you can learn to do this yourself.

Instructions

- Place the headstand bench close to a wall and kneel in front of it. Position your shoulders on the far end of the bench and lift your knees. Check with your fingers that you have between ½ inch and 1 inch of the rubber strip behind your shoulders (figure 8.2-11). The back of your head should touch the rubber strip; keep this contact as light as possible. It is essentially for maintaining the length in your neck.
- Allow your upper back, in the area between your shoulder blades, to relax. Direct your breathing to this area, and allow the upper back to sink in deeper with every exhalation (compare figures 8.2-12a and 8.2-12b). When we jump up from the bent spine (see figure 8.2-12a), we move from our habitual tension. Figure 8.2-12b shows us how to initiate the first two steps of Critical Alignment: relaxation and movement. These are the first two steps of Critical Alignment: relaxation and movement.
- Secure the relaxed position of your back by connecting your upper arms with your shoulder blades (see chapter 6.3.4).
- Pull lightly on the legs of the headstand bench to actively connect your shoulder blades to your rib cage. This way, your ribs also support the relaxed position of your spine (see the arrows in figure 8.2-13). The traction of pulling on the legs absorbs the movement of the jump, allowing your upper back to remain relaxed and mobile.
- Move one foot a little closer without changing the position of your back, and swing the other leg up so you can jump. Bring your body weight directly into the area between your shoulder blades.
- Movement is directed to this area of your upper back, which can now be extended further. The weight of your legs and pelvis will push your upper back straighter. Bend your knees and place your feet against the wall as shown in figure 8.2-14.

8.2-13

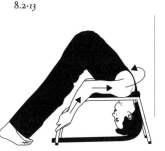

8.2-14

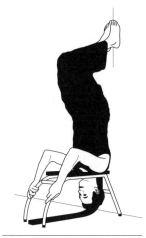

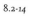

> **Note:** When you jump, observe whether your hands *pull* on the legs of the headstand bench or start to *push*. If you keep pulling, your shoulder blades will support your back, maintaining stability during your jump. If you start to push, this will allow your back to move into its habitual position, which means you will end up with a bent back. Your hands tell you precisely what is happening in your back.

- After jumping, pull on the legs of the headstand bench with your hands to align your upper body. Your ribs should gradually move toward your abdomen, and your pelvis should be positioned so that your abdomen feels spacious and relaxed. Once you feel stable enough, take your feet off the wall and stretch your legs straight up, one at a time.
- Once your body is balanced and aligned, it will feel a little unstable and wobbly. This is a sign that the deeper postural muscles are activating and starting to bear your weight. This is the third step of Critical Alignment: strength and coordination.
- Breathe deeply and slowly; relax your shoulders and neck.
- Do not stay in this pose too long in the beginning. Once the pressure on your shoulders lessens, you can extend the time to 5, 10, 15, and even 20 minutes.

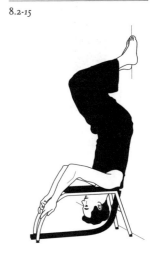

8.2-15

☞ Warning
Read the warnings under Method 1.

☞ Key points
After you jump into position, two situations can occur:

1. Your head may lose contact with the rubber strip (figure 8.2-15).
This occurs when pulling on the legs of the headstand bench turns into pushing, causing your back to bend and your head to move forward (see the arrow in figure 8.2-16).

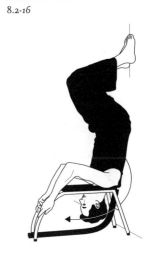

8.2-16

Solution
Push the back of your head firmly against the rubber strip and support this action when jumping by pulling on the legs of the headstand bench. Visualize the inward movement of your spine between your shoulder blades before you jump. It is important to jump high in order to extend your back. Do not "roll" yourself up with a bent back.

If this does not help, use the support of the strip and the backbender first. Jump up on an exhalation, direct your breath to your upper back, and keep your head stable as described above for Method 1. As you get stronger, try again without the support of the backbender.

2. Your lower back may become excessively concave (figure 8.2-17).
In this case, your hands have continued pulling on the legs of the headstand bench, and your head still has contact with the rubber strip, but your body weight has been "caught" in your lower back. This can have two causes:

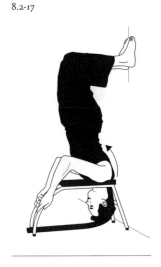

8.2-17

Your upper back is stiff.
Your diaphragm moves forward, instead of your upper back.

Solution
Mobilize and invigorate your upper back with special exercises (lying on the rubber strip, described in chapter 6.3, connection 4; or lying on the backbender, described in chapter 11, coordination exercise 1) before using the headstand bench. See if your mobility increases enough to allow your back to become straighter. If you do not feel any improvement, keep using the support of the backbender and the strip, and increase the pressure on the strip against your spine by activating your inner tube and pushing your ribs backward.

When you are balanced on the headstand bench, try to relax your shoulders, initiating

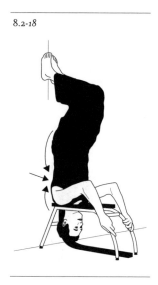

8.2-18

a movement toward your upper back. You will now be standing with a *downward* pressure from your legs and pelvis directed toward the area of your back around the strip and an *upward* pressure from your shoulders directed to the same area (see the arrows in figure 8.2-18). The only thing you can do now is accept the pressure. When you exhale, try to relax in the areas where the pressure is the greatest. Supported by the pull of your hands, imagine your upper back moving inward during inhalations. Ultimately, your back will release its tension, allowing your spine to straighten.

It is daunting to let go of the tension in your back, because it stimulates the "Help, I'm going to fall" feeling.

If your hands keep pulling on the legs of the headstand bench, your shoulders will support your back in the correct position so the weight of your legs and pelvis can move into your upper back. Then your back receives enough support from your hands that it can accept the movement and relax. This is a strange situation, because the back normally tightens when it has to bear weight, as when standing or sitting. It can never adopt the correct position gradually in Sirsasana because there is a critical juncture in this movement where the back is erect—exactly between the points of a bent back and an overextended back. It is a critical juncture because it's either "there" or "not there," and you cannot build up to it slowly. If you could watch it in slow motion, the action of moving from a bent to a straight back would follow the progression in figures 8.2-19a through 8.2-19e. In this movement, the bent back (in 8.2-19a and 8.2-19b) "falls" into a straight position (in 8.2-19c and 8.2-19d; it is in 8.2-19d that the feeling of falling occurs), and the necessity for tension in the back is eliminated. Because it is so accurately aligned, the back only needs muscular support from the postural muscles to maintain balance. They are the strongest muscles in the back but produce a feeling of lightness.

The fear of falling can hamper the practice of this asana. I regularly see students' doubt and uncertainty, despite the fact that they want to break through their movement restrictions. They begin to sweat, their breathing falters, and they hesitate: Shall I? Shall I not? There is only one way to break through this fear—just do it. When you perform the pose without tension, your body will manage it without a problem. This shows that from

8.2-19a–e

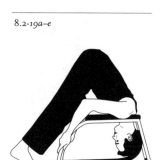

a

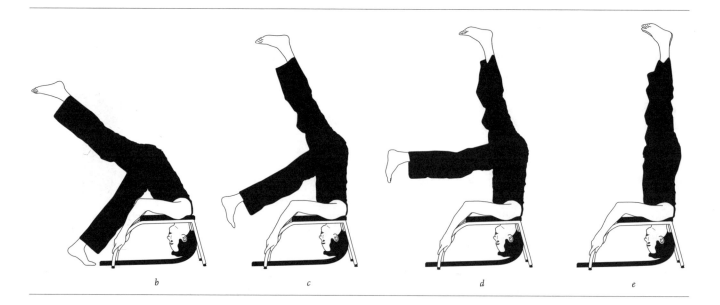

b   c   d   e

all the choices we have about how to interpret a movement or pose, only *one* method really works: relaxation.

Solution

Practice close to a wall while keeping the mental image of the movement in your mind's eye. Visualize the image of movement into your back before jumping; that is, try to imagine the feeling of the movement and exactly where it will take place.

This exercise can have a big impact and should not be underestimated. Admittedly, I have suggested that it is all about the relatively simple problem of fear of falling. In truth, more is involved. I am talking about the psychological and social causes that have led to the stiffening of your upper back. There are strong indications that emotions such as grief, anger, and frustration, as well as such issues as stress—all of which have a social cause—make an important contribution to tension and stiffness in the upper back (see chapters 2 and 3).

It is not the objective of Critical Alignment to analyze what these causes are (see chapters 3 and 4). Critical Alignment confronts the tension directly in order to restore mobility. During this process, however, it is possible that strong emotions associated with the stiffening of your upper back may be released, and you must experience them. They are a part of you. It is only by allowing relaxation to take over, that you take away their ability to control your movements. It is a way of purifying yourself.

After some time, you will notice improvements as you do this asana. These improvements are initially small and difficult to see. Only an experienced eye will be able to see the changes taking place.

Sirsasana variations

2. Parsva Sirsasana on the headstand bench

Parsva means "side"; in this variation we rotate to the sides, hence the translation Rotated Headstand.
In this variation, you turn from left to right on the headstand bench. Because your upper back is extended and rotated in this exercise, it is useful for increasing the mobility of your spine.

Rotations are all about the transfer of movement from one vertebra to the next. This transfer makes the rotation uniform, and uniformity requires mobility and balance. (This will be discussed further in chapter 12; see also the coordination exercise in chapter 12.2.)

When the vertebrae are stacked correctly, the lumbar vertebrae are not designed to rotate because of the angle of their facet joints (see the arrows in figure 8.2-20). The angles of the facet joints in the thoracic vertebrae (see the arrows in figure 8.2-21) and the

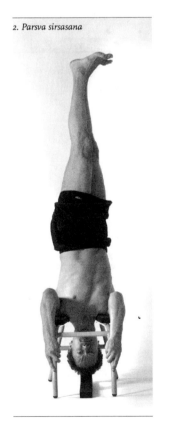

2. Parsva sirsasana

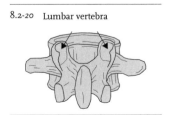

8.2-20   Lumbar vertebra

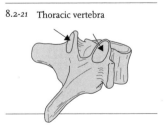

8.2-21   Thoracic vertebra

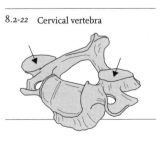

8.2-22   Cervical vertebra

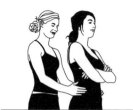 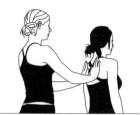 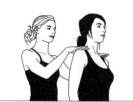

cervical vertebrae (see the arrows in figure 8.2-22) make rotations possible in these sections of the spine. The areas of these different joint clusters are illustrated by the teacher's hands in figure 8.2-23, which highlights the lumbar vertebrae; figure 8.2-24, which highlights the thoracic vertebrae; and figure 8.2-25, which shows the cervical vertebrae.

If the lower back is straight when sitting or standing, it allows the postural muscles to align and stabilize the upper back. Without a good foundation (the lower back), the upper back will collapse, or the movement muscles will take over to "pull" the back straight. When the movement muscles contract, it is at the expense of the freedom of the upper back and will obstruct the ease of rotation. During inversions like Sirsasana, the opposite is true; the upper back becomes the foundation for the lower back.

In Parsva Sirsasana, the lower back must be erect in order to transfer the rotation that has been initiated from the pelvis. The lower back can obstruct the movement if it is too concave (figure 8.2-26) or too convex (figure 8.2-27). The coordination exercise on the roll, described in chapter 12.2, demonstrates the correct rotation and is a good preparatory exercise.

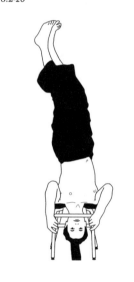

Instructions

- After standing for a few minutes in Sirsasana on the headstand bench, determine whether your upper back is straight and your balance light and mobile. Slowly turn your pelvis to the right, without disturbing your balance. Stay in this position for 30 seconds.

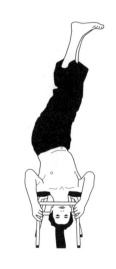

- Rotation on the headstand bench improves the mobility of the area below your shoulder blades. That transfer of movement happens in the previously mentioned coordination exercise, but in this asana, the movement develops even more and toward the neck. It enters the higher thoracic spine up to T1, T2, and T3. When your spine becomes straighter, this rotation develops pressure on the sides of your spine, against your ribs. When you rotate your pelvis to the right, the left side of your spine—just between the vertebrae and your left shoulder blade—receives the pressure and starts to straighten out more. Use this movement to release more tension in your left shoulder.
- Keeping the area on the left side of your spine straight, pull with your left hand and slowly turn back to center. Breathe in and out a few times, then repeat the rotation to the left.

Note: Your weight should not fall forward (toward your hands and collarbones) during the rotation. Keep it on the back of both shoulders.

If you can maintain your balance, you can gradually increase the speed of the movement. Remain in the end pose for a few seconds before turning to the other side. Ultimately, this can become a fluid movement to the left and right, without stopping. Keep your weight off your hands.

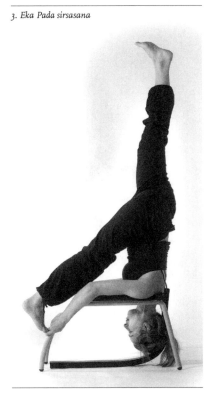

3. Eka Pada sirsasana

3. Eka Pada Sirsasana on the headstand bench

Eka means "one"; *pada* means "foot," because the pose involves putting one foot down to the floor while in sirsasana.

In this variation, one leg is lowered while the other remains extended and aligned with the back. During this exercise, it is important to remember the difference between using your upper lower back through the use of the quadratus lumborum muscles at the sides of your lower back and stabilizing the complete arch of your lower back with its postural muscles situated in the center line (see also chapter 6.3, connections 7 and 9). While lowering one leg, the arch of your lower back must remain strong. Maintaining this extension, you need to control the gradual bend in your lower back, which is the job of the elevated leg. Your pelvis moves slightly with the lowering leg, but the elevated leg prevents a loss of alignment in the spine.

Instructions

Read "Stretching the upper part of the lower back," in chapter 6.3, connection 7.

- After standing in Sirsasana on the headstand bench for a few minutes, rotate your legs inward and stretch your knees. Pull lightly on the legs of the headstand bench to prevent your upper back from bending.
- Keep your left leg in place and slowly lower your stretched right leg. The lowered leg often bends so that the knee leads and not the foot; allow your foot to lead the movement. During this first stage, the arch of your lower back remains straight. At the same time, you will feel an end to the movement of the leg that you are lowering. The stretch to the hamstrings produces the end movement.

> **Note:** When you are lying on the rubber strip (see chapter 6.3, connection 8), the movement stops because your pelvis remains in contact with the floor. In Eka Pada Sirsasana, your pelvis can move farther.

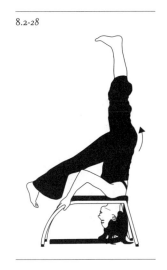

8.2-28

- Keep your left leg in the exact same position and move your right leg a bit further in order to release the quadratus lumborum. This will create space in the pelvic area of your lower back. Keep your left leg in line with your spine; this helps you keep your lower back in a stable bend position. Your pelvis tilts slightly backward (figure 8.2-28).
- Remain in this position and breathe regularly for 10 to 30 seconds.

> **Note:** Keep your right leg precisely in front of your right shoulder. A lot of incorrect rotations develop during this pose, the most common being where the extended (left) leg rotates out, pulling the right foot toward the left shoulder.

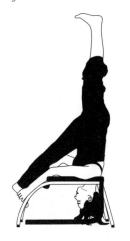

The neck often shortens in the end position. To prevent this, stretch your neck out along the rubber strip before you initially lift your leg. It is important to learn this now, as it will make it easier to do traditional Sirsasana, in which your head is on the ground with your neck supporting your weight.

· Repeat the pose on the other side.

During this variation, extra pressure builds at the back of the shoulders. Try to accept this pressure and notice whether your shoulders are relaxed at the end of the exercise.

Variation

When you feel confident enough in this pose and have developed enough length in your hamstrings, you can intensify the position by pulling your foot farther down with your hand (figure 8.2-29). Be careful to keep the extended leg in position. This pose is an interaction between pulling with your hand, stretching your leg, stretching your lower back, and relaxing your hamstrings and hips.

4. Parsvaika Pada Sirsasana on the headstand bench

Parsva means "side"; *pada* means "foot," because it involves lowering one leg to the side during a headstand.

In this variation, one leg is lowered laterally (to the side). This asana can be done after Eka Pada Sirsasana.

Instructions

· From Sirsasana, turn your right foot laterally and lower your right leg.

Note: Be careful to distribute your weight evenly on both shoulders when lowering your leg; do *not* end up with more weight on one shoulder. See the differences in figure 8.2-30a (which shows equal pressure on both shoulders) and figure 8.2-30b (which shows too much weight on the right shoulder). The tilted pelvis prevents the left side of the lower back from supporting the position. To avoid the distorted position of figure 8.2-30b, you must strongly activate the muscles on the left side of your pelvis. Compare this position with Trikonasana (see chapter 9.3, numbers 8 and 9) and Ardha Chandrasana (see chapter 9.4, number 12).

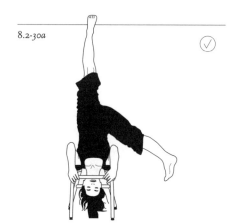

8.2-30a

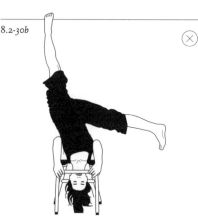

8.2-30b

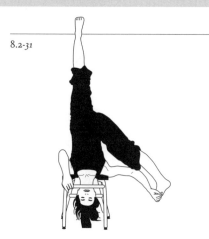

8.2-31

- Remain in the end position for 10 to 30 seconds, then repeat the movement to the other side.
- If you can hold your foot with your hand, do the variation as in the previous exercise (see figure 8.2-31).

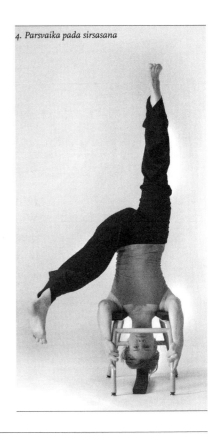

4. Parsvaika pada sirsasana

5. Urdhva Dandasana on the headstand bench

Urdhva means "above"; *danda* means "stick." Hence, the name **Inverted Staff Pose.**
By keeping your back, especially your lower back, well extended, your upper body will not move backward. It will remain totally straight and in balance with the wall behind you.

Instructions

- Do this variation after spending some time in Sirsasana on the headstand bench. If you are doing the entire cycle of variations, do them in the order given here.
- Make sure that your lower back is erect and that your inner tube is activated, connecting your lower ribs with the arch of your lower back. Stretch and rotate your legs inward. Lower both legs to a 90-degree angle.
- As the pressure to the back of your shoulders increases, use it to release deep layers of tension in your shoulders.
- Lengthen your neck as much as possible.
- Remain in this end position and breathe regularly for 10 to 60 seconds.
- Make sure to extend your neck before starting to lift your legs, and use your hands to fix your shoulder blades firmly against your ribs. Keep your inner tube active throughout the entire movement, relaxing the front of your hips at the end.
- You can repeat this movement three to five times.
- Instead of remaining static in the end position, you can also "rebound," in which you drop into the end position and your legs immediately bounce back up. Your hamstrings create the end of the movement. If you do not feel an end movement, you have bent your lower back too much. You can repeat this ten times.

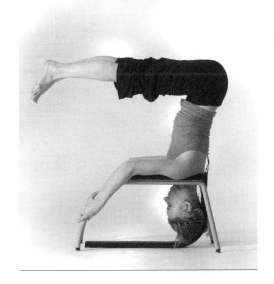

5. Urdhva dandasana

Variation

You can also alternate this with the following variation:

- Lower your feet to the floor, keeping your back as straight as possible (figure 8.2-32). Maintain the strength in your back and immediately lift your legs back to vertical. If you have kept the strength in your bent back, you will be able to lift your legs; if you have lost this strength, you will not be able to get back to vertical. If this happens, lower your legs a little less the next time. This movement is similar to that of lifting your legs into Halasana (see chapter 8.3, number 14).
- Repeat this movement three to five times.

8.2-32

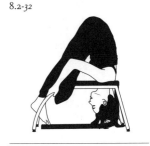

Note: Here, too, stretch your neck before lifting your legs. This exercise strengthens your lower back and the coordination between the lower back–hips–legs connections (see chapter 6.3, connection 7). It develops your inner tube and gives your shoulders a strong, extra stimulus to relax.

6. Jatukasana on the headstand bench

Jatuka means "bat"; hence the name Bat Pose.
While standing in Sirsasana on the headstand bench, try to mobilize your upper back by blocking movement in your neck. The coordination for this movement is best learned in the following exercise and looks like a bat hanging from the ceiling. You can learn the asana in two movements.

Instructions

- After standing in Sirsasana on the headstand bench for some time, slowly lessen your grip on the legs of the bench. See if your body can take over the balance without losing the extension in your neck. Keep pushing the back of your head against the rubber strip, but keep this pressure minimal.
- When you have found your balance, lay your arms on top of each other on the headstand bench (figure 8.2-33). Try to carry your weight on your shoulders.
- When you have succeeded in this, you can place your arms, one at a time, against the sides of your legs (figure 8.2-34). If you feel that you are about to lose your balance, do not try to recover by contracting your neck muscles: allow your back to recover the balance. Lengthen your neck and remain stable there. The pressure of the back of your head against the rubber strip should remain constant.
- Stay in this end position for 10 to 60 seconds or longer.

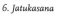

6. Jatukasana

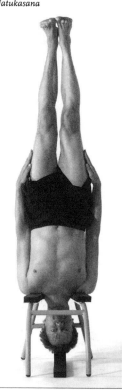

8.2-33

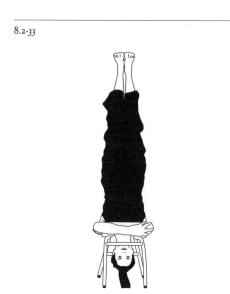

8.2-34

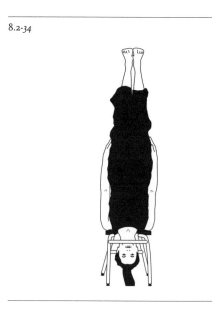

7. Salamba Sirsasana I

Salamba means "with support"; *sirsa* means "head."

The biggest difference between Sirsasana on the headstand bench and Salamba Sirsasana is that the postural muscles of your neck must develop enough strength to carry your body weight through the extended position of your neck. Your shoulders must develop the strength necessary to support your body actively in the same way as on the headstand bench.

Otherwise, all of the previous instructions relating to Sirsasana on the headstand bench apply to this asana. The support comes from the arms and shoulders.

Personally, Sirsasana has become a part of my life. Initially, I practiced irregularly and no longer than 5 minutes at time. Now I do this pose daily for 20 minutes, but I have also had periods in my life when sessions lasted up to an hour and a half.

A personal story

I was eighteen when I started to practice Sirsasana. At first, I did it sporadically and only when I felt like it. I did the same with all the other asanas in my practice. It was only later, after reading that you should practice regularly (even when you don't feel like it) that I developed more consistency. At that age, in my late teens, I was strongly influenced by my emotions, and I was regularly confronted with confusing feelings during the exercises. My practice was influenced by this, and instead of becoming calmer when practicing, I felt more like I was fueling negativity and insecurity.

During this period, my neck began to hurt during Sirsasana, and the accompanying uncertainty disturbed me even more. Occasionally, as if by accident, I could stand in the pose with no problems, and I held on to those moments. Later, I began to focus on the technique of the exercises, so I could try to ease the physical pain. This helped, as it gave me something to concentrate on so I could start to distance myself from my feelings. I tried all sorts of adjustments to relieve my neck pain. After a while, the uncertainty about how long I was standing became a source of disquiet. A kitchen timer provided the solution to that; I could finally see how long I was standing. It was often not as long as I thought; there were actually huge differences in time. Sometimes I could stand easily for twelve minutes, but the following day, I had to come down after only two minutes because of the pain in my neck. The enthusiasm of one day became a source of tension for the next—evidently enthusiasm is also related to muscle tension.

Then I started to "neutralize" my feelings and recollect previous sessions. I made myself think about the technique *before* lifting my legs instead of adjusting once I was up. That helped. My movements became quieter, and my attention stabilized. I became conscious of the fact that focusing on technique could reverse my moods and that the feelings generated through Sirsasana were becoming increasingly pleasant. I tried to commit to memory the feelings I had at the end of the pose. If it went well, I felt alert and would try to recall that feeling at the start of my next session.

By consciously recalling that experience, I could detach from my normal everyday feelings, and I began to experience a change in my emotions as a whole. The positive feelings generated by Sirsasana began to linger. At first, I retained them only for a short time directly after practicing, then eventually I could hang onto them for longer periods. The stress lessened and the pleasure increased; practicing became less of a chore. Then I

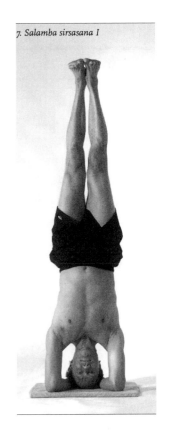

7. Salamba sirsasana I

started to work out more aspects of the pose, like the use of breathing, perfecting balance, the order in which corrections should be done, and so on. For me, this asana has become a never-ending practice and is never tedious. I once heard someone say that she watched television during Sirsasana because those twenty minutes were so boring. I cannot imagine that: for me, the pose has always had a "laboratory function." Many new concepts have been developed for me while I practice it.

The emotions and feelings I experienced during Sirsasana corresponded with the events of my life. For instance, you can feel unhappy or angry when your practice does not go as you plan or want. However, with the passing years, I realized that such reactions are counterproductive and certainly do not add anything positive to the overall practice. Because of this, I became increasingly detached from the results of my practice, and it was only when I felt better that I tried to analyze why that was.

I began to see more and more correlations with processes that took place during my daily life but occurred over a much longer period than the processes I experienced during headstand. However, this recognition made them more manageable. Understanding Sirsasana gave me more balance in my daily life. If life could be described as prose, then Sirsasana would be poetry. I once had a discussion with a friend who was studying medicine, and he told me about the fluctuations in concentration he experienced when studying for periods of ten to twelve hours. It was identical to what I had experienced during twenty minutes of Sirsasana. Now, the pose has become a meditation for me. There, I experience lightness, space, and pleasure. That's what it's all about.

✐ Key points

1. The support that your upper arms give your shoulder blades is extremely important for supporting your neck (see chapter 6.3, connection 4 for more information). The correct connection depends on the shape of your back. If your upper back is bent, it would be sensible to start with Sirsasana on the headstand bench and to practice Salamba Sirsasana afterward. This way, your shoulders and back are "preformed."

2. Do not be hasty when increasing your time. It is much better to practice regularly and have shorter sessions than to push yourself too far too quickly. The preceding personal story covered a period of many years. Timing your pose is pleasant and worthwhile, because through timing you are able to measure what you have done.

3. If you are plagued by recurring problems, seek the advice of a teacher (preferably one who works with the Critical Alignment method).

4. Use a wall for support when you begin to practice until you can stand for 5 to 10 minutes. This will help you stay calm and give your neck time to become stronger. When you can stand for 5 to 10 minutes, start to practice without the wall. If you are afraid of falling to the side, practice in a corner (figure 8.2-35).

5. Do not see Sirsasana as a trick; it is a symbol of yoga. Make a ritual of placing your mat and gathering your thoughts.

6. Think before you act! Contemplate the movement before you jump up, and do not forget your intentions when you start moving. One good intention—for example, "I will keep my neck relaxed and extended"—is more important that fifteen separate

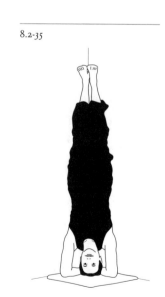

8.2-35

instructions. Use the knowledge you are developing to make choices relevant to you. When you keep your focus on one point, it becomes possible to see if your point of attention is successfully maintained during the entire session. When your attention wanders, try to discover why that happened. This is your learning process.

The feeling of lightness you can experience in Sirsasana is mostly dependent on the connection between your upper arms and shoulder blades. I will now discuss this connection for a seated position in which your neck is unburdened. You can then practice this connection actively during Sirsasana.

The connection of the upper arms with the shoulder blades

Instructions

· Sit on a chair and fold your hands so that a tennis ball can fit between them (figure 8.2-36). Lift your arms to shoulder-height and bend your elbows so your arms form a right angle.
· Keep your elbows shoulder-width apart and raise them above your head (figure 8.2-37). Push your hands as far as possible away from your head. This will pull your upper arms into your shoulder blades.

> **Note:** Moving your elbows out to the side will contract the muscles in your shoulder girdle (figure 8.2-38) and obstruct the transfer of movement in your back. Then your shoulders will retain the movement of your arms, preventing the movement from reaching your shoulder blades. This often occurs during Sirsasana and is a major source of neck pain and overload.

· If you push your little fingers farther away than your thumbs (see the arrow in figure 8.2-37), then your elbows will be pulled more securely toward your shoulder blades. Your shoulders are low, and the base of your chest and diaphragm should feel relaxed. This allows you to breathe without restriction from your stomach to your chest (see chapter 6.3, connection 8).
· Allow your upper arms to sink deeper into your back. Extend your neck and place the back of your head lightly against the base of your palms (figure 8.2-39).

8.2-36

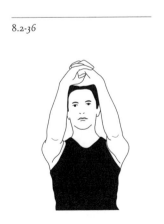

8.2-37

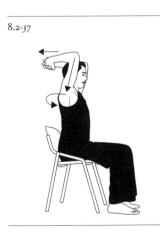

8.2-38

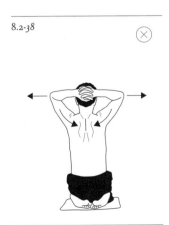

8.2-39

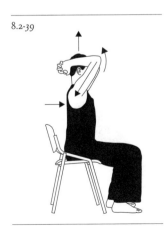

- Keep your shoulder blades and upper arms actively low, and push your elbows slightly higher. This is the final movement that ensures your shoulder blades keep pushing your ribs and chest forward.
- Stay in this position for as long as you can; keep your breathing deep and relaxed. This will soon become taxing for your upper arms, but this is exactly the strength you need to support yourself in Sirsasana.

Jumping up with one leg

Preparation

It is best to use a sticky yoga mat for this exercise, with a firm blanket underneath for comfort. I use a felt mat that I have designed specifically for this purpose. It is a firm, soft material and very durable. Place your mat against the wall and kneel on it.

Instructions

- Place your fingers on your shoulders and your elbows on the floor directly under your shoulders.
- Fold your hands and place them on the floor an inch from the wall. Once again, keep enough space between your hands for a tennis ball (figure 8.2-40).
- Push your wrists against the floor. This helps you to make the connection between your upper arms and your shoulder blades.

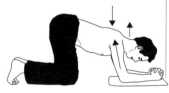

- Connect your arms with your shoulder blades by allowing your upper back to sink deeper between your shoulder blades. This creates the relaxation that is necessary for movement. Walk in a little with your feet and stretch your legs (figure 8.2-41). Be careful not to bend your back when you stretch your legs.
- Placing your head on the floor is the most difficult part of the movement. If you keep the extension in your back, your head will be just above the floor (see figure 8.2-41).

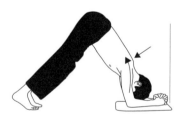

- Actively lower your shoulders. When you place your head on the floor (moving from figure 8.2-41 to 8.2-42), feel that your arms connect with your shoulder blades and thus slide deeper into your back. Feel the contact between the back of your head and the base of your hands (the juncture between wrist and hand—your palms and fingers do not touch your head) and do not walk any closer (see figure 8.2-42). You will now be carrying a lot of weight on your arms, which allows you to keep your neck relaxed.

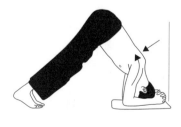

8.2-40

8.2-41

8.2-42

- Extend your neck by releasing its movement muscles and actively push the crown of your head into the floor. The pressure toward the floor can be exerted by the postural muscles of your neck. This downward pressure creates an upward movement toward the spine above your neck. This creates a proper support for your upper back.
- Move one foot closer; keep your upper back straight and your upper arms well connected with your shoulder blades. Swing one leg up; the other will follow. The upward strength of your upper arms and the extension of your neck receive the movement. Place your feet against the wall (figure 8.2-43).

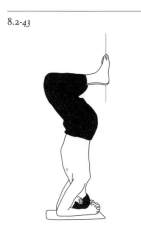

Note: To help your neck relax, you can initially carry more weight on your forearms than on your crown. When you have placed your feet against the wall, maintain the strength in your arms and the connection with your shoulder blades. At the same time, feel your weight being transferred slowly from your lower arms to your crown. During this transfer, your neck should remain relaxed and extended, allowing its postural muscles to carry your weight, although the vertebrae of the neck will also receive increasingly more weight.

You now have a foundation that is comparable to that on the headstand bench: your arms push your ribs forward via your shoulder blades, and your neck controls your midline. When your foundation gets straighter and stronger, you can gradually increase the amount of weight you carry on your crown. This was described in Sirsasana on the headstand bench (see page 146) and requires the correct placement of your lower ribs. This movement straightens your upper back.

Note: You can assist your shoulders by elevating your elbows slightly. Special wooden planks have been developed for this, but a firm mat (as shown in figure 8.2-44) or an extra blanket that is about ½ inch thick will do as well. Practice this variation close to the wall, as the extra height of your shoulders will make the position feel unsteady at first.

☞ Key points after the jump

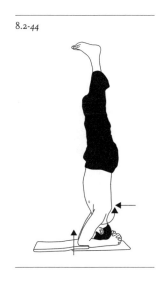

1. Once in Sirsasana, check that your elbows have remained in the same position; one or both will often move laterally. This happens when the muscles of your shoulder girdle contract during the jump (see figure 8.2-38). If this happens, you can correct yourself by shifting your elbow(s) in toward your head, but it would be better to come back down and try to come up again without tension in your shoulder girdle.
2. When you are standing with your weight on the crown of your head, push your crown directly into the floor without moving it forward or backward. The part of your head that is touching the floor is its highest point. In Sirsasana, the back of your head should not move toward your neck, and your forehead should not move toward the floor. Do not extend your neck so much that it becomes convex. This will cause tension and pressure in your throat. To identify the exact point of balance on your head, stand as straight as you can with your back against a wall and place a book on your

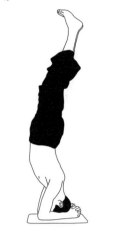

head. (See chapter 6.3, connection 3, for a detailed description of how to position your neck and head.)

3. Keeping your shoulders high will initially push your lower ribs forward, creating tension in your middle and lower back (figure 8.2-45). You can correct this by moving your pelvis and ribs backward a little to relieve the pressure on your lower back. But remember that the position of your chest and pelvis is always the result of your jump. Your posture improves when your body can make the connections that lead to relaxation. This applies to the practice of all asanas. The coordination required for the different movements develops gradually and is a slow process. After jumping up, you should not be thinking, "I must straighten my back, pull my shoulders up, straighten my neck, just do this, just do that." If you have jumped up with attention, you will already be in your best position. After that, you should not move at all, because every movement will disturb your position. The adjustments that occur in Sirsasana are small and subtle and are done through breathing. Do not try to correct your position constantly; try to develop a greater feeling of space in your present position—not by losing your structure but by relaxing within that structure. Maintaining your structure, not allowing your shoulders to sag, or not losing your inner tube, and so on develops strength. This is an improvement.

Standing without the support of a wall

Do not be in a hurry to stand without the support of a wall. Just remember that your body should not be leaning against the wall. The necessary support should be provided by bending your knees; only your feet should touch the wall. Remain standing in this position for 5 to 10 minutes before straightening your legs; this develops the correct strength in your arms and neck. Other corrections, like the accurate extension in your lower back, will be discussed later. It is important to create a stable foundation first. You should, however, ensure that your lower back does not hold on to the movement of your pelvis. Move your pelvis back toward the wall by releasing the quadratus lumborum muscles so you can feel your lower back (partially) transfer movement through the midline of your spine to your upper back. The extension of your upper back determines how deeply the movement will penetrate the area between your shoulder blades. When your spine is straight, it will be able to transport your body weight vertebra by vertebra until it reaches your neck.

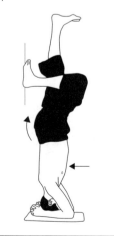

Instructions

· Take one foot off the wall and stretch that leg parallel to the wall, as shown in figure 8.2-46. When you are in balance, extend your other leg. The position of your legs is initiated from your thighs and not your feet. Your thighs are connected to your shoulder blades; they "stand" stacked on top of your shoulder blades.

· When you stretch your legs, you lift your back into extension. This only works if the movement is powered from inside. Begin by moving your lower ribs backward. Then use your stomach muscles to extend your lower back toward your tailbone and end by straightening your legs (see the arrows in figure 8.2-46).

· The position of your legs helps your pelvis relax. By turning your thighs inward, your pelvis can broaden around your sacrum. Push your knees together and position your ankles and feet as if you were standing on them.

Note: Tension often develops in the lower back when standing (this also applies to standing in inversions), and one side is frequently tighter than the other. Rotating your legs inward can help your lower back relax. But this will only be effective if you realize beforehand why you are turning your legs and where the relaxation should occur. When you have this image in your mind's eye, rotate your legs and consciously allow your lower back to relax. It is possible to turn your legs inward and still hold on to the tension in your lower back. Remember that relaxation must always be coupled with awareness. It does not happen automatically.

· When you start to practice Sirsasana without the support of a wall, your balance often changes dramatically, making you feel that you have to start all over again. This is due to carrying more weight on your elbows than your head. If you notice this happening, gradually transfer more weight to your crown without contracting the muscles in your neck and shoulders. Keep your shoulders high and your neck lengthened. The moment that your crown carries your weight, it will feel as if all the weight is off your elbows. Do *not* panic when this happens; you will fall. (When your body is correctly aligned standing on the headstand bench, it can feel as if you are going to fall, but that is exactly the point where you want to be.) From this alignment, actively stretch your lower arms and elbows as you did in the seated preparatory exercise described earlier. Then your shoulder blades will press strongly against your ribs, providing support to your back and creating space in your chest.

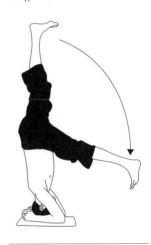

8.2-47

Note: Learning to balance on the exact point of your head is the first step. After accomplishing this "weightless" state, the next step is to develop the correct movement in your arms, shoulders, and neck. At this stage, there is a distinct difference between strain and strength. Although strain gives a certain feeling of control to the pose, it blocks rather than stimulates free movement in your body. This occurs when you carry excessive body weight on your elbows. When you press your elbows down without losing the weightless state in your balance, it develops strength in your arms and shoulders that stimulates the free movement toward your shoulder blades and spine. This movement is not controlled. It is the result of an open state of mind. Be sure to breathe freely.

8.2-48

· Remain standing for as long as you feel comfortable. This can be anywhere from a few minutes to 20 minutes. If your neck starts to hurt, do not come down immediately; try to correct yourself and find out why it is hurting. If that does not work, come down.
· Come down one leg at a time to start with, as seen in figure 8.2-47. Do not lift your head immediately; wait until the pressure there has normalized. If you stand up too quickly, you may become dizzy.
· When you have practiced Sirsasana for some time, you can come down with both legs together. Try to maintain the extension in your lower back as long as possible; otherwise, your neck will collapse (see the arrows in figure 8.2-48).

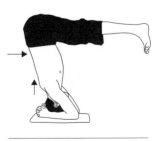

Note: When you lower both legs together, the last part of the movement almost always ends with a drop. This is caused by too much tension in the quadratus lumborum muscles of your lower back. To create a smooth movement, you must steadily bend your lower back from the strength in the midline of the arch. This will allow your pelvis to tilt backward with control. Lower your legs gradually during exhalations. Keep your shoulders elevated and maintain the length in your neck. Practicing asanas that are specifically aimed at increasing the flexibility of your hips and legs (see chapters 9 and 10) will make this movement easier. If you can come back down with broad shoulders and a relaxed neck, then you can also go up with both legs together.

Lifting both legs together

Do not be in a hurry to practice this version. Many people can lift their legs together with ease, but it is very difficult to maintain the connection between the upper arms and shoulder blades and to retain the upward strength that the neck must pass on to the spine. And it is exactly the smooth transfer of these connections that determines your end pose. For this reason, only attempt going up with both legs together when you are confident of your ability.

Instructions

8.2-49

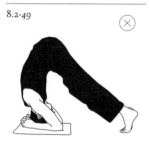

8.2-50

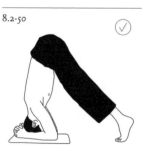

- Follow the earlier instructions for jumping up with one leg, up to the point that your head touches the ground.
- Extend your lower back as much as possible and walk in with both legs, getting your feet as close as you can. If your lower back does not push your pelvis higher, your weight will be pushed into your shoulders and neck, as seen in figure 8.2-49. If your lower back is in a position to coordinate the correct movement, then your shoulders and neck will be spared from trying to support too much body weight and able to maintain their upward strength (see figure 8.2-50).
- Initiating movement from the muscles that connect your pelvis and lower back, lift your legs and pull them halfway in, as shown in figure 8.2-51a. Do not lift your legs all

8.2-51a–e

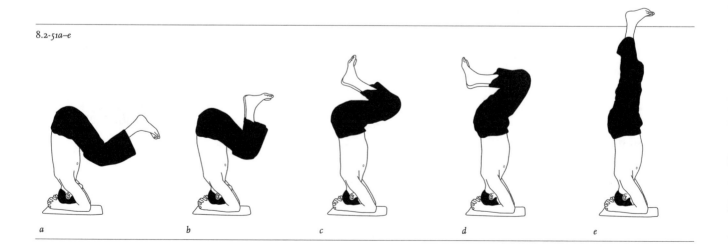

a   *b*   *c*   *d*   *e*

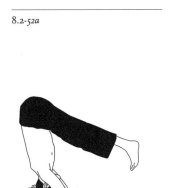

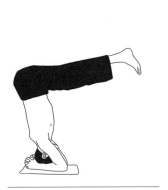

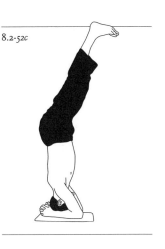

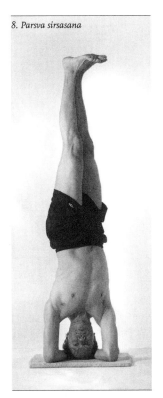

8. *Parsva sirsasana*

the way up; first, establish the correct balance on the crown of your head. From that balance, extend your neck and push your upper arms and shoulder blades high. Now lift your legs higher, but remember that your neck and shoulders should move faster than your legs! Follow the movements in figures 8.2-51b through 8.2-51e.

· When you can lift your legs easily, you can try doing the same thing with straight legs, as shown in figures 8.2-52a through 8.2-52c. End this movement with your legs directly above your back.

Variations in Sirsasana

8. Parsva Sirsasana

Parsva means "side."

Instructions

· Read the instructions written for Parsva Sirsasana on the headstand bench (see page 151).

· Stand for some time in Sirsasana. Make sure you keep both of your shoulders high. When rotating to the right, pay particular attention to your right shoulder: it must remain stable and not rotate with the movement. Keep your breathing steady as you turn your pelvis to the right. Allow the movement of the rotation to continue as far as possible into your upper back.

· Stay in this position for 30 seconds, turn back to center, and find the exact alignment where you can balance on your head without tension. Repeat the movement to the left.

9. Eka Pada Sirsasana

Eka means "one"; *pada* means "foot."

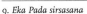

9. *Eka Pada sirsasana*

Instructions

· Read the instructions written for Eka Pada Sirsasana on the headstand bench (see page 153).

· Keep both legs straight and lower your right leg, allowing your toes to touch the floor. Do not allow your left leg to move forward during this movement.

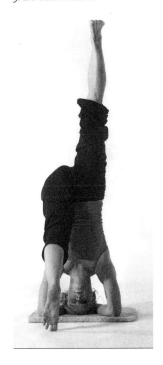

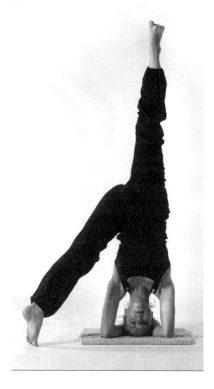

10. Parsvaika pada sirsasana

- Your neck will receive extra weight in the beginning, because your shoulders will not be able to absorb the extra movement adequately. This also occurs on the headstand bench when the backs of your shoulders receive extra weight. Keep this in mind before lowering your leg, and actively lift your shoulders. This is a good exercise to prepare for lifting both legs up into Sirsasana. Your shoulders and neck become stronger in this variation, and even though they collapse a little, they should not lose their upward strength.
- When your hamstrings become more flexible, this position will become easier. Thus, even if your foot does not touch the ground, be content. If you allow your body to move forward so your toes can reach the ground, you will lose the integrity of the asana.
- Remain in this position for 20 to 30 seconds. Extend your neck and shoulders before lifting your leg.
- Remain for some time in Salamba Sirsasana to recover your balance. Repeat to the other side.

10. Parsvaika Pada Sirsasana

Parsva means "side"; *eka* means "one"; *pada* means "foot."
Do this variation after Eka Pada Sirsasana. Here, the leg is lowered out to the side.

Instructions

- Read the instructions for Parsvaika Pada Sirsasana on the headstand bench (see page 154).
- Keep both legs straight and rotate your right foot outward. Keep your right shoulder very firm and high, as it will receive an extra load during the movement of your leg. Slowly lower your right leg to the side, allowing your toes to touch the ground.
- Keep your left leg firmly in line with your back.
- Remain in this position for 20 to 30 seconds before slowly lifting your leg back up.
- Remain for some time in Salamba Sirsasana, then repeat the movement on the other side.

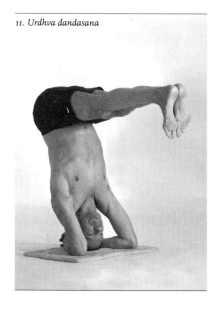

11. Urdhva dandasana

11. Urdhva Dandasana

Urdhva means "up"; *danda* means "stick."

Instructions

- Read the instructions for Urdhva Dandasana on the headstand bench (see page 155).
- Stand in Sirsasana for some time, then straighten your legs and rotate them inward. Lower them halfway to the ground.
- If the variation with straight legs (figures 8.2-53a and 8.2-53b) is too difficult, bend your knees as shown in figure 8.2-54, or do not lower your legs as far.

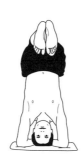

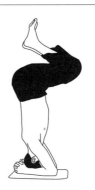

- If your shoulders are not well prepared, this variation will exert pressure on your neck. Urdhva Dandasana is a demanding position. Therefore, take your time and build up to the end pose slowly. Your Sirsasana will become lighter with the strength that you acquire here. This variation also helps you build the strength required to lift both legs together into Sirsasana.

In the lesson plans (chapter 14), the variations following Parsva Sirsasana are called the Sirsasana series.

12. Salamba Sirsasana II

The palms of the hands are placed on the floor under the edge of the headstand mat, directly under the elbows, one shoulder-width apart. Thus, the direct support of the shoulders is gone, and the neck must become more active in its support. Practice this variation only when you can complete Salamba Sirsasana I (page 157) without any problems in your neck. (This variation can also be found in chapter 11, with the balancing asanas.)

Instructions

- Lay a felt mat on top of your yoga mat and slide your hands halfway under the front edge. Place your head on the mat so that it forms a triangle with your hands; extend your neck.
- Elevate your shoulders and connect your arms to your shoulder blades. Walk in and extend your lower back as much as possible so that you feel a strong connection between the extension of your neck and your lower back. It should feel as if your back forms a line that you can stretch right to your sit bones (see figure 8.2-55).
- Lift your legs, one at a time, maintaining the extension in your neck. End with your feet together.

  Or

- Lift both legs together without straining your neck. Your neck may bend slightly during this movement, but through the activity of your neck's postural muscles, you can still push with your crown so that your neck extends as soon as your legs leave the floor. Here, too, you need to effect the movement of your neck before the full movement of your legs.

12. Salamba sirsasana II

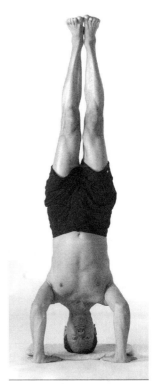

8.2-55

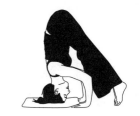

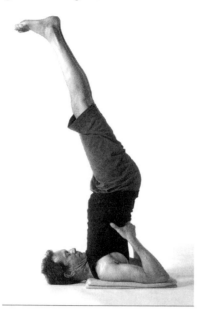

13. Salamba sarvangasana

- Slowly transfer your weight from your hands to your neck. It will now become obvious how demanding it is to carry your weight there. Remember that in Salamba Sirsasana I, your crown carries the same amount of weight.
- Remain in this position for 1 minute. Come back down with your legs straight, either one leg at a time or both together.

8.3 Inversions with a flexed neck

These asanas increase the relaxation of the movement muscles in the back and the strength of the postural muscles around the spine. Salamba Sarvangasana with its variations and Halasana belong to this subgroup.

13. *Salamba Sarvangasana*

Salamba **means "with the support of";** *sarvanga* **means "all parts of the body."**
In Sarvangasana, we attempt to maintain stability through the deeper postural muscles, but the manner in which we achieve this deviates from the Critical Alignment concept of relaxation, movement, and strength and coordination (see chapter 2.4.1). There are no rules without exceptions. In Sarvangasana, we strengthen the superficial movement muscles in such a way that they increasingly "draw" the strength into the midline of the body. We finally reach an end position where the relaxation of the movement muscles can intensify and the postural muscles along the spine can become increasingly active. This makes the back strong and straight.

This strength is essential for a straight back in daily life. Yoga makes this possible, but it is a slow process to develop a straight back from a stiff and/or bent one. During the change process, stability is essential. This is one of the important functions of Sarvangasana: while other asanas relax and mobilize the lower back, it provides stability.

According to Critical Alignment, the lower back is the center of strength. If the lower back is straight and strong, the rest of the body will benefit, allowing us to experience more openness and relaxation. But what do we do if we have not reached this place? Practice Sarvangasana.

The importance of a strong lower back

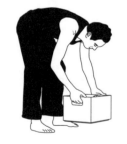

8.3-1

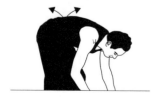

8.3-2

Imagine a person with disc problems in the lower back that have resulted from constantly loading the back in preferred habitual positions (figure 8.3-1). Instead of keeping his back compact and stable when lifting heavy objects, he increases the bend in his back at the precise moment that he applies strength for the lift (figure 8.3-2). His stomach muscles actually push his back outward. This is a risky movement. Lumbago and certain forms of spinal disc herniation can arise from such an instable position. Many exercises, such as lying on the lower back roll and backbends, allow the lower back to move the other way. These exercises all have excellent results for recovering the mobility of the vertebrae, but they do not build up the strength necessary to change habitual postures.

Let us assume that the person in figure 8.3-1 has long, stiff lower back muscles that prevent him from keeping his lower back in an adequate natural arch. Lying on the lower back roll is a good passive exercise to allow the back to relax and extend. But in daily life, it is important that the lower back muscles become *shorter* and *stronger* and that the intervertebral discs be brought into a position where they can absorb and transfer the pressure of body weight.

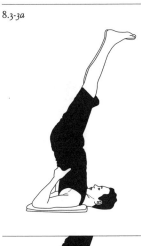

According to Critical Alignment, the person in question must practice as shown in figure 8.3-3a to achieve the required turnaround in form and strength. The position of the legs is essential in this pose. They place the pelvis in the correct position to load the lower back. At the same time, the angle of the legs acts as a lever, pulling the lower vertebrae up so the discs can return to a balanced position (see the arrows in figure 8.3-3b).

The big advantage of Sarvangasana is that it lets you isolate the movement of the lower back easily in order to build up strength, because the neck and the base of the sternum are kept stable. The body frequently compensates in these two areas. For example, the forward shifting of the lower ribs during Sirsasana will cause the lower back to lose its proper alignment and strength. Because this is not possible during Sarvangasana and the lower back muscles must work hard when positioned correctly, this is quickly experienced as a fiery band across the breadth of the lower back (caused by the increase of strength in the movement muscles) that is difficult to endure. But as always when developing strength, if you practice consistently, you will improve slowly. This process is very important for the person in our example, because he must learn how to keep his back compact in everyday situations. Then, if he can also make the arms–lower back connection (see chapter 6.3, connection 6), his back will remain stable during lifting.

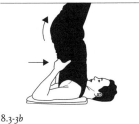

8.3-3b

After a few weeks (or months) of practice, the back will slowly start to straighten. This corresponds with a narrowing of the area where the strength is increasing (the

Note: The body is able to contract a muscle and then slowly release that contraction. This capacity for slow release controls the moment of bending and is necessary in the act of lifting (see figure 8.3-1). A sudden release causes a break in the bending movement that can be very harmful.

Before the slow release, there must be strength in the whole arch of the lower back as discussed in chapter 6.3, connections 7 and 9. When we stabilize the strength in the arch of the lower back by using the quadratus lumborum muscles, there is no strength in the lower lower back, so we are unable to release those muscles slowly. From the perspective of Critical Alignment, this causes most lower back problems.

The correct order to coordinate the moment of bending the lower back is as follows:

1. Release the tension, then mobilize and extend the whole arch of the lower back.
2. Build up strength in the postural muscles around the arch by correctly coordinating the core muscles.
3. Once you have enough strength, even in the L4 and L5 vertebrae, slowly release the strength in the muscle to stabilize the bending movement.

Now the whole arch is protected, and there will be a proper interaction between the postural muscles and the movement muscles of the lower back.

When bending is performed this way, the lower back keeps the column in the stomach area intact, creating support from the front during lifting.

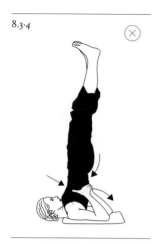

8.3-4

fiery band). This means the middle of the back is beginning to build a concentration of strength. Eventually, the shape and position of the vertebrae in the lower back will change, allowing the lower back to reposition itself. The curvature in the back will return to its correct shape—a normal lordotic curve. When this happens, the pain will disappear, and the deeper postural muscles will support the weight of the body. This process traverses the entire spine; once the lower back has the correct alignment, the midback will be addressed. In this way, the spine will develop the correct strength and be brought into alignment vertebra by vertebra.

Sarvangasana is an intense exercise that literally holds the body (especially the lower back) together.

There are as many "correct" ways to take Sarvangasana as there are styles of yoga. Many styles do not encourage correct alignment in Sarvangasana. Since this pose is held for long periods of time, incorrect alignment can have serious consequences.

When carried out correctly, Sarvangasana is an excellent answer to the "criticism" the medical world sometimes has regarding yoga; namely, that the stretching and relaxation done in asanas can weaken the structure of the body. Many yoga styles align the legs with the body in Sarvangasana, as shown in figure 8.3-4. This eliminates the alignment and strength from the posture and feels relaxing. But Sarvangasana, according to the Critical Alignment method, is not relaxing—it is hard work!

The consequences of aligning the legs with the body this way are disastrous: tension increases in the lower back, because L4 and L5 are pushed so far forward that the rest of the lower back has no opportunity to preserve its natural form and extension. This, in turn, has serious consequences for the position of the diaphragm and sternum, both of which are held in constricted positions. This has consequences for the load on the upper ribs near the collarbones; they fall inward, as the arrows in figure 8.3-4 indicate. The upper back can no longer extend but falls back into its habitual bent shape, and the hands can no longer provide the necessary support. But the most disturbing factor is that a bend forms in the midback, which compresses the base of the sternum. This area, the heart gravity point, is a feeling center and should be open in all asanas (see chapter 6, connection 1). If this area becomes constricted, it will hamper the emotional connection with the body, which blocks the sensory feelings of lightness and space. It literally pushes away the positive connection with the body. Assuming that body and mind are one, this impinges on the feeling of lightness and ease within ourselves and our interaction with the space around us.

8.3-5

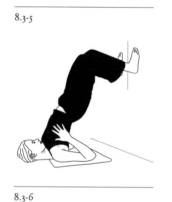

8.3-6

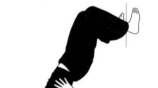
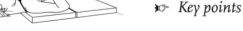

➤☞ *Key points*

1. Do Sarvangasana with Halasana (see number 14 later in this chapter). I learned from my teacher to always practice Halasana as preparation for Sarvangasana, because the former stretches the superficial movement muscles, allowing a deeper penetration into the spine during Sarvangasana, which is beneficial. However, I have added another variation here that has an immediate effect on the position of the spine and chest and stretches both areas maximally (figure 8.3-5).

2. Use shoulderstand blocks sparingly (figure 8.3-6). Using too many allows your lower ribs to dominate and eliminates the strength in your lower back (figure 8.3-7). On the other hand, if your neck muscles are short, extra blocks can be useful for developing space in your chest. When you use shoulderstand blocks, adapt the height to position

8.3-7

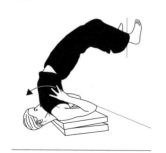

your diaphragm so that it ends in equilibrium. Your lower ribs should not point out to the front, but neither should they feel compressed. Take your time and experiment.

The exercise described in method 1 consists of the following: Sarvangasana with feet against the wall, Halasana, and Salamba Sarvangasana.

For this exercise, you will need a yoga mat and two shoulderstand blocks (each of them measuring 16 × 20 × 2 inches). When Sarvangasana becomes easier, you can exchange the blocks for a blanket or two felt mats.

Place the long side of one block against the wall with the second block butted up against the first (figure 8.3-8).

Method 1

Salamba Sarvangasana with feet against the wall

Instructions

- Lie down with your shoulders on the edge of the second block and your feet against the wall. Place your arms along your sides (see figure 8.3-8). Be aware of the free movement of your ribs and sternum based on your breathing.
- The following movement consists of two phases:
  1. Use your legs to push your pelvis up, allowing your lower back to follow until you feel your weight resting on your shoulders. Although the strength to produce this movement comes from your legs, move up on an inhalation as if the space around your sternum is raising your body off the floor. Imagine your inhalations are able to extend the vertebrae between your shoulder blades as mentioned in chapter 6.3, connections 1 and 2.
  2. As soon as you feel your weight on your shoulders, move them under your body as far as possible. The next movement is made by your upper back. Extend your back from C7, and lift your chest as high as possible toward your chin.
- Place your elbows behind you at shoulder-width and your hands on the sides of your chest (figure 8.3-9).

> **Note:** This is the correct contact between your chin and chest. Your chest should move upward and forward in relation to your throat (see the arrows in figure 8.3-9). Then your neck and throat can remain relaxed, and maximal space can be created around your upper ribs and collarbones. Try to penetrate this area with deep breaths. This is an important stretch for improving the circulation to your arms. Circulation is often reduced due to habitual postures in which the shoulders—and thus the collarbones—slump forward (see chapter 4.6 regarding RSI and CANS). Your back now forms a quarter circle above the ground. When you do this correctly, the strength will be distributed over the entire arch of your back. What often happens, however, is that the lower back moves much more easily than the rest of the back, causing your pose to look like figure 8.3-10. This is comparable to that in 8.3-4; your chest will fall inward. To correct this, extend your upper back so that it moves deeper between your shoulder blades, and allow your pelvis to move slightly back toward the wall (figure 8.3-11). Your pelvis works like a rudder in this movement.

8.3-8

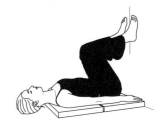

8.3-9

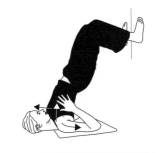

8.3-10

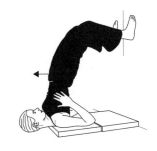

8.3-11

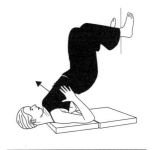

· Your upper back must maintain this posture without the help of your hands. Search for the correct coordination in the movements of your pelvis, abdomen, and chest. This will provide maximal space at the base of your sternum.
· The pressure on the front of your shoulders will increase steadily as your chest opens. Allow your shoulders to relax into this pressure.

8.3-12

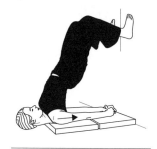

· After 2 minutes, place your hands behind you and stretch your arms toward the wall. Your arms pull your shoulders farther under your body, increasing the relaxation in your shoulders. Pushing your elbows into the floor causes your shoulder blades to elevate and develops more space in your chest (figure 8.3-12). In this way, you make connection 4 (see chapter 6.3).
· Remain in this position for 3 to 5 minutes, and try to breathe right up to your collarbones. The rhythm of your breath allows the tension in your chest to dissolve.

Look at figure 8.3-13, and compare the man sitting at the computer with a bent back with the woman in this variation of Sarvangasana. It is obvious that her pose is the complete opposite of his collapsed posture. I have summarized the main differences in the following table; the man's characteristics are given on the left, and the woman's are listed on the right.

Sarvangasana variation on the headstand bench
This Sarvangasana variation is the opposite of what most of us do all day long—sit. Because of this, many people think that the pose feels unnatural when they do it for the first time. This is understandable, since it is so contrary to their habitual posture.

Collapsed posture	Sarvangasana variation
Passive legs	Active legs
Collapsed lower back	Erect, active lower back
Collapsed chest	Erect, high chest
Inadequate, superficial breathing	Deep breathing
Tense shoulders	Relaxed shoulders
Collapsed, tense neck	Stretched, relaxed neck
Arms turned in toward the front of the body	Arms turned out toward the back of the body

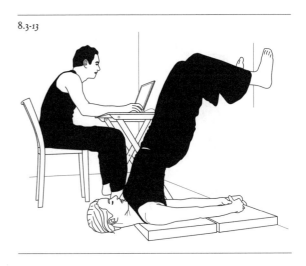

8.3-13

This pose is similar to the one you just did, only here your shoulders are supported on the headstand bench. This variation gives an extra stretch to your sternum (see the similarities to figure 8.3-14), because your neck and head are free and do not restrict the movement. Therefore, this is an excellent addition when you are working to mobilize your upper ribs, shoulders, and upper back.

Use the arrangement of the headstand bench, rubber strip, and backbender shown in figure 8.3-15.

Instructions

- Place your shoulders against the backbender without touching the back of your head to the rubber strip. The strip should push firmly against your upper back. Take hold of the legs of the headstand bench.
- Jump up on an exhalation, and place your feet against the wall (figure 8.3-16). Your shoulders should not shift away from the backbender. Remain in this position for about 30 seconds, and use your exhalations to release the tension from your shoulders.

8.3-14

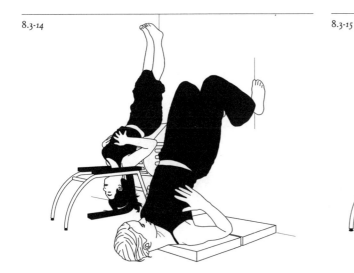

8.3-15

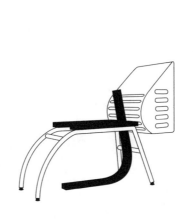

8.3-16

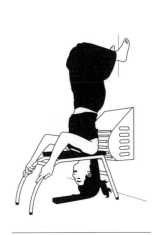

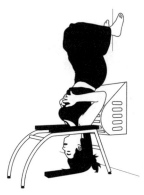

- Place your hands on your lower ribs, and during your exhalations, slowly start to move your pelvis backward (figures 8.3-17a and 8.3-17b). Pause during inhalations and breathe into the uppermost part of your chest.

> **Note:** Your upper back must pass the movement on to your pelvis; your pelvis should not take over the initiative. This slows the movement down. Follow the correct sequence to get the most out of the movement.

- If you feel a lot of pain or pressure in your lower back, prepare for this exercise by lying on a lower back roll first.
- When you have reached the end position (figure 8.3-17b), stay there for 2 to 5 minutes. Keep your breathing slow and deep. Your back may feel "blocked" when you move back to the erect position (see figure 8.3-16), because the discs and vertebrae have received a substantial impetus to move inward. That can make the return feel a bit wooden, but it is a positive sign that your back has started to move.
- For this reason, return to your erect position slowly, on exhalations, and take your time.

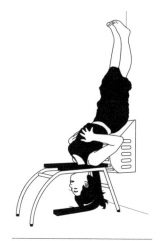

Both this exercise and the previous Sarvangasana variation isolate the upper part of your sternum like no other exercise can. Circulation to the upper part of your lungs is stimulated, and your upper chest develops flexibility. This is necessary for backbends, twists, and standing poses and will increase your enjoyment of these asanas. Therefore, practice this variation sometimes before you do Adho Mukha Vrksasana.

From Sarvangasana with feet against the wall, you can now move into Halasana.

14. Halasana

Hala means "plough."

Halasana is often (but not always) used as a preparation for Salamba Sarvangasana. It can also be combined with forward bends. It is discussed in this book in two ways. First is the movement from Salamba Sarvangasana with feet against the wall using the space already developed in your chest and abdomen and the extension in your back. Try to maintain as much space as possible in the front of your body while keeping your back compact.

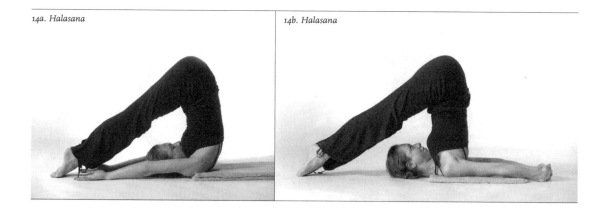

14a. Halasana

14b. Halasana

☞ *Key points*

1. Two bothersome situations can arise when practicing Halasana, especially if your feet cannot touch the floor. In the first, too much pressure develops at the base of your sternum; in the second, there is too much pressure on your throat. Both situations cause you to feel breathless.

2. Too much pressure to the base of your sternum is caused by your midback collapsing. If you cannot keep it erect when lowering your legs to the floor, rest your legs on a headstand bench or a stool (figure 8.3-18). When your hamstrings become more flexible through practicing forward bends (chapter 10) and standing poses (chapter 9), you can again try to practice Halasana without the headstand bench.

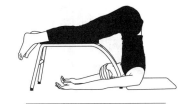

8.3-19

3. Excessive pressure in your throat is due to the collapse of your entire back. This causes your sternum and chest to fall inward toward your throat. The muscles around your throat resist and contract, causing feelings of suffocation. An extra block (or some blankets) under your shoulders can provide more space to your throat. If that does not help, try resting your legs on a headstand bench or use a combination of both props (figure 8.3-19).

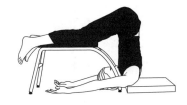

8.3-20

4. Pressure may also develop in the back of your head. This occurs because your neck muscles contract when you move your legs over your head. Try to keep your neck relaxed. Focus on the point where the muscles attach to the back of your head. If your neck remains relaxed, the back of your head will move away from your neck as described in the release of the atlas (see chapter 6.3, connection 3) and will not be pulled into your neck or the floor. This will lessen the pressure on the back of your head immediately.

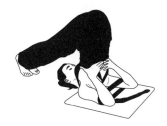

8.3-21

Two important tools: the belt and the rubber strip
These two props can greatly facilitate your progress in Sarvangasana. They will not be discussed in the instructions for the pose; you can decide for yourself if they are necessary.

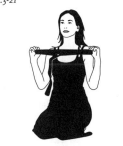

8.3-22

1. The belt
When you start to support your back with your hands, your elbows often compensate for stiff shoulders and/or upper back by moving sideways. When this happens, your shoulder blades lose the support from your arms, and your shoulders contract around your collarbones. This is precisely the area that you must stretch in Halasana. Place a belt around your upper arms (figure 8.3-20) to prevent your elbows from shifting. Pay attention to the following points when using a belt:

a. If the belt is too tight, the nerves and blood vessels in your arms and/or shoulders can become compressed, making your arms and hands numb. Experiment with different widths so you get the right support without compression. Shoulder-width is generally the correct distance (figure 8.3-21).

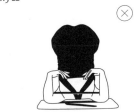

8.3-23

b. If the belt is too tight, your hands will lose their strength. They will still be touching your back, but they will not receive adequate support from your wrists and forearms (figure 8.3-22). Loosening the belt allows your forearms and wrists to transfer the movement to your index fingers so they can push your back higher (figure 8.3-23).

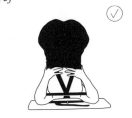

Pay attention to these corrections. The strength and position of your hands are often the weakest link in the chain of movements that constitute Sarvangasana.

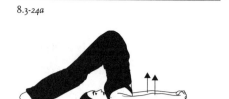
8.3-24a

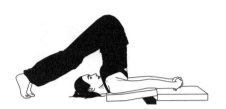
8.3-24b

2. The rubber strip

Sometimes your upper arms, shoulders, and back are so stiff that they prevent your elbows from touching the block when you bring your legs over your head (figure 8.3-24a). If this is the case, place a rubber strip under the block at the level of your elbows (figure 8.3-24b). This is an important support; the extra height under your elbows makes it easier to carry your body weight on the front of your shoulders. Without this support, your body will have to fall back for your elbows to reach the floor.

Instructions

·   After standing for 3 to 5 minutes in Sarvangasana with your feet against the wall, place your hands against your lower or midback. Support your back with your hands, and recall the difference in invoking strength from the lower and higher parts of your lower back. (This was included in the discussion of Eka Pada Sirsasana on the headstand bench (see page 165).

·   Actively press C7 into the block and maintain the extension of your back from this vertebra. Take your feet away from the wall, and bring your legs over your head toward the floor. Let your spine bend, but it should not relax; your back retains its strength in order to maintain the space to the front of your body.

·   As the position of your upper body changes, it has consequences for the amount of stretch on your neck muscles. Your entire body is now positioned at an angle over your shoulders, and your weight rests on the front of your shoulders (toward your collarbones). Be careful to maintain an active stretch from C7, as well as from your hands. Observe how your neck reacts to the constantly changing position, and give it time to relax. As soon as you feel more space in your neck and shoulders, move your hands a little lower (toward your shoulder blades) and use them to push your body higher without losing the pressure on your shoulders. Your upper body tilts farther over your head, stretching your neck muscles even more (figures 8.3-25a through 8.3-25c).

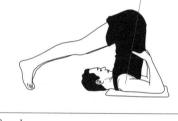
8.3-25a

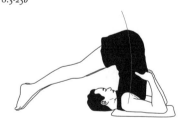
8.3-25b

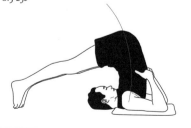
8.3-25c

Note: If you move too fast, your neck muscles will not be able to relax, then your back will bend and lose its structure. You can prevent this by observing your neck and only moving farther when your neck relaxes.

Ideally, your little fingers should almost reach your shoulder blades, and your hands should support your midback (the same place where you lie on the midback roll). Your index fingers, wrists, and forearms are dynamically active in this movement (figure 8.3-26).

When your neck muscles have relaxed and lengthened and you have placed your hands as close as possible toward your shoulder blades, return your feet to the wall without losing the strength in your wrists and hands. Instead of relaxing your hands, try to relax your *back* under your hands. Then, just like jumping up on the headstand bench, the movement from your legs and pelvis help you to extend your back (figure 8.3-27).

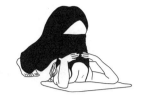

8.3-26

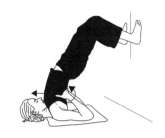

8.3-27

Note: If your hands give substantial support to your back and your back relaxes when returning your feet to the wall, the support from your hands will change. When you move your feet back toward the wall, your spine pulls your ribs together, causing your back to narrow. This movement is transferred to your hands, causing them to narrow also and your fingers to overlap. If your back is erect under your hands, it will feel as if you can lift your entire spine up and forward with the tips of your little fingers.

Consider what happens when you support your back correctly with your hands. Anatomically, your ribs angle inward to form the costovertebral joints (see figure 9.2-2a), so when your hands push your spine forward, the vertebrae pull your ribs deeper, narrowing your back. With your hands supporting your midback (at the level of the midback roll), your lower ribs can move slightly backward over your hands (toward the wall). This creates space in your upper chest that can respond by moving forward (see the arrows in 8.3-27). This is the ideal position for your upper body.

- You can now position your pelvis and lower back directly above your hands in the following manner. Bring your right leg over your head, and position your lower back and pelvis so that your inner tube is activated (figure 8.3-28a). When you feel that your back has found its correct balance, straighten your left leg without changing the shape of your back. You will now be standing as shown in figure 8.3-28b.

Note: When your feet were resting against the wall, your back was passive. It is now active, and if you have made the transition from the wall to standing erect correctly, the shape of your back will be the same. However, the midback frequently bends at the level of the hands during this transition, because this is its habitual position when actively loaded. When you still have one foot against the wall, the muscles in your back will feel soft under your hands, but the moment you take your foot away, your back muscles will become active.

Be very aware of the shape of your back under your hands when you bring your legs together. Your legs should meet approximately halfway, ending as in figure 8.3-3a. Move slowly, maintaining your balance on the front of your shoulders.

8.3-28a

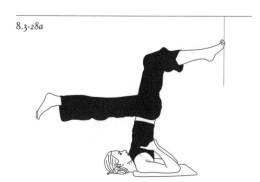

8.3-28b

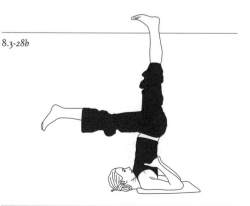

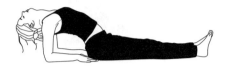

8.3-29

- Stay in this position for 5 to 20 minutes. Keep your breathing deep and relaxed.
- To come out, place your feet against the wall while keeping your chin tight to your chest. Stretch your arms behind your head, keeping your neck long and relaxed. Return with your spine to the floor, vertebra by vertebra, with exhalations.

You can make the opposite movement to neutralize your back and neck (figure 8.3-29).

I would like to discuss the following movement in more detail, as it is important for practicing Halasana. It can best be experienced when the legs are supported by the head-stand bench (figure 8.3-30). The advantage of this position is that the chest can remain spacious and open when the back relaxes, and it is easy for beginners to practice.

When asked to extend the back from a relaxed position, many students contract the lower part of the lower back from the quadratus lumborum muscles. Then the pelvis is pulled toward the lower back and the feet move toward the ceiling, because the movement releases the hamstrings (figure 8.3-31). This is incorrect and causes strain in the movement muscles of the lower back at the sides (the quadratus lumborum) instead of strength in the postural muscles connected to the vertebrae. This occurs because many people associate a straight back with tension in the lower back. The rest of the back is pulled up slightly through this movement; therefore, it looks straighter but remains in-active. The exact opposite should be happening: the *lower* back should be relaxed at the sides, and the strength should be well coordinated in the rest of the back starting at C7. If the back is extended this way, it will transfer the movement to the pelvis, and the pelvis will transfer movement through to the legs. When the neck muscles lengthen, the legs move in the direction of the arrow in figure 8.3-32. If the lower back contracts, as in figure 8.3-31, then the pelvis is pulled toward the lower back, and the movement from the spine to the pelvis and legs will stagnate.

Note: The movement just discussed (contraction of the lower back) is often persistent. The back is frequently used this way, as in a swaybacked posture (see chapter 2.3). It is very difficult to change such a habit, because when the tension in the lower back is released, it feels like you are doing nothing. The correct coordination can also be difficult to understand and experience, and that can cause irritation. If you recognize yourself in this description, take your time and try to

8.3-30   8.3-31   ⊗   8.3-32   ✓   8.3-33

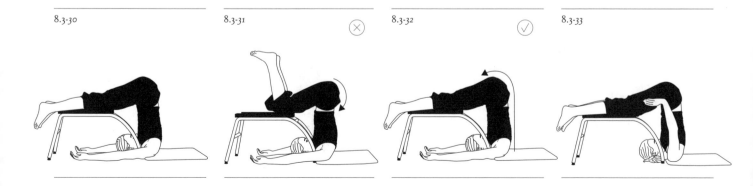

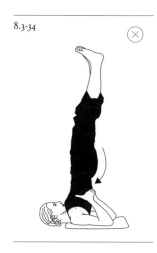

relax into the feeling of doing nothing. Just "hang" in this position for a while without taking any initiative. Then slowly start to press C7 into the block, and follow the upward movement through your whole spine until it reaches your lower back. Let your feet be heavy, and visualize the correct movement through the center line of your lower back before you start to contract the specific muscles. These muscles flatten the bend in your lower back, producing an intense feeling of strength in the corresponding areas of your spine. This pose develops cohesion and strength in the weakest spots of your spine when it is bent. This makes the exercise very valuable, because you can draw on this strength during normal daily activities like sitting behind a desk or lifting, when the spine generally loses its stability. Therefore, it is advisable to hold this position as long as you can to build awareness and strength.

Pushing your hands against your thighs (figure 8.3-33) can help by allowing the quadratus lumborum muscles to relax immediately. This release makes it possible for the midline of your lower back to support the movement. If you cannot correctly complete the movements and connections as described, then your pose will look like that in figure 8.3-34, with all its serious consequences. In figure 8.3-34, the lower back is active, but the rest of the back has collapsed. For more information about this, see the instructions for Sarvangasana at the beginning of this chapter.

Method 2

From Halasana to Salamba Sarvangasana

This is the method taught to me by my teacher. It is the preferred method if your feet can touch the floor. The same props discussed in method 1 can be used here.

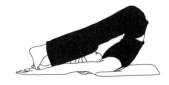

8.3-35a

Instructions

- Lie on your back with your arms stretched over your head. Lift your legs 90 degrees and, on an exhalation, bring your legs over your head.

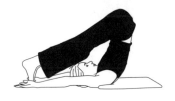

8.3-35b

Note: If this is not possible, place your hands next to your thighs and help your legs to come up and over by pushing your hands into the floor.

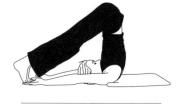

8.3-35c

- A lot of concentration is necessary to follow what happens in your back when you bring your legs over your head. Frequently, the end pose assumes and accentuates all of the back's habitual postures. The following movement makes it possible to reestablish the correct movement. With your arms lying on the floor, allow your body to fall back toward the floor without losing the contact between your toes and the floor. This creates space in your chest, throat, and lower back (figure 8.3-35a). Your back and the front of your body are in an ideal position; try to maintain it when you start extending your back. Push your chest up from C7 and let your midback and lower back follow the movement (as described earlier when your legs were supported on the headstand bench) shown in figures 8.3-35a through 8.3-35c.

- The upper part of your lower back will now push your sit bones toward the ceiling, and that activates your legs (see chapter 6, connection 10). When these connections are correct, the end pose feels as if your back is pushing your thighs up. Your thighs, in turn, are lifting and extending your back.

> **Note:** Correct movement is often supported this way: one part of the body stimulating and activating the other, and vice versa. The different parts of the body and their movements start to form a sort of closed system. This can clearly be experienced in the arms, shoulders, and hands during Sarvangasana.

- The increasing relaxation in your neck and shoulders allows your back to push your feet farther away from your head and lifts your shoulder blades farther off the floor. The higher your shoulder blades, the easier it is for your hands to connect to your midback.

> **Note:** The extension of your back pushes your feet farther away from your head. Do not reverse this movement by moving your feet first. If your feet take over the initiative, your back will bend, and the front of your body will collapse.

- Allow your inhalations to broaden the area between your shoulder blades. Use your breath to stretch and massage the muscles in this area.
- Remain in this position for 1 to 2 minutes, keeping your breathing as regular and relaxed as possible. Allow yourself to become absorbed in the rhythm of your breath. Try to develop a feeling of spaciousness through your breathing.
- Stretch your arms out behind you. Lace your fingers together and pull your shoulders, one at a time, farther under your body by lifting them up and sliding them back.
- The beauty of this support is that it (admittedly, from another angle) uses the connection between your arms and shoulder blades without having to use your back muscles as in the previous exercise. The strength you need to bring your shoulder blades together is provided by your arms and the relaxation of your shoulders, not by the muscles between your shoulder blades.
- This support will help you stabilize the upward movement of your spine between the floor and the area where your hands will give support to your spine in the next stage. Remain in this position for a minute, breathing as freely as possible.
- Place your hands against your ribs as close as possible to your shoulder blades. Push firmly with your index fingers and feel the support given by your forearms and wrists. Maintain the strength in your hands and bring your feet in (figure 8.3-36).

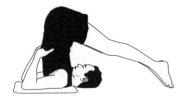

8.3-36

> **Note:** Compare the position of your chest before and after you bring your feet in. Before this, your sternum pushes the movement toward your throat. Afterward, your lower back lifts your sternum away from your throat. When lifting your legs, make sure you keep your chest lifted; it should not collapse back into your throat.

- Your back should narrow under your hands when you bring your feet in. Your lower back is not yet straight, but it is a dynamic problem. Activate your lower back muscles *as if* you are going to lift your legs.
- When you start to lift your legs, the extension to your lower back is the most important modification to your pose. Initially, it is better to lift your legs one at a time. After your back becomes stronger you can practice lifting both legs, straight and together. When you feel that your lower back has straightened, pause; otherwise, your back will lose its strength. Feel how your lower back transfers the weight of your pelvis to your midback where your hands support it (figure 8.3-37).
- Slowly lift your legs into Sarvangasana and stay there for 5 to 20 minutes.
- When you have found the correct balance on your shoulders, try to release the tension there without losing the strength in your hands. Unfortunately, relaxation in the shoulders is often paired with diminishing support from the hands. Relax your shoulders and feel how you can actively pull the tops of them under you by stretching your upper arms and elbows farther back. This movement transfers the action to your forearms and wrists, which can then push your back higher (from your index fingers) and extend it (through the narrowing of your back). Because your body is in balance, there is enough freedom for your back to react positively to the pressure of your hands and the extension of your back. Deep breathing opens your chest, and this helps your shoulders to carry their load more effectively and relax. Then the cycle of movement can begin again. The movement chains you have created have formed a closed system where one movement stimulates and strengthens the next.

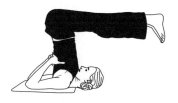

Note: If you feel that this pose is hard on your hands, ensure that you are not *leaning* on them and that your weight is carried on your shoulders. If your back is bent and out of balance, it cannot provide enough strength. In this case, push your back higher, positioning your pelvis directly above your hands. This makes your back work harder and alleviates the strain on your hands. If this does not work, put more support under your shoulders. That will automatically lift your shoulder blades higher and lighten the load on your hands. Your hands and wrists may be weak and require some time to build up strength.

In method 1, we saw how the hands can lose their strength when the wrists shift out to the sides. The opposite can also happen: the wrists are placed uselessly against the (lower) back, as shown in figure 8.3-38. In this position, they cannot transfer movement to the hands. The sequence for developing strength in your hands is as follows: Initially, your index fingers should keep pushing your back higher, so your hands can be placed closer to your shoulder blades in your midback. When your back can rise higher and straighter, your index fingers can also assist in narrowing your back. Every time your midback becomes a little straighter, another finger can actively support and assist in narrowing your back until the little fingers are finally involved. When your little fingers are close enough to your shoulder blades, your chest will be able to stretch fully and relax. The latter is dependent on the relaxation of your shoulders. Even when your back is ideally stacked, there should be some space remaining between your palms and your back.

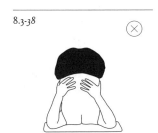

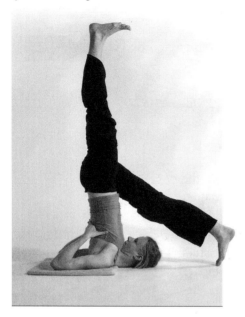

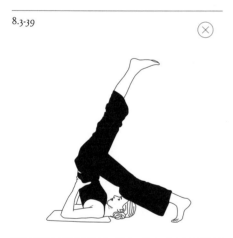

8.3-39 ⊗

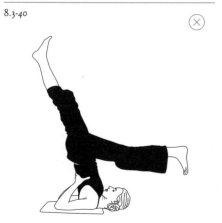

8.3-40 ⊗

Sarvangasana variations

15. Eka Pada Sarvangasana

Eka means "one"; **pada** means "foot." So the pose is called **One Leg Down Shoulderstand.**
In this variation, one leg is lowered to the ground, while the other remains aligned with the back.

Instructions

- After standing in Sarvangasana for some time, rotate both your legs inward and lower your stretched right leg to the floor. Do not change the shape of your back.
- The left leg remains connected with the area between your hands and keeps your back straight. Your back supports the weight of your body. Your weight should not follow the leg that lowers (figure 8.3-39), and your upper leg should not be used as a counterbalance (figure 8.3-40).
- Your pelvis moves slightly with the leg that has been lowered. This gives a feeling of space and relaxation in your back in the area of the iliac crest (at the top of the pelvis). When this area relaxes, your leg will be able to lower beyond halfway.
- Maintain the end pose for 20 to 30 seconds. Keep your breathing regular.
- Repeat with the left leg.

In this variation, an attempt is made to use the entire spinal column. If your back bends in the end pose, your hands will slide toward your lower back (see figure 8.3-39). If this happens, recover the position of your hands after you have completed one side.

16. Parsvaika Pada Sarvangasana

Parsva means "side"; **pada** means "foot." So the pose is called **Sideways One-Legged Shoulderstand.**
In this pose, one leg is lowered laterally while the other maintains alignment with the back.

Instructions

- After completing Eka Pada Sarvangasana on both sides, rotate your left leg inward and your right leg outward. Lower your right leg out to the side, letting your toes touch the floor. Do not use your left leg as a counterbalance; it should not move to the left. This will disturb the balance in your spine.
- The support of your right hand is very important here. When your hamstrings are tight, your back will prefer to collapse under your right hand, and this will cause pressure to your heart region. You can prevent this from happening by focusing on the release of your

hamstrings. Keep your right hand firmly in place, ensuring an erect and compact position in this part of your back.

· Remain in this position for 20 to 30 seconds, breathing regularly.
· Repeat the pose to the left.

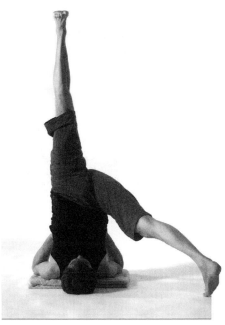

17. Urdhva Dandasana in Sarvangasana

Urdhva means "above"; *danda* means "stick."
This variation should be done at the end of the Sarvangasana series. If you cannot complete the previous two variations, use this one to build up the necessary strength.

Instructions

· In Sarvangasana, rotate and stretch both of your legs inward, then lower them halfway toward the floor.
· Keep your entire back erect so that the middle of your spinal column carries your weight.
· Slowly build up the amount of time that you stay in the end pose from a few seconds to 1 minute. Then come back down slowly into Halasana. You can repeat this variation five or ten times, holding the end pose for short periods.

Note: Two significant problems can arise during this variation:

1. Your body angles away from your shoulders, making your hands carry your weight (figure 8.3.41).
2. Your weight moves over your shoulders toward your neck, causing tension in your neck and throat and pressure on the back of your head.

When you are able to carry your weight in the middle of your back, this variation will build strength in your entire spinal column.

Note: If it is too difficult to lower your legs when they are straight, let them bend (figure 8.3.42). Practice this way until you have developed enough strength to keep your legs stretched out.

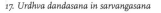
17. Urdhva dandasana in sarvangasana

8.3-41

8.3-42

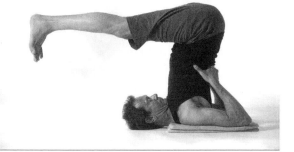

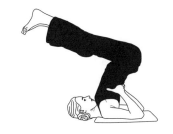

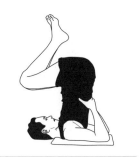

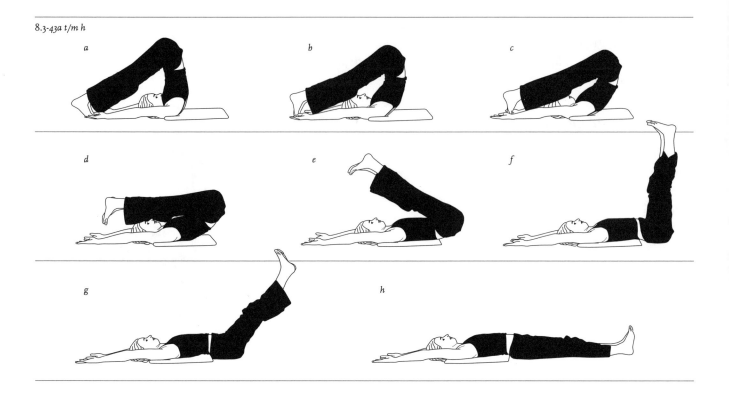

a   b   c

d   e   f

g   h

18. Adhomukha vrksasana

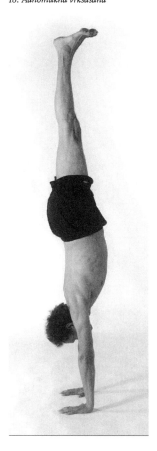

Returning from Halasana

·   After Sarvangasana, lower your legs over your head, placing your toes on the floor in Halasana.

·   Stretch your arms over your head and roll your back onto the floor, vertebra by vertebra. Keep your neck lengthened and your arms stretched on the floor (figures 8.3-43a through 8.3-43h).

·   When your legs are perpendicular to the floor (see figure 8.3-43f), try to keep them straight when lowering them toward the floor.

8.4 Inversions with an arched (concave) neck

Adho Mukha Vrksasana and Pincha Mayurasana strengthen the muscles of the arms and the deep postural muscles of the shoulders. Both asanas support the extension of the midline of the spine by giving support to the ribs at the sides, via the shoulders and shoulder blades. Adho Mukha Vrksasana and Pincha Mayurasana belong to this subgroup.

18. Adho Mukha Vrksasana

Adho mukha means "with the face downward"; *vrksa* means "tree."

The connections between the arms, shoulder blades, and back (see chapter 6.3, connection 4) form the foundation of this asana. It is preferable to learn these connections before practicing Adho Mukha Vrksasana. An easy, step-by-step buildup is given here so that students who have difficulty jumping up can practice specific exercises to make this easier. Critical Alignment specifies that the weight of the body should be supported by the entire spinal column during inversions. However, movement is often held in the lower back. Critical Alignment ensures that movement can be transferred to the upper back, where the position of the head, arms, and shoulders provides stability.

Instructions

Step 1

- Begin by practicing the arm–shoulder blade connection described in chapter 6.3, connection 4. Start slowly and gradually increase your speed until you finally allow your arms to fall into their end pose. Your hands do not touch the ground in this exercise. This allows you to experience space in your chest and increases your confidence in the strength of the connection.
- Keeping your arms connected to your shoulder blades means they will end in a stable position so that even when you "bounce" your arms up and down slightly, the connection will not be disturbed. You will experience this bouncing as pressure toward your shoulder blades. Your shoulder blades will exert pressure on the ribs that are attached to your spine. Therefore, the cooperation between your arms, shoulders, and shoulder blades supports the extension of your spine between your shoulder blades from the sides.

You can feel the unstable position by stretching your arms away from you and allowing your hands and arms to rest on the floor. In this case, the movement breaks in your shoulders, and you lose the connection with your back. This often occurs when students learn Adho Mukha Vrksasana; they cannot stand without the support of a wall because of the lack of connection with the back.

Step 2

8.4-1

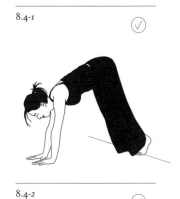

- Stand on your hands and knees, with your feet against a wall and your hands under your shoulders. Relax your upper back so that your arms and shoulder blades can connect. Spread your fingers. Place your thumbs approximately 3 inches apart.
- Keep your back well extended when lifting your knees from the floor (figure 8.4-1).

> **Note:** The shoulders and upper back are often pushed upward, causing them to harden (figure 8.4-2). This immediately breaks the connection with the shoulder blades.

8.4-2

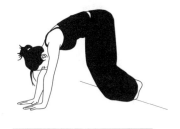

- Relax your hamstrings, allowing your lower back to form its natural lordotic curve. Connect your ribs with your abdomen to stabilize your inner tube. Lift your knees. Maintain your inner tube, and move toward the wall in a position similar to Adho Mukha Svanasana (see chapter 9.2, number 4), leading with your pelvis. Your arms, shoulder blades, and back are in a stable position. If you move your upper body up and down slightly, you will also feel the elastic connection of your arms, shoulder blades, and back.

Step 3

- Raise your feet one at a time onto the wall without losing the central connection to your back. As soon as you have done this (figure 8.4-3), move your chest toward the wall and lift your head toward your upper back.

> **Note:** This coordination is difficult for many students. When they move the upper part of the chest toward the wall, they often lower the head (causing the shoulders to lose their connection and "bend"). If the head is lifted, the shoulders remain integrated (allowing them to retain their strength). Practice this coordination correctly when moving from figure 8.4-4 to figure 8.4-5; keep your chest forward and your head high.

- Your body should now be at an angle toward the wall, moving away from your shoulders (see figure 8.4-3), and your arms should be at right angles with the floor. Now you can work on connection 5 from chapter 6.3. Push the palms of your hands and your fingertips into the floor. This will tighten the ligaments in your wrists and supply structure and stability. The back of your hands should be flat, allowing your wrists to remain relaxed.

Step 4

- Slowly straighten your legs, positioning your pelvis above your shoulders (see figure 8.4-5). Feel how your weight is accepted into the stable end position of your shoulders.
- Check the following points in your end position:
  1. The back of your head is still connected to your upper back.
  2. Your ribs are connected to your abdomen.
  3. Your arms are at right angles to the floor.

This position is a good alternative if you cannot jump up into Adho Mukha Vrksasana alone. It will develop needed strength in your arms due to the erect position of your lower back, which pushes the weight of your body precisely into your arms. Part of your weight is still carried by the wall where your feet are placed. Because you can move slowly, it is easier to keep your wrists relaxed.

8.4-3

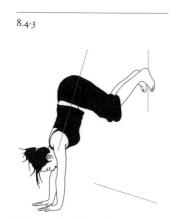

8.4-4

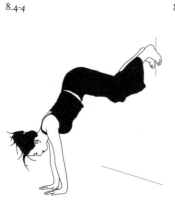

8.4-5

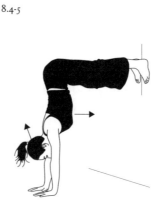

8.4-6

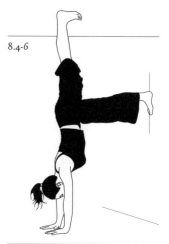

Note: If the load on your wrists is excessive, elevating them slightly (such as with a rubber strip) will reduce the pressure.

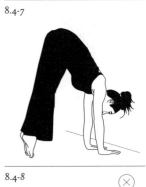
8.4-7

- Now you can practice the variation seen in figure 8.4-6, in which you alternately raise each leg.
- Remain in this end pose for as long as you can to build up the required strength in your arms. You must be confident of your strength before moving on to the next step.

Step 5: jumping up against the wall

- Place your hands on the floor, shoulder-width apart, approximately 6 inches from the wall. Your arms should be perpendicular to the floor. Stretch your fingers and press your fingertips lightly into the floor. If you have problems with your wrists, place a rubber strip under them (see earlier note).
- Allow your upper back to fall deeply between your shoulder blades, making the connection between your arms and shoulder blades. Move your feet closer without losing this connection. As you walk in, move your chest forward, stretch your lower back as much as possible, and lift your head toward your upper back (figure 8.4-7).
- Keep your head at exactly the same height and feel how your arms give a counter-pressure to your shoulder blades. Remember the instructions "chest forward and head high" before you jump up. Visualize how your pelvis will end above your shoulders in your jump.

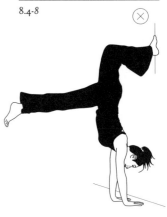
8.4-8

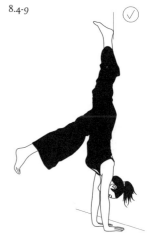
8.4-9

Note: When jumping up for the first time, nearly everyone jumps with their feet (figure 8.4-8). The feet cannot lift the pelvis, and the lower back will remain inactive. For this reason, only jump up with a straight leg that connects to your pelvis in the movement. Then your lower back will be activated, and it will be able to pull your pelvis and legs above your shoulders. The difference between this and the first jump is that the leg that jumps up remains slightly forward (figure 8.4-9) and does not go "over the top." If you have learned to jump up with your feet, your end pose will look like figure 8.4-10, with tension in your shoulders and lower back. Then there is absolutely no possibility of transferring movement. Unfortunately, this occurs frequently in Adho Mukha Vrksasana and causes tension to build up in the lower back and shoulders.

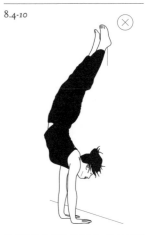
8.4-10

Note: Nearly everyone who jumps up moves their head forward. This is incorrect, as it prevents the upper back from accepting the movement. The movement then ends up in the shoulders, causing the pose to destabilize. Keep your head in the same position (elevated) during your jump. Only then can you make a stable arms–shoulder blades–back connection, allowing your upper back to accept the movement.

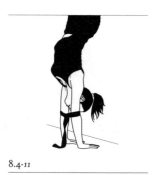

8.4-11

- Stretch your arms and jump up with one leg, allowing the other leg to follow. Stand with one foot against the wall for as long as you can. Do not try to stand without the support of the wall at first. Use the support to build up your strength until you can stand for approximately 1 minute.

Note: If you are unsure about the strength in your arms, place a belt around your upper arms (at shoulder-width), as shown in figure 8.4-11.

- Slide your lower ribs back and use your stomach muscles to position your pelvis above your shoulders so your inner tube is activated.

Step 6: standing without the support of a wall

- When you feel confident about how to carry your weight correctly, you can start to move away from the wall. Control the position of your head, your inner tube, and the balance in your hands while lifting your feet, one at a time, away from the wall. You must trust in the end movement that is formed by the arms–shoulder blades–back connection and the correct position of your head.
- Once you are experienced in Adho Mukha Vrksasana, you can try jumping up with your legs together (figures 8.4-12a through 8.4-12c).

19. Pincha Mayurasana

Pincha means "feather"; *mayura* means "peacock."
This asana resembles a peacock with its tail lifted and spread. The positioning of the arms in this pose makes the connection between the arms and shoulder blades easier than in Adho Mukha Vrksasana. However, the constraint can sometimes be so great that jumping up is hindered. If this happens, increase the flexibility to your shoulders with the following exercises.

8.4-12a   8.4-12b   8.4-12c

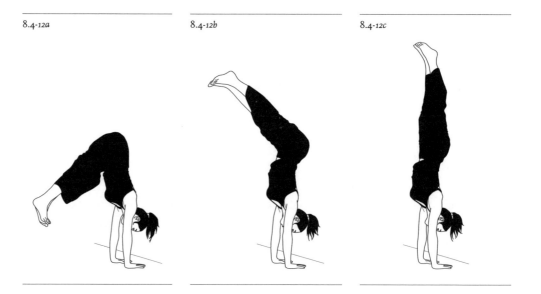

Instructions

- Place the headstand bench (or a chair) in front of you with the straight legs facing you. Kneel on a felt mat and place your elbows on the rubber strips of the bench. Lace your fingers together but keep your hands and wrists apart. If your shoulders are stiff, your wrists will move toward each other in the end position. This prevents the movement from being transferred from your arms to your shoulder blades.
- Lower your upper body and move your pelvis back. End with your pelvis above your knees and keep your wrists spread (figure 8.4-13). The headstand bench keeps your elbows a shoulder-width apart. If your elbows are too wide, then your shoulders will end up in an unstable position, creating pressure in them rather than transferring the movement from your arms to your back.
- If the movement is very painful in your shoulders, stay within your pain threshold when lowering your upper body. Then focus on providing length by pushing your elbows forward and your pelvis back. This will create space in your shoulders and in the area between your shoulder blades.
- Keep your breathing deep and regular. Use every inhalation to broaden the space between your shoulder blades. When exhaling, extend your back and allow your upper back and shoulders to relax.
- Stay in this position for 1 to 2 minutes, then come out slowly.

Instructions: *Pincha Mayurasana against the wall*

Use a belt and a wooden block to maintain the correct position of your elbows and hands.

- Fold your yoga mat a couple of times to create a soft base. Kneel in front of the mat and place the wooden block against a wall. The belt should be just above your elbows and at shoulder-width. Place your hands on the floor at either end of the block near the wall. Your forearms should be parallel to each other (figure 8.4-14).

Note: When you become accomplished in this asana, you can practice without one or both props, but do not be in a hurry to do this.

- Lift your knees from the floor and push your arms up into your shoulders so that your shoulders remain high. Lift your head.
- Keep your shoulders high, and swing your legs up one at a time. Allow your heels to rest against the wall.

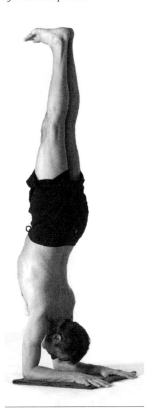

8.4-13

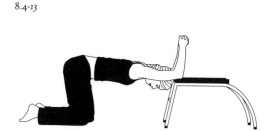

8.4-14

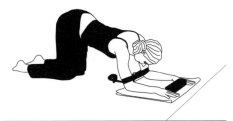

Note: If you do not feel comfortable jumping up, you can place the crown of your head on the floor as in Sirsasana. Once your legs are up, you can lift your head from the floor. This can feel safer, because your shoulders do not have to absorb the jump. You can try to jump up later, when your shoulders are flexible enough to accept the movement.

- Many students end up with an excessively concave lower back. Correct this by using your stomach muscles to position your pelvis correctly above your shoulders. This movement requires flexibility in the shoulders and upper back (figures 8.4-15a through 8.4-15c).
- Remain in this position for 20 to 60 seconds.
- When you are accomplished in this asana, you can try jumping up with both legs together.

8.4-15a 8.4-15b 8.4-15c

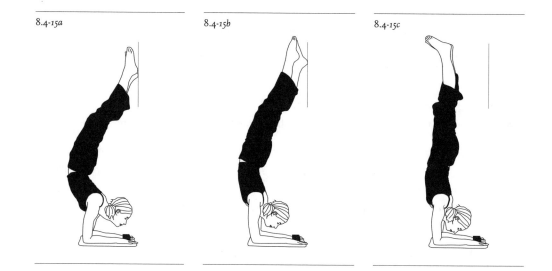

9

STANDING POSES

9.1 Introduction

Stability through the midline of your lower back, which is achieved by extending your lumbar spine and correctly positioning your lower ribs, allows the weight of your body to transfer through the last lumbar vertebra into your sacrum. The movement splits in the sacrum through your SI joints to your hips, which are loaded in different ways, depending on the pose. Every pose loads your legs in different ways, as your body constantly moves from one plane to another. Your neck transfers the weight of your head to your upper back.

The first noticeable result of standing poses is increased mobility around the large joints of the lower body, including the lumbar vertebrae, SI joints, hips, ankles, and feet. The active practice of these asanas stimulates the postural muscles around these joints, which leads to better mobility.

Tight leg muscles cause the lower joints to function poorly. The vigorous and varied challenges of standing poses stretch and strengthen the leg muscles. Developing length and strength creates a new alignment in the legs that can support freer movement of the large joints.

Another noticeable result of standing poses is that they prepare us for all the other groups of asanas. They illustrate how movement must be seen in a larger context: stretching the lower back, for example, can only take place when the hips and hamstrings can relax. These compound movements (connections) were discussed in detail in chapter 6. Based on their unique characteristics and the preparation they provide for other asanas, standing poses can be divided into the following subgroups.

1. Back stretches

Back stretches are a good preparation for forward bends and inversions. The back is constantly placed and held in an erect position with the aim of strengthening the spinal column through the midline so there can be a strong interaction between the postural muscles and the movement muscles. This provides the correct control during forward bends and inversions.

Tadasana, Utkatasana, Dandasana (standing), Adho Mukha Svanasana I and II, and Virabhadrasana II belong to this subgroup.

2. Twists

In this type of standing pose, the upper body is rotated, with the spine functioning as the axis for the rotation. Because the upper body is typically placed in a diagonal or horizontal position, the strength of the lower back is constantly challenged, making this subgroup an ideal preparation for seated twists. In seated twists, the end position must also be supported by the lower back; unfortunately, there is often a tendency to "hang" in the lower back, as it does not have any strength to control the extension.

Utthita Trikonasana, Parivrtta Trikonasana, Utthita Parsvakonasana, and Parivrtta Parsvakonasana belong to this subgroup.

3. Leg stretches

The leg stretches done in standing poses are an ideal preparation for seated forward bends. If the hamstrings cannot stretch properly during these bends, the cause is often a combination of an inadequate stretch in the lower back and stiffness in the hips. The lower back must be strong to break through these patterns, and the necessary strength is developed during standing poses.

Dandasana (standing), Utthita Trikonasana, Parivrtta Trikonasana, Parsvottanasana, Adho Mukha Svanasana II, and Ardha Chandrasana belong to this subgroup.

4. Standing backbends

Standing backbends are good preparation for backbends. The inner tube—consisting of the diaphragm, lower back, and pelvis—is dependent on the strength of the stomach muscles to create free movement in the hips and thighs. This makes it possible for movement to be transferred to the pelvis and legs instead of becoming caught up in the lower back. Standing poses emphasize the development of strength in the legs, and it is precisely this strength that must be used during backbends. Emphasis is often placed on the back and shoulders when practicing backbends, mainly because they are often stiff and demand all our attention.

Virabhadrasana I belongs to this subgroup.

Strength in the legs provides free movement in the large joints in standing poses. This theme pervades all the standing poses, and there is an athletic aspect to it. You will quickly experience how tired and hot you can become when practicing standing poses, especially in the variations where one leg is held at a right angle. The heat and fatigue occur when the leg muscles contract, compressing the blood vessels just at the moment when the muscles need more blood for their energy supply. The body reacts by temporarily increasing blood pressure so that more blood can reach the muscles; in the long term, this increases the number of blood vessels. Temporary high blood pressure creates the same type of heat and increased circulation you experience when running. The positive aerobic effect that sports have on blood circulation also occurs in standing poses.

9.2 Standing poses: back stretches

Tadasana, Utkatasana, Dandasana (standing), Adho Mukha Svanasana I and II, and Virabhadrasana II form a subgroup within the standing poses and emphasize the development of strength in the spinal column. They do this by extending the back in an erect position, thus establishing the basis for forward bends and inversions.

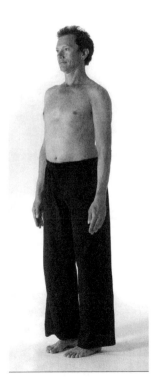

1. Tadasana

1. *Tadasana*

Tada means "palm tree."
The name of this asana can be summarized as a metaphor for the exercise itself: when you look at a palm tree, you see not only a firm connection with the earth but also how the crown of the head rises toward the sky. Tadasana has a firm foundation in the lower body and legs, while the upper body and crown stretch into the space above. When the weight of the body is carried by the postural muscles of the back, the movement in the spine is constant and light, the way a palm tree moves with the wind.

In Tadasana, your abdomen is controlled by the transverse abdominals (see chapter 6.3, connection 8) and activates the inner core. This distributes your body weight to your pelvis, legs, and feet (which are planted firmly on the floor). Standing like this can allow a feeling of lightness to develop above the diaphragm.

During this asana, the two most important gravity points—the lower abdomen and the heart region—are brought into balance.

Instructions

- Standing with your feet in line with your hip joints, turn your heels slightly outward. Ensure that the toes of both feet are all in a line. This allows you to turn your thighs

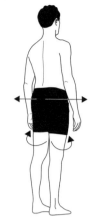

inward (toward your hips and groin) and align your legs with your hips. The inward rotation of your legs broadens the back of your pelvis (see the arrows in figure 9.2-1).

· Position your pelvis by relaxing the lower part of your lower back and the front of your hips. This will provide extension to your lower back and space to your lower abdomen. To facilitate the release of tension in your lower back, bend your knees slightly and feel how your pelvis moves away from your lower back. Feel the connection between your lower ribs and the arch of your lower back. Pull the area 1 inch under your navel upward to activate your transverse abdominal muscles (see chapter 6.3, connection 8). Slowly stretch your legs. Bearing your weight on the front part of your heels will help the front of your hips remain relaxed.

Note: The connection between the lower ribs and the arch of the lower back is the most difficult movement to realize in a standing position, because it is hard to determine whether or not the pelvis is in its neutral position. Therefore, it may be helpful to start Tadasana from a sitting position, as described in chapter 6.3, connection 9. When the pelvis is in contact with the chair, it is easier to find its neutral position and make the connection with the arch of the lower back. Once you have found that position, stand up slowly and repeat the same movements with straight legs.

Note: The balance on the front part of your heels is important. It is necessary in all of the standing poses and helps relax the muscles around your hips and your lower back. Do not stand absolutely still in Tadasana, as this makes it difficult to judge whether or not the movement muscles of your lower back are relaxed. Make small, irregular movements with your upper body to generate a feeling of release in the arch of your lower back. Try to find the precise balance in the midline of your spine. This may help release the tension in the movement muscles of your lower back. After this release, you may perceive a feeling of individual movement in the vertebrae. When you experience this, you can stop the movements and hold your balance for a while.

· Your diaphragm should be positioned in such a way that your weight is transferred toward the SI joints in your sacrum. Do not lose your normal lordotic curve or the upward pull in the area below your navel during this movement. The latter keeps your inner core active.

Note: Your legs, pelvis, diaphragm, abdomen, and lower back are now correctly positioned. This alignment allows a relaxed feeling of space to develop in your lower abdomen. Limit your breathing to your abdomen in this phase and feel how your lower ribs broaden during slow, deep inhalations. Try to experience solidity *and* relaxation here.

Do not worry about the position of your upper body at this stage. We generally initiate movement with our head (getting up out of a chair, for example), and there is often a tendency to lead with the head during Tadasana. This results in a forced pose, resembling the military principle of "shoulders back, chest forward." Such a buildup disturbs our inner tube, and the inner tube is exactly what is required to keep our pose well coordinated from the postural muscles in the lower back so that the movement muscles can remain relaxed.

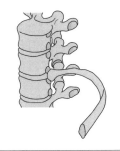

- Do not think about muscular strength when you are aligning your upper body. Use your breath. Figures 9.2-2a and 9.2-2b illustrate how the ribs connect to the vertebrae and the sternum. Try to imagine how inhaling lifts your sternum and automatically pulls your thoracic vertebrae into a straighter position via your ribs. This depends on you having sufficient mobility in your upper back. Keep your back and shoulders as relaxed as possible.
- The movement of your sternum, ribs, and back places your neck and head directly above your back. Try to make this neck movement (see chapter 6.3, connection 3) as light as possible.

9.2-2b

Spine with ribs and sternum

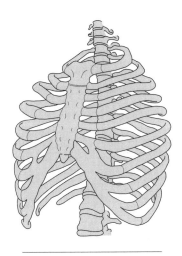

Note: The movement is directed toward your sternum and not your lower ribs. Make sure your diaphragm remains stable during the movement; it should not shift forward and/or upward. If this occurs, the alignment in your lower back will be distorted.

- Become consciously aware of your heart gravity point. Use your inhalations to develop a feeling of lightness in this region. When this feeling becomes tangible, allow it to circulate through your entire body and support full awareness.
- You can now connect the two gravity points—the heart region and the lower abdomen—with your breathing. At the same time, remain conscious of the feelings of relaxation in your lower abdomen and lightness in your chest.

2. Utkatasana

The starting point of all standing poses is the establishment and maintenance of correct balance between these two gravity points. Only when you have that balance can you consciously use your breath to develop relaxation in your lower abdomen and lightness in your chest. When you monitor these points and correct yourself consistently, your body will be able to relax in the areas to which the movement is directed. For example, stiffness in your back or hips will relax more easily, allowing your body to find its natural balance in the asana. When this happens, you will experience the standing poses (which are actually very strenuous) as light and relaxed.

2. Utkatasana

***Utkata* means "strong" or "forceful."**
Utkatasana is the first exercise that increases strength to the lower back. There is a strong interaction between the postural and movement muscles there, because the spine is held in a diagonal position. Once mobility has improved through practice on the lower back rolls, it is possible to begin strengthening the lower

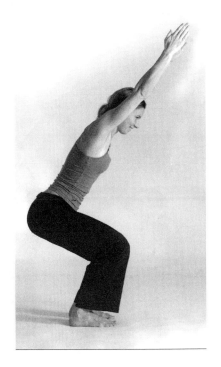

back. Because the knees are bent, tight hamstrings do not hinder the free movement of the pelvis. This makes Utkatasana accessible for everybody.

The mobility of your vertebrae defines how you can use your lower back. If you lead a sedentary life and your lower back is often in the position shown in figure 9.2-3, it will most likely develop a preference for this position. It will also stiffen in this shape. Children often sit with a bent back, but they usually relax into an "end pose" where they cannot go any farther. This creates much less tension than the half-collapsed back shown in figure 9.2-3. When the back is half collapsed, the muscles have to work continuously. Stress increases tension in the back as well.

The result of this is that you cannot use your lumbar vertebrae correctly when standing erect. They cannot move beyond the position seen in figure 9.2-4. To stand up straight, other areas of the back must compensate for this insufficiency. One alternative to this is shown in figure 9.2-5: the swayback. Men often have a penchant for this posture. Another alternative is shown in figure 9.2-6, where the diaphragm is shifted forward and the chest is lifted. Women are more inclined to this posture. Both variations cause tension to increase around the lumbar vertebrae, often predominantly to one side. Observe how people stand when they are waiting in line. Figure 9.2-7 shows how such a waiting posture increases tension to the right side of the lower back. This has serious consequences for the mobility of the lower back, right hip, and right leg. (For more information about this, see Trikonasana in chapter 9.3, number 9, and Virabhadrasana II in chapter 9.2, number 7). These preferences will have an effect on Utkatasana and all standing poses. The first variant (the swayback) will cause the chest to collapse and constrict the heart gravity point (see chapter 9.2, number 1), making it impossible to experience a light posture. Thus, the person with the posture shown in 9.2-8a ends up in the pose shown in figure 9.2-8b.

The second variant (see figure 9.2-6) will build up tension in the midback, causing the inner tube to lose its stability. Thus, the person with the posture shown in figure 9.2-9a will end up in the pose shown in figure 9.2-9b. This weakens the lower back and makes it impossible to experience the relaxation achieved from a balanced hara gravity point. Thus, this person will always experience standing poses as forced instead of relaxed.

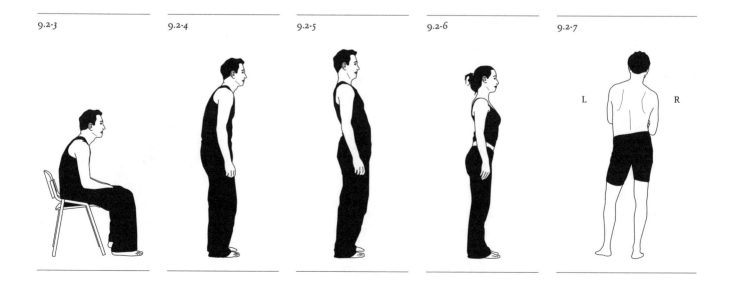

9.2-3   9.2-4   9.2-5   9.2-6   9.2-7

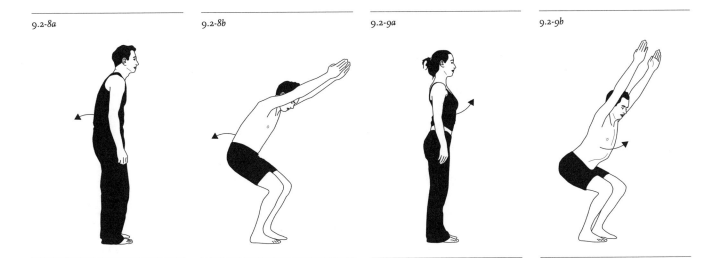

9.2-8a   9.2-8b   9.2-9a   9.2-9b

Practicing Utkatasana is the first step toward breaking these patterns (see the instructions in chapter 6.3, number 10). If you have problems bending your hips, you can use the exercises there as preparation.

Instructions

- Stand in Tadasana, turn your palms outward, and lift your arms overhead without losing your grip on your inner tube (see chapter 8.3, number 8). Bend your knees and allow your upper body to move forward diagonally.
- Try to determine whether your hamstrings have relaxed or contracted as you bent your knees. If your lower back has rounded and you feel no pressure in your hips, your rounded back may be caused by stiffness in your hamstrings, hips, and lower back; it can also be the result of habit. Ice skaters, for example, learn to bend their knees while contracting their hamstrings and pulling their sit bones toward each other. If this occurs automatically during Utkatasana, then it is a coordination problem: the correct movement is possible, but the body doesn't do it because it has developed other preferences. Contracting the hamstrings pulls the sit bones (their point of origin) toward the knees and causes the lower back to round. When the hamstrings are relaxed as the legs bend, the sit bones can move back up, allowing the lower back to maintain its balanced position.
- Carry your weight on the front of your heels and feel how that affects your hips. The weight of your upper body is transferred toward your hips. However, the muscles located under the creases formed at your groin (see the arrow in figure 9.2-10) can resist this pressure. Balancing at the front of your heels helps soften this resistance. Then you will feel your hips move deeper and your sit bones move farther back.
- When your knees point straight ahead, they provide an even pressure to the inside and outside of the creases. If your knees fall to the sides, the outside of the crease will be pushed deeper, causing tension to your groin. The opposite will happen when your knees move too far inward. The correct balance in your knees also affects the position of your feet. There, the pressure should be spread evenly over the inside and outside of each foot. The power line will then return to the midline as seen in figure 9.2-11.

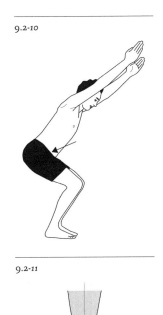

9.2-10

9.2-11

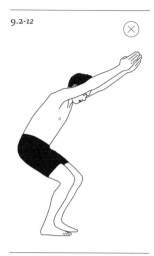

9.2-12

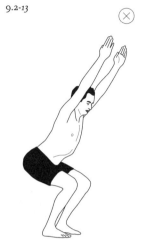

9.2-13

Note: Two important movements that are often made to compensate for a lack of mobility in the lower back were discussed in the introduction to this exercise. These same compensations are also possible in Utkatasana. Figure 9.2-12 illustrates how bending the lower back increases its tension, while figure 9.2-13 shows how the midback compensates. Both problems can be avoided by practicing the pose in the following manner.

· Stand with your back against a wall and your feet approximately 1 foot away from it. When your ribs are connected to the arch of your lower back, there will be just enough space between your lower back and the wall to slide one hand between them. Your lower ribs are connected to your abdomen, and your pelvis moves away from your lower back (figure 9.2-14). Stabilize this position from the front by pulling the area just below your navel up toward your navel. This will innervate your transverse abdominals.

· Bend your knees and slide your pelvis down the wall (figure 9.2-15). Feel the contact of your pelvis with the wall. Lean forward with your upper body while lengthening your hamstrings. Do not lose the active connections in the back itself. The contact of your pelvis with the wall will change: first, you will feel it against the back of your pelvis, but the farther forward you lean, the more the pressure will move toward your sit bones. As long as you feel your pelvis moving against the wall, your back is in the correct position (figure 9.2-16). If your pelvis stops moving but your trunk continues, then your back will bend. This is exactly what you are trying to avoid.

Note: This break often happens because the hamstrings start to contract. Try to find out for yourself whether your hamstrings started to contract because of tightness in the muscles or because of poor, unconscious coordination. Maybe your hamstrings started to contract because they wanted to protect your hips. The continuation of the movement will produce more pressure in your hip joints, and when your hips are stiff, your body will activate precautions in advance. Maybe your hamstrings started to contract because they are stronger (or tighter) than the quadriceps at the front of your thighs. In that case, you need to break the pattern and seriously build up the strength in your quadriceps. Coordinating the movement from your hamstrings will undoubtedly pull your lower back into an unstable position.

· Push yourself away from the wall with your hands while maintaining your pose (figure 9.2-17).

· Lift your arms and make the connection with your shoulder blades (see chapter 6.3, number 4).

Note: If you cannot lift your arms high enough to complete the pose, it would be wise to practice the shoulder exercise on the rubber strip regularly (see chapter 6.3, number 4).

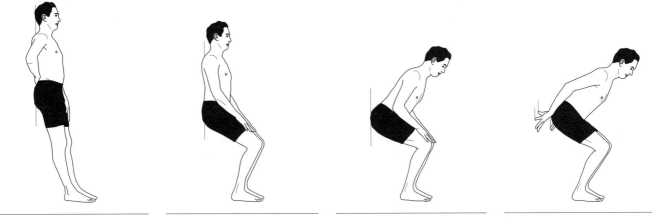

3. Dandasana (standing)

***Danda* means "stick."**

Dandasana can be done after Utkatasana. The main difference from Utkatasana is that this pose also stretches the hamstrings. To reach an angle of 90 degrees in the hips with an extended lower back requires length in the hamstrings. This asana also further strengthens the lower back.

3. Dandasana

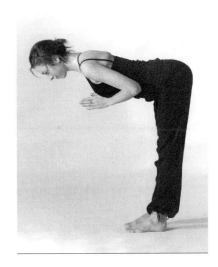

Instructions
From Tadasana

· Place your hands together in front of your sternum. Turn your thighs inward and contract your quadriceps to straighten your legs. Envision that the strength required to lift your kneecaps comes from the superior part of your quadriceps, near your hips, and not from the area just above your knees, as if your leg muscles are passing the dynamics of the movement from your knees to your hips.

· Your hips are the driving force in the continuation of the movement. Without changing the shape of your back, bend your trunk at the hips, ending in a 90-degree angle. Maintain your balance on the front of your heels (see the following instructions for the correct method).

Note: If your lower back remains erect, the movement will be arrested by your hamstrings. If you do not feel your hamstrings stretching in the end position, check the shape of your back in a mirror. If it looks like that shown in figure 9.2-18 and you are unable to change it, initiate the movement as follows (from Utkatasana). That will provide greater freedom of movement to your hips and allow your hamstrings to relax.

9.2-18

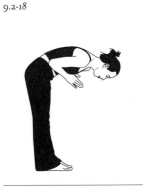

· When your lower back is straight, align your neck on a deep inhalation so your thoracic spine straightens between your shoulder blades and supports the space of the heart gravity point behind your thumbs.

- Keep your breathing free. Inhale from your lower abdomen (hara) to your heart region. Relax your shoulders, keep your neck at the same height, and feel the ribs in your back narrow with your exhalations.
- Remain in this position for 30 seconds to 2 minutes.

From Utkatasana

- Stand in Utkatasana and maintain your balance on the front part of your heels; this helps your hips relax and move farther back. Be sure to maintain the correct balance on your feet when moving so you can bend freely from your hips and activate the deep postural muscles that stabilize them. The movement of your hips allows your sit bones to move farther back, causing them to protrude. Be careful not to tighten your hamstrings when standing with bent knees.

> **Note:** Your hamstrings attach to your sit bones. When you contract them, they will change the position of your pelvis in such a way that it will round your lower back. After the release of your hamstrings, your sit bones can move away from the backs of your knees. Through this release, your pelvis rotates forward, which will help you extend your lower back. This movement has strong consequences for the use of your leg muscles. Bending your knees with the release of your hamstrings means that your quadriceps rather than your (tight) hamstrings must carry your body weight.

- Perform the following movement to learn how to stabilize your core in this position. When you feel the release of your hamstrings and the resulting extension of your lower back, place the tips of your fingers on your lower ribs. Overarch your lower back by pulling your shoulders backward. Make sure your whole lumbar spine is moving inward. Keep your pelvis in the same position. Do not contract your hamstrings when you bring your lower ribs down again. When your lower back does not lose its extension, there will be a break in the movement of your ribs, indicating that the movement has reached your pelvis. After feeling this break (as described in chapter 6.3, connection 7), contract the area 1 inch below your navel upward. This will activate your transverse abdominals and often happens automatically as soon as your lower back extends fully. Now your core is stable, with the column at the front, the neutral extension of your lower back, your diaphragm, and the muscles of your pelvic floor all properly connected.

> **Note:** When you are not quite certain about the connection of your core, it is advisable to use this technique in standing poses. First, overarch your lower back to make sure it is well arched. Then lower your ribs to make the connection. When this movement is performed well, there will *always* be a stop in the movement of your ribs. When you do not feel that stop, your lower back is not properly arched.

- Place your hands on your upper thighs and pull the *skin* up toward your hips. Follow this movement with your muscles so that they slowly lift your kneecaps and stretch your legs. Visualize this happening again when you straighten your legs. The upward movement of your knees is transferred toward your hips via your quadriceps.

- When your legs are stretched, a groove remains that runs through your lower lower back (L4 and L5) into your sacrum; it is caused by the activity of the extensor muscles that run on either side of the vertebrae. You can easily feel how the action of contracting your quadriceps, together with lengthening your lower back, converges in your hips.

4. Adho Mukha Svanasana I

Adho mukha means "face downward"; *sva* means "dog."
Adho Mukha Svanasana is, coordination-wise, a difficult exercise. Many of the connections can fall apart in this pose—particularly, the inner tube (see chapter 6.3, number 8); the connection between the lower back, hips, and legs (chapter 6.3, numbers 7 and 10); and the connection between the arms and shoulder blades (chapter 6.3, number 4).

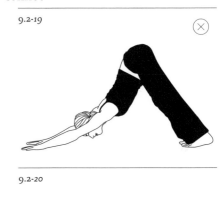

9.2-19

The extension of the lower back has an important role in this asana. The lower back, pelvis, and hips form the highest point of the body in this pose, and as such, the pelvis and hips are not burdened with the weight of the body. That can become a disadvantage, because the muscles are not required to hold the body up as in Utkatasana. Often the extension of the lower back is displaced due to overextension in the shoulders, as illustrated in figure 9.2-19. It is important to bear this in mind, because preferential movements may become strengthened rather than challenged. Because the lower back is minimally engaged and no particular flexibility is necessary for this asana, it can be practiced easily. But it is a difficult exercise to complete with the correct coordination. To eliminate incorrect coordination patterns, it is important to move slowly, carefully, and with constant attention when practicing this pose. These problems will be discussed during the description of the exercise.

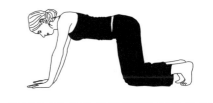

9.2-20

Your starting position can vary; you may start with your hands and knees on the floor or by jumping back. The best starting point is the former, as shown in figure 9.2-20.

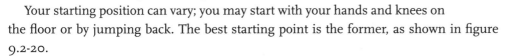

| 4a. Adho mukha svanasana I | 4b. Adho mukha svanasana I |

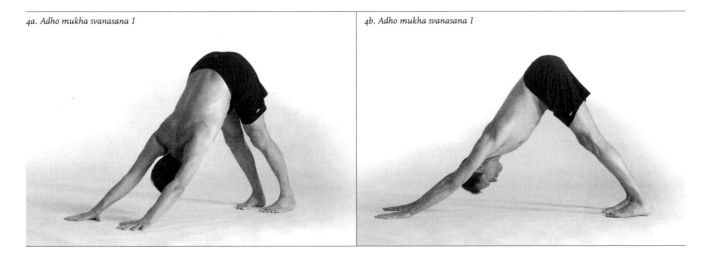

Instructions

- Kneel with your hands at the front of your mat and your knees under your hips. Your feet should be at hip-width and your thumbs approximately 6 inches apart.
- Relax your hamstrings and allow your sit bones to move upward. Now your lower back is able to relax and move downward.

Note: If your hands are too far apart, it will become difficult to make the correct connection with your shoulder blades. The movement will then most likely terminate in your shoulders, causing them to bend deeply (see figure 9.2-19).

Note: The inward movement of the curvature of your lower back and the straightening of your upper back is achieved through relaxation. It is not something you can do actively; you simply allow gravity to do the job. Local mobility will increase over time when you practice exercises directed to specific areas, such as lying on the lower back roll, lying on the rubber strip, doing hip stretches, and so on.

- Repeat the contraction and release of your hamstrings several times; notice that the contraction of your hamstrings does not feel like a contraction at all. It is actually difficult to ascertain from the muscle itself. It can be determined only by observing its *result*. That result is the downward movement of your sit bones, the forward rotation of your pelvis, and the bending of your lower back. The release of your hamstrings produces the opposite movements.
- After a full release of your hamstrings, your lower back will probably feel overextended. Do not worry about that at this stage of the movement, but use the extension to pull your lower ribs in as explained in the previous exercise (standing Dandasana). This will produce a break in the movement of your ribs if your lower back does not lose its extension. Hold your lower ribs in this neutral position by contracting your upper abdominal muscles lightly.
- Pull the area below your navel upward. Now the column between your diaphragm and lower abdomen becomes active, which means your core is connected. Breathe into that column and try to experience a feeling of relaxation.

Note: In this position, your lower back does not carry any body weight. Nevertheless, your core feels like a firm frame. The stop in the movement of your ribs and the pressure on your hips are good signs for this connection. Keep monitoring those areas during the movement, making sure you do not lose the connection, which occurs through the use of the postural muscles. That is why, in this asana, we talk about the stabilization through the inner core.

9.2-21

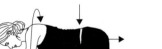

- The lordotic curve of your lower back will activate your upper thighs dynamically.
- At the other end of the connection, relax your upper back to connect your arms with your shoulder blades. Study the arrows in figure 9.2-21 carefully.

- Make sure you keep your upper back deep and straight and the muscles in your shoulder girdle totally relaxed as you lift your knees and start to carry your weight with your arms. Start moving back slowly as if someone behind you is pulling on your upper thighs (figure 9.2-22a). Do not allow your core to relax. The column produced by your transverse abdominals should support the curve in your lower back throughout the movement and, as a result, transfer movement and pressure to your hips and thighs.

9.2-22a

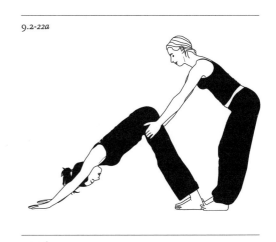

Note: It is much easier to practice this movement with bent legs in the beginning. This will keep your hamstrings relaxed and enable you to keep your sit bones in the same upward position. This, in turn, keeps your inner core stable. When your trunk has finished the movement, slowly straighten your legs without releasing the pressure in your hips.

9.2-22b

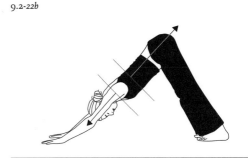

- At the same time, move your arms toward their end position, where your arms and shoulder blades "lock" into your ribs. In this position, there is also an end to the movement. Your shoulders are low, as described in chapter 6.3, number 4. Your elbows are high, and there is pressure to the inside edge of your hands.
- To lengthen your upper back, push your hands and hips away from each other as far as you can. Keep the image of lengthening your upper back in your mind's eye.

Note: When working out this extension, ensure that your shoulders do not collapse toward the floor, as this will break the connection to your back (see figure 9.2-19). Try to maintain the same alignment as when you felt the end of the movement (figure 9.2-22b).

- Relax your forefoot and ankles; lower your heels as far as you can toward the floor.
- Keep your breathing deep and relaxed, breathing from your abdomen to your chest. Allow your back to broaden when you inhale and to narrow when you exhale. Maintain the pose for 30 seconds to 1 minute. Occasionally, you can extend the time to 5 minutes.

5. Adho mukha svanasana II

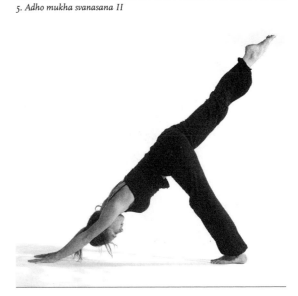

5. Adho Mukha Svanasana II

This asana is a good exercise for strengthening the lower back extension that can be difficult to achieve in Adho Mukha Svanasana I. You will not feel the extension in your lower back immediately, and you will feel it first in your hips. A strong pressure is directed to your hips in this variation, which prompts your body to bend correctly from your hips rather than from your lower back.

Instructions

- Stand in Adho Mukha Svanasana I and lift your right leg. Maintaining your inner tube keeps your lower ribs connected to your abdomen. When you lift your leg, your lower back will be pushed deeper, and your midback will remain stable.

> **Note:** Do not lead with your foot when lifting your leg; lead with your thigh. This was discussed with jumping up in Adho Mukha Vrksasana (see chapter 8.4, number 18). Keep your knee extended. Do not rotate the left side of your pelvis upward; keep it level with the left side.

- Give extra attention to your left ankle, which is now carrying the weight of your body. The added weight makes it easier to relax. Take advantage of this, and relax your calf, forefoot, and ankle.
- Remain in this pose for 20 seconds, then repeat on the other side. Or continue to the next exercise.

6. *Virabhadrasana III*

Virabhadra is the name of a warrior from Indian mythology.
Virabhadra was created from the armpit of the god Shiva (the lord of yoga). Together with the demon Ganas, he destroyed Daksha's sacrificial ceremony. Daksha's daughter, Sati, had committed suicide because of the insult of her father failing to invite her and Shiva to the sacrifice.

The order of the Virabhadrasanas in this book differs from the traditional sequence, because the poses here are categorized in another manner. Virabhadrasana III and II are discussed in this section, while Virabhadrasana I is discussed with backbends in chapter 9.5.

The following pose is described starting from Adho Mukha Svanasana II.

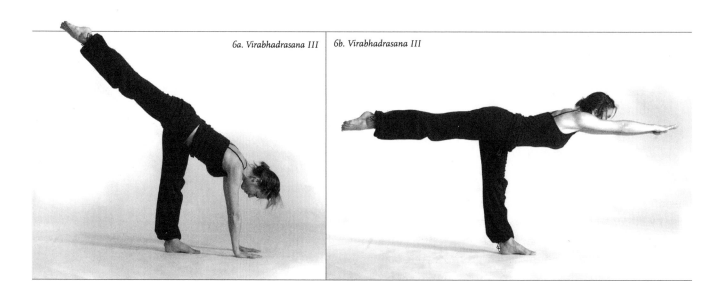

6a. Virabhadrasana III   *6b. Virabhadrasana III*

Instructions

- From Adho Mukha Svanasana II, with your feet together and your hands on the floor, move your right foot forward about 4 feet and push your abdomen against your upper thigh to activate your lower back. Place your fingertips on the floor next to your right foot, extend your neck, and look at the floor.

> **Note:** Almost everybody looks to the front and contracts their neck muscles after assuming the required foot position. This reflex, which tightens the neck muscles, occurs during many of the standing poses. It is possible to lift your head and look to the front without creating excess tension in your neck. To do this, you must extend your neck and connect it with your upper back (see chapter 6.3, numbers 2 and 3). If you do not establish this connection, the tension created in your neck will be maintained for the duration of the movement. This point will be worked out in detail in the following instructions.

- Bear your weight on the front part of your right heel and relax your right hip. Simultaneously relax your right hamstring. Your right sit bone will move up. Lift your left leg, aligning it with your back so that it supports the extension to your lower back. Your upper body also connects to your lower back and thus strengthens it when you reactivate your inner tube by correctly positioning your lower ribs.
- Your supporting leg is initially bent. Straighten it without losing the unity to the rest of your body, as shown in figure 9.2-23. Remember the guidelines given for the alignment of your leg in chapter 6.3, number 11.
- You can turn this into a balancing exercise by placing your hands together in a namaskar in front of you with your thumbs lightly touching the base of your sternum. Concentrate on your right foot and its balanced contact with the floor. When your leg is correctly aligned and your foot relaxes, the deep postural muscles of your ankle will activate and stabilize.
- In the traditional end pose, your arms are stretched out to the front with your eyes looking out over your thumbs. Hooking your thumbs together will help you relax your shoulders.

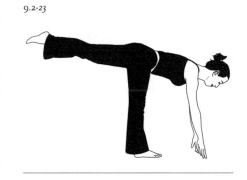

9.2-23

> **Note:** Now try to lift your head by connecting the back of your head to your upper back in the following manner. When you inhale deeply, your sternum will move toward the floor, which will lengthen your upper back. It is as if the movement of your sternum pulls your upper back inward. During an exhalation, allow your upper back to sink even deeper and connect to the movement of lifting your head and arms. This gives you the best chance of connecting your arms to your shoulder blades, and you will feel your neck align with your upper back all the way through to the area between your shoulder blades.

- Hold the end pose for 20 to 30 seconds. Bend your supporting leg and place your fingertips back on the floor. Move your left foot to the back of the mat and step back into Adho Mukha Svanasana. Repeat the movement on the other side.

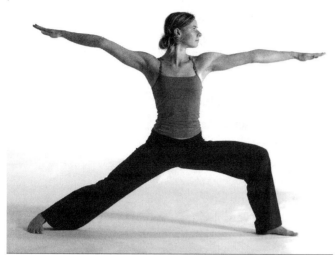

7. *Virabhadrasana II*

This is the second variation from the Warrior series.
This asana also presumes that supple hips are a necessity for a free and stable positioning of the pelvis and lower back. Virabhadrasana II focuses on the relationship between the inside thigh and the hip of the bent leg and the outside leg and hip of the stretched leg.

Before discussing the end pose, I will introduce two preparatory exercises that will prepare the insides of your legs. These are regularly used in the Indian dance tradition and in ballet training. I learned these exercises during my training in the Bharata Natyam dance tradition.

Groin stretch 1

Passive

9.2-24

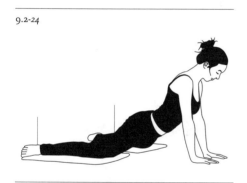

- Place two blankets in front of a wall and kneel on them with your knees wide apart. Place the soles of your feet against the wall at the same level as your knees and, with straight arms, lean on your hands (figure 9.2-24).
- Reengage your inner tube by activating your abdominals. Feel how your lower ribs move toward your abdomen and how contracting your lower abdominals up to your navel causes the area around your coccyx to become heavier. You will then feel the weight (pressure) of your upper body transfer into your coccyx instead of getting stopped in your lower back. When you feel your groin and inner thighs relax, slowly lower your pelvis. When your pelvis lowers, it should move toward the wall, not away from it. This will push your knees wider apart.
- When your pelvis nears the floor, you can lean on your elbows. Be careful to lead with your lower abdomen when moving toward the floor, not with your lower ribs, which have a tendency to move away from your pelvis.
- Remain in this pose for 2 to 3 minutes and then come up slowly. Follow immediately with the standing variation.

Groin stretch 2

9.2-25

Active

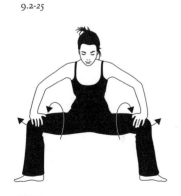

- Stand with your feet and knees approximately 3 feet apart and turn your feet out. Place your hands on the insides of your knees, bending your knees until your pelvis is level with them. Keep your balance on your heels. Using your hands, pull the insides of your knees up and push them farther apart (figure 9.2-25).

Note: Pulling the insides of your knees up rotates your thighs externally, which helps the hip area relax and allows your pelvis to lower. To understand this, study the arrows in figure 9.2-25.

- Keep moving the backs of your hips down while slowly lifting your trunk. The pressure you applied with your hands should be taken over actively by your legs. When you can spread your knees adequately, more of your weight will be borne on the outer edges of your feet.
- When your hips are flexible enough, your pelvis will be able to finish the movement and thus connect your diaphragm with the arch of your lower back and your pelvic floor. If the adductor muscles on the inside of your thighs are stiff, then your lower back will stay tense (figure 9.2-26a) or it will become jammed or strained (figure 9.2-26b). Your back will receive more freedom to align with your pelvis when your adductor muscles have more flexibility.
- Place your hands in a namaskar in front of your chest and try, even during these strenuous conditions, to experience the quality of relaxation that deep abdominal breathing provides. Remember the athletic and circulatory benefits of maintaining strenuous poses described at the beginning of this chapter.
- Carefully examine the angle that your thighs have made with your pelvis. Your bent leg will make the same angle during Virabhadrasana II. Keep actively spreading your knees apart.
- Remain in this pose for as long as you can. Repeat a couple of times if necessary.

When trying to lower your pelvis to the level of your knees, you will experience a strong limitation in the movement of your pelvis. The hara area of your lower abdomen and your knees rarely reach the same level. The advantage of this is that it becomes easier to isolate your pelvis in the end position, allowing you to engage the arch of your lower back properly. Virabhadrasana II is, therefore, eminently suitable to work out your lower back extension right up to your SI joints.

Virabhadrasana II can be initiated from Tadasana or Adho Mukha Svanasana.

From Tadasana

- Stand in Tadasana and jump your feet apart approximately 4 feet. Your heels should be even, level, and turned slightly outward.
- Place your hands on your hips, as shown in figure 9.2-27, and push your left thumb against the left greater trochanter, which is located on the outside of your thigh (figures 9.2-28a and 9.2-28b).

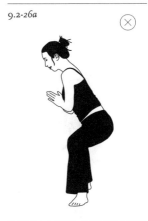

9.2-26a

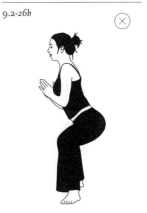

9.2-26b

9.2-27

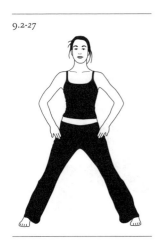

9.2-28a 9.2-28b

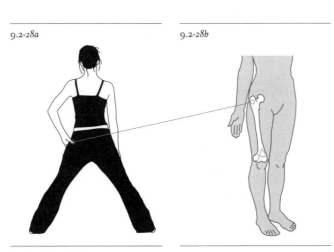

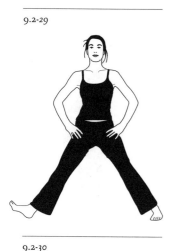

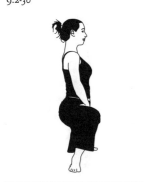

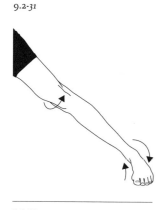

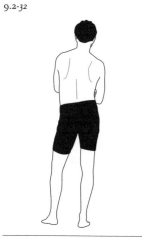

· Pivoting on your heel, turn your right foot out 90 degrees, and turn your left foot in 45 degrees. Do this without changing the position of your pelvis or rotating your upper body. Keep your right foot lifted (figure 9.2-29), as this will help you keep your pelvis level.

· Push your left thumb against the greater trochanter, as if you are initiating the movement from this pressure. Bend your right leg and gently lower your foot to the floor. Your left greater trochanter moves deeper and lowers when your right knee moves into a 90-degree angle. A crease will develop under your left thumb and index finger where your thigh meets your pelvis. It will become more pronounced as this area relaxes. Your pelvis remains balanced in the frontal plane.

· If you observe the position of your right thigh, you will see the same angle it made in the active groin stretch (figure 9.2-30). Energetically activate your right leg and move your knee out to the side as far as you can, without moving the greater trochanter under your left thumb forward or upward. The stretch to the inside of your right thigh will develop gradually. If your thigh falls inward, adapt the angle of your foot to follow the position of the thigh. After a time, when you knee can move farther, allow your foot to follow that movement.

· As you lower into the position, your left leg remains in contact with the outside edge of your left foot. The inside arch of your foot remains actively lifted. This movement toward the outside edge of your foot is initiated from the inside of your knee (see the arrows in figure 9.2-31).

Note: There may be problems in this pose if habitual lower back preferences are maintained (figure 9.3-32). When these occur, the greater trochanter of the thigh will move forward and up rather than backward and down. Then the right knee can easily be positioned above the ankle, but if the position is completed in this way, the lower back will tighten and limit the possibility of developing the position further. Look at the differences in the position of the pelvis and lower back in figures 9.2-33a with 9.2-33b.

· Keep your diaphragm in balance on top of the neutral arch of your lower back. Do not lift your lower ribs when you extend your upper back; follow the movement of your sternum, which originates from the inside out with a deep inhalation. At the end of your inhalation, position your neck effortlessly above your spine; do not feel that your back muscles have to engage for this.

9.2-33a

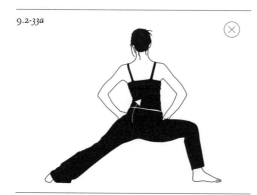

9.2-33b

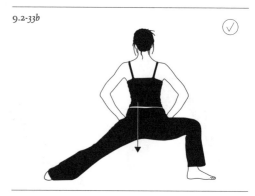

- Keep your core muscles engaged when you spread your arms; the insides of your elbows face forward. Relax the muscles between your neck and shoulders and broaden your shoulder girdle in the following three ways:
  1. With your arms horizontal, extend your thumbs away from your chest so your pectoralis major muscles consciously release and your collarbones broaden.
  2. Extend your little fingers away from your back so your shoulder blades broaden as if they were sliding doors being pulled open.
  3. Extend your middle fingers away from your neck, allowing the tops of your shoulders to broaden away from your neck. This is the area where your body weight rests on the headstand bench. When you turn your head to the right, maintain the connection between your neck and upper back.

Note: To become more conscious of the position of your head and neck, you can do the following coordination exercise: Fold your rubber strip in half and put it between your shoulder blades. Lie on it as described in chapter 6.3, connection 4. Relax for a while, making your spine heavier with each exhalation. Inhale slowly to the top of your sternum. Visualize your spine being pulled inward at the end of your inhalations. Stabilize this inward movement during your exhalations by pressing the back of your head against the strip. It will produce a feeling of lengthening of your spine. This movement can be imitated during standing poses when you face straight ahead. Imagine the rubber strip behind your head, giving a constant imaginary pressure.

The second variation can be used when your head rotates to either side. This happens in almost all standing poses, usually when there is no awareness of the connection between the head, neck, and spine. Indeed, the neck is often strained and contracted when rotated, especially in positions where the body is in a diagonal position, such as the poses described in chapter 9.3.

Rotate your head to the right and become aware of the pressure of the right edge of the strip in the area between your spine and your right shoulder blade. Imagine your inhalation will pull the ribs on that side of your spine farther in. Press the side of your head softly against the strip during your exhalations to stabilize the extension. Remember the spot on the side of your head touching the strip, and lengthen the side of your neck and spine by exerting pressure on the strip. This movement can be imitated in every standing pose where the neck is rotated to one side. It will create an awareness of the interaction between your breath, the extension of your spine, and the stable support of your neck that pulls the length in your spine and distributes the weight of your head in the area between your spine and shoulder blades.

Read about the release of the atlas muscle, described in chapter 6.3, connection 3.

- Keep your attitude relaxed and open, as if you are looking from the back of your head without tension in your eyes; feel that your eyes rest deeper than usual in their sockets.
- In the end position, connect your two gravity points while remaining conscious of lightness, space, and relaxation. Connect yourself to the space around you via your breathing, as if you are breathing through your skin; feel that you are filling the space around you and that the space around you is filling your body.

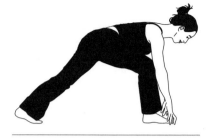

- Remain in this position for 20 to 60 seconds, straighten your bent leg, turn both feet to the front, lower your arms, and repeat on the other side.

From Adho Mukha Svanasana

- From Adho Mukha Svanasana I or II, take a large step forward with your right foot. Press your abdomen against your right thigh and lift your torso until your shoulders move down away from your neck and your fingertips rest on the floor (figure 9.2-34). Think about where your gaze will be in the end position, so your eyes can move fluidly toward that point. This will make the movement feel confident and open.
- Extend your lower back and lift your left arm. In one movement, allow your left arm to sweep up and back over your left foot so that the weight of your body is carried by your left hip and leg as described earlier.
- Try to complete this movement in a light, direct way. Feel the difference between moving hastily and moving directly with control. The latter occurs when you combine your movement with your breathing and remain conscious of the space around you.
- Remain in this position for 20 to 60 seconds, then place your hands back on either side of your right foot without pulling your shoulders up. Allow your lower back to carry your weight. Return to Adho Mukha Svanasana I or II, and repeat on the other side.

9.3   Standing poses: twists

Utthita Trikonasana, Parivrtta Trikonasana, Utthita Parsvakonasana, and Parivrtta Parsvakonasana are standing poses that all involve a rotated upper body. They strengthen the lower back and thus provide an ideal preparation for seated twists, where the rotation and the end position should be guided from the lower back.

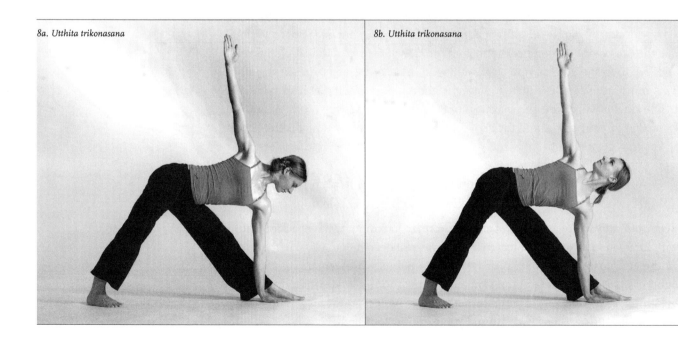

8a. Utthita trikonasana

8b. Utthita trikonasana

8. Utthita Trikonasana

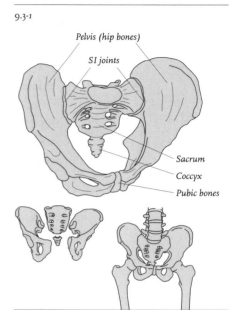

Utthita means "standing erect"; *tri* means "three"; *kona* means "angle."
Trikonasana focuses on strengthening the extension of the midline of the lower back that transports the body's weight to the sacrum and SI joints. The SI joints will distribute the body weight to the hips. This pose is meant to mobilize the SI joints (figure 9.3-1) that connect the sacrum with the two halves of the pelvis (hip bones). The following example illustrates how this area can become stiff (this was already shown for Virabhadrasana II and Utkatasana).

Many people develop the habit of standing on one leg, causing the lower back to collapse (figure 9.3-2), when they do such things as wait for the bus. The result is that the lower back becomes cramped in the quadratus lumborum muscles at one side of the spine. The position of the lower back and pelvis becomes asymmetrical, and the crunched hip stiffens. The weight of the body is not passed on to the SI joints; the lower back just above the pelvic rim bears the weight and becomes tight. Therefore, there is no proper distribution of body weight to the lower lower back (L4 and L5). These vertebrae are no longer part of the free chain of movement, making them stiff and rigid. These habitual positions are nearly always incorporated into Trikonasana, causing the asana to look like figure 9.3-3a. Compare this to figure 9.3-3b, where these patterns have been broken.

Movement in the area of the SI joints cannot be fully exploited because of tension caused by this postural preference. This can have serious consequences for walking in a free, energetic manner. If you walk with active SI joints, the energy for each step develops around these joints (figures 9.3-4a and 9.3-4b). This energy is generated by the elevation of the back leg. When the energy is passed on to the SI joint, your next step feels light and effortless. If the joint cannot move, which is often the case in elderly people, then walking becomes a careful shuffle.

When posture is stabilized from the side (see figure 9.3-2), preventing the free transfer of movement, tension increases in the SI joints. The movement stops at the iliac crest. Trikonasana focuses on strengthening and extending the properly arched lower back. This is important for people with a weak, painful lower back who find it difficult

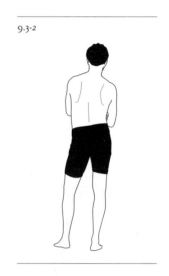

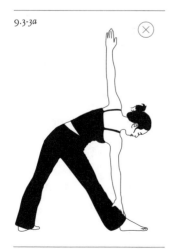

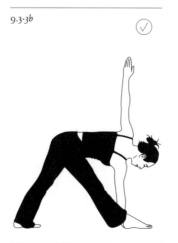

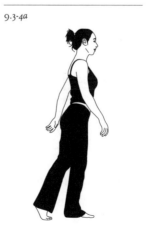

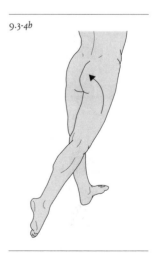

to stabilize this area in the standing variation of Dandasana (see chapter 9.2, number 3) because they are scared they will "put their back out." Releasing the tension to the side of your lower back is safe when your midline is strong.

When your correctly positioned lower back and pelvis can carry your body weight, the tension in your lower back will be replaced by strength in an extended, well-arched lower back. You will quickly realize that this also strengthens your legs. Some people flinch from the confrontation with tension and stiffness, while others shy away from building strength. Do not be surprised at the effort required by your legs; they must "carry" the relaxation of your back. Remember that strength stimulates free movement of the body, whereas tension oppresses the body and causes stiffness.

To stimulate relaxation in the quadratus lumborum muscles (see figure 6.3-53b) at the sides of the lower back and strengthen the midline of the lower back, I favor building this pose up from Adho Mukha Svanasana (see chapter 9.2, number 4). You can use Tadasana (see chapter 9.2, number 1) after you've gained enough practice with Adho Mukha Svanasana.

This asana is complicated and, as such, will be developed in stages. It is important when learning the pose that you stop at each step to allow the movement to work into your body. After some practice, you will be able to move fluidly.

From Adho Mukha Svanasana

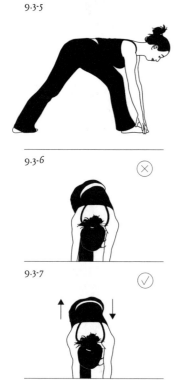

9.3-5

9.3-6 ⊗

9.3-7 ✓

· From Adho Mukha Svanasana, move your right foot about 3 feet forward and place your hands on either side of it. Do not hang with your trunk over your leg; immediately push your abdomen against your thigh so that your body weight shifts from your hands into your right hip. Raise your chest so that your shoulder blades are lowered (figure 9.3-5). Activate your lower back quickly after stepping forward; this will make the movement light and open.
· The pressure applied to your right hip allows it to relax, as in Utkatasana (see chapter 9.2, number 2), by allowing the muscles in the transition area between your thigh and abdomen to relax more. To stimulate this, carry your body weight on the front of your right heel and not on the ball of your foot. When your hip moves farther back, it will create more space in your SI joints. Take time to feel this.
· Turn your left heel in slightly and place it on the floor without losing the relaxation in your lower right back.

Note: Tension often develops in the lower back when the left foot is positioned, because this movement pulls the pelvis crooked, as shown in figure 9.3-6. For this reason, after turning your heel in, immediately rotate the left side of your pelvis forward so that your right hip is pulled back (see arrows in figure 9.3-7). Maintain this forward movement of the left side of your pelvis as you develop the pose further.

Note: Do not allow your right knee to rotate outward when turning your left heel in. Try to move your knee inward, creating a backward pressure in your groin.

- Place the palm of your right hand against the inside of your right ankle and the back of your left hand on your upper lower back precisely at the spot where your lower back feels most bent. Lift your upper body until you feel the extensors form a groove in your back under your left hand. After bringing your lower back into its neutral arched position, pull your lower ribs inward *without losing the extension in your spine.* Then pull the hara area up to your navel. Now your core is connected. This will increase the pressure on your right hip. Remain in this position and immerse yourself in it. Keep your weight on your right heel.

Note: Before you pull your lower ribs in, make sure the arch of your lower back is well extended. You can overextend the arch by making it as hollow as possible to learn the movement. That makes it easier to experience the break in the movement when your lower ribs move downward and connect your core.

- Without losing the extension in your lower back, straighten your right leg. To do this, dynamically engage the upper part of your thigh, feeling the thigh transfer the movement of your knee to your hip. Contract your thigh muscles and lift your kneecap. There should be an even distribution of pressure to the inside and outside of your right foot.
- Feel the presence of your inner tube. It should feel relaxed when you direct your breath there.
- Place your left hand on your heart region and feel the connection between your neck and this area (also see the coordination exercise mentioned under Virabhadrasana II, number 7, in this chapter). Breathe a feeling of lightness toward the area under your hand, and try to unite feelings of relaxation and lightness to the experience of breathing.
- Keep pressing your right hand against the inside of your right ankle, and rotate the area under your left hand upward.

9.3-8

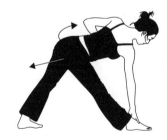

Note: A reflexive tension often develops in the lower right back the moment you start to rotate your chest upward, as shown in figures 9.3-3a and 9.3-6. This is an important moment for coordination. Be careful when turning your chest upward that the left side of your pelvis keeps moving forward. This allows the right side of your pelvis to move back, keeping your SI joints relaxed and mobile, as shown in figure 9.3-8.

9.3-9

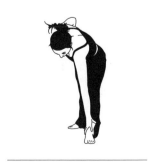

Keep your face exactly above your right foot; do not let it turn with your trunk. It is much easier to determine whether or not you are aligned when you keep your face stable. If your face is pushed forward during the rotation (figure 9.3-9), then your lower back is probably bent, although some students also bend in the midback, just under the shoulder blades. In that case, try to keep your face above your foot by straightening your back. Do not rotate your head up right away; instead, follow the instructions on page 209 in detail. Otherwise, the movement will create tension in your neck.

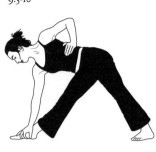

9.3-10

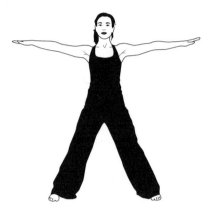

9.3-11

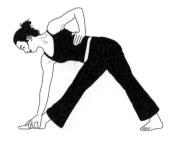

9.3-12

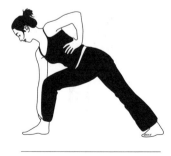

9.3-13

- Place your left hand on your waist, as shown in figure 9.3-10; allow the muscles in your left side to pull your ribs in so that your side becomes concave. Now you have created two types of activity, (the back and the side of the lower back) both having their own function: the strength in your side ensures that your weight is transferred to your right hip, while the groove in your lower back makes free rotation possible. If your lower back is bent, then it is impossible to rotate your upper back freely. (For instructions about how to rotate and the use of your hand, arm, and shoulder, see chapter 12.3, number 1.)
- There is still a balanced distribution of weight between the inside and outside of your foot. Your kneecap is aligned with the midline, pointing directly toward the middle of your foot.
- The development of this end position is directed toward stretching your hamstrings. When you feel that your hamstrings have lengthened, you can move your hand closer to your foot or to the inside of your foot. It should not lose the pressure to initiate the rotation. Elevate yourself so the muscles in your right side become active again and transfer pressure to your hip. Never lean on your hand; carry your weight with your legs and the superior left side.
- Lift your left arm and align it with your right arm. Keep your shoulders low, and feel your neck extend your back when you move your crown forward. Rotate your head and look at your left hand. Make sure your neck does not pull back and become tense during this movement (see the coordination exercise mentioned earlier).
- This pose will produce an extension in your hamstrings. When they start to release their tension, you can bring your right hand farther down. Always contract the muscles in your left side immediately after moving your right hand to convince yourself that the left side of your core remains stable.
- Maintain this pose for 30 to 60 seconds; allow your breath to circulate freely through your body (see chapter 5).
- Bend your right leg, rotate back to center and place your hands in front of you on the mat, and step back to Adho Mukha Svanasana. Repeat on the other side.

From Tadasana

- From Tadasana, jump your feet apart about 3 feet. Turn your heels slightly outward and straighten your legs. Extend your arms sideways at shoulder-height (figure 9.3-11).
- Rotate your right foot 90 degrees outward from the heel, and turn your left foot in slightly. Allow the left side of your pelvis to turn in slightly, but keep your shoulders in the same position above the baseline between your heels. Your chest should remain stable and not turn with your pelvis.
- Lift your right arm and place your left hand on your left side, just below your ribs. Pivot your upper body around your right hip and rotate, as explained earlier, with the left side of your pelvis forward so that your right hip can move backward freely. When your upper body is parallel with the floor, without losing control in your left side, bring your right hand against the inside of your right ankle and position your face above your right foot (figure 9.3-12).
- Check the space and relaxation in your two gravity points, and do not lose your alignment when you rotate your chest up to the left.

- Move sideways toward your leg as already described, but now keep your right leg bent. When you are deep enough, take hold of your ankle with your right hand and look at your foot (figure 9.3-13).
- Contract the muscles in your left side so you feel that you can lift your foot with your right hand. The ribs under your left hand are clearly pulled into your side. This will increase the pressure on your right hip, through which you can release the tension in your lower right back—a liberating feeling for stiff backs!
- Straighten your right leg without losing the traction of your hand on your right foot or the pressure in your right hip.
- If you do lose the pressure in your hip, rotate the left side of your pelvis farther forward.

From this point, follow the instructions given earlier for moving from Adho Mukha Svanasana.

- To return, place your left hand back on your waist. Lift your right arm until you feel your weight falling back into your right hip, and move from your pelvis back to a standing position.
- Turn your feet forward and repeat to the other side.

9. Parivrtta Trikonasana

9. Parivrtta trikonasana

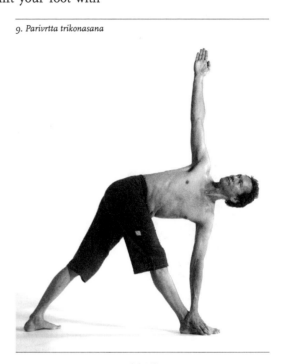

9.3-14a

Parivrtta means "rotated"; *trikonasana* means "triangle." (This is the rotated version of Utthita Trikonasana.)

Parivrtta Trikonasana is no mean feat with regard to coordination, flexibility, and technique. It is a difficult posture. If you are a beginner, take plenty of time to follow the steps described. If you are an experienced yoga practitioner who knows this pose, you must ask yourself if you tend to do it passively. By this I mean, do you lean on your hand, or are your legs and lower back bearing your weight. There is a world of difference between active and passive performance, and for this reason, I advise you to do this pose as if for the first time.

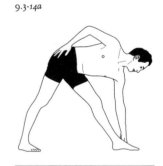

9.3-14b

The engaged use of your lower back and the relaxation of your hips are central here, but Parivrtta Trikonasana goes further than Utthita Trikonasana. It increases the rotation and therefore the flexibility of your spine. Another difference is in the position of your pelvis. In Utthita Trikonasana, it is positioned diagonally, but in Parivrtta Trikonasana, it is brought to a parallel position by the movement of your upper body. This increases the pressure to your right hip and the stretch to your hamstrings (figures 9.3-14a and 9.3-14b). If your hamstrings are stiff, this pose is a good preparation for seated forward bends, because it frees your hips and lengthens your hamstrings.

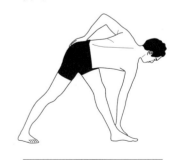

The pose will be built up from Adho Mukha Svanasana I or II, and then from Tadasana.

From Adho Mukha Svanasana

9.3-15a

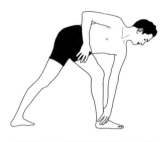

9.3-15b

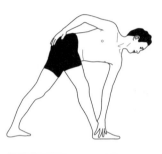

9.3-16a ⊗

9.3-16b ✓

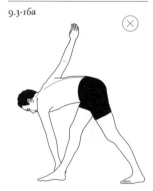

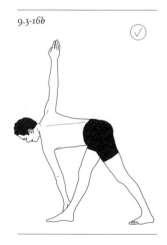

- From Adho Mukha Svanasana I or II, bring your right foot about 3 feet forward. Do not move it too far, as this will make it difficult to extend your lower back in the end position. Immediately place your hands on either side of your right foot and push your abdomen against your thigh to shift the gravity point into your pelvis. Keep your shoulders lowered. Remain here for some time, allowing the pressure to work into your right hip. (For some people, relaxation comes immediately, but those with stiff hips should stay a little longer and allow relaxation to develop slowly.) Try to relax the muscles in the fold between your thigh and abdomen by carrying your weight on the front of your right heel. This will allow the deeper postural muscles to stabilize your hip.

- Place your right hand on your thigh and take hold of your right lower leg or ankle with your left hand (figure 9.3-15a). Raise your body until your lower back feels well arched. It will be impossible to create a free rotation later if you do not give proper attention to the movement here. Lengthen your abdomen as much as possible by lifting your upper body, then pull your lower ribs inward. This will connect them with the arch of your lower back. Remember that the contraction of your abdominal muscles only works when your lower back has already been extended. This will initiate a passage of movement through the midline of your lower back. Pull the area under your navel upward to engage your core completely.

- After stabilizing your core, rotate the left side of your abdomen as far as possible toward your right thigh. Position your face above your right foot and straighten your right leg slowly (figure 9.3-15b). Visualize the lengthening of your hamstrings and the upward movement of your right sit bone when you stretch your leg. This release of your upper leg muscles will keep your core stable.

- Carry your weight increasingly with your lower back instead of your hand, and maintain your balance by turning your right leg in and pushing the inside of your foot firmly into the floor. Your right leg turns inward, and the inside of your foot pushes your groin backward.

> **Note:** Your hips and hamstrings need a lot of flexibility to carry your weight with an extended lower back. For beginners, this position becomes the end pose. The rotation can be developed further only when your extended lower back and legs are able to carry your weight. Take time to stabilize your body in this position before moving on. If you try to rotate too soon, your back will return to its habitual position, which usually means that the twist develops from a bend in the lower vertebrae. Then the lower back loses its stability. Remember that the normal lordotic curve of the lower back is its stable position. To see this, compare figures 9.3-16a and 9.3-16b.

Problems that can develop with this pose and ways to deal with them are as follows:

1. If you find it difficult to maintain your balance, broaden your stance, place your back heel diagonally against a wall, or both (figure 9.3-17).

2. If you find it difficult to carry your weight with your lower back, place your hands on a chair or yoga block and slowly allow your lower back to take over. You do not have to

do this all at once. You can start by dividing your weight between your hand, back, and legs. Do not use the all-or-nothing strategy; allow the strength to develop gradually in your lower back and legs.

3. The upper body often ends diagonal to the baseline (the line that runs from the front heel to the back heel) when the lower back is asked to carry the weight. Then the hip and lower back revert back to their tension-related habitual postures (figure 9.3-18). The correct use of your hip is important here. Try to maintain your upper body exactly above the baseline and extend the upper part of your lower back. This will ensure that your face remains directly over your front foot. Then your body will be in a good position to start rotating.

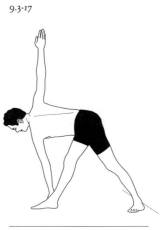

9.3-17

· Place your left hand against the outside of your right ankle. Connect your left upper arm with your shoulder blade and rotate your chest up to the right by pushing your hand against your ankle. This rotation is much greater than in Utthita Trikonasana and can be taken farther. The development of the rotation is synonymous with the development of the extension of the upper back. Therefore, it will have an effect on the extremities of the spine: your neck will lengthen, and your hip will extend farther back. To follow the movement of your hip, you can place your right hand on your right buttock to feel if movement occurs there (see figure 9.3-15b).

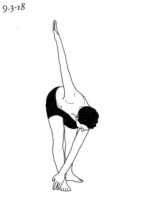

9.3-18

· Keep turning your right leg inward as you increase the rotation to your upper back. The ankle often collapses outward at this point, causing students to fall. Your back leg should be straight and pressure applied to the outside of your left foot. By carrying your lower back actively, the movement is brought back into the center of your body (the hara). That does not mean both legs will carry the same amount of weight. More weight will be transferred to your back leg when that hip can assimilate the movement better. This will create more stability, but most of your weight will be carried by your front leg and foot.

9.3-19

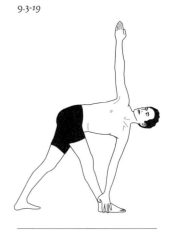

· When the rotation of your chest is complete, stretch your right arm straight up, aligning it with your left arm. Finally, turn your face toward your right hand (figure 9.3-19).

· When your lower back has provided space to the hara and you are able to relax into your breathing, you can connect your neck to your heart gravity point. Try to develop

Note: Compare figure 9.3-16a with figure 9.3-16b from the perspective of the position of the upper arm and shoulder. In the first figure, the upper shoulder is strained. There is no connection with the shoulder blade. In the second figure, the shoulder blade gives the upper arm an open foundation to "stand on." The arm and shoulder blade are well connected, and there is a free passage of movement in the shoulder. This gives the extension of the arm an open feeling of being strongly connected to the space you are in. From this point of view, the arm functions as an antenna that receives a feeling of space that can fill your entire body.

The image of an antenna may be helpful. It can be used in all standing poses where the arms are extended and properly connected to the shoulder blades. The extension of your legs can be used to develop a strong feeling of moving in space as well. Because you are able to lengthen the lines of your body in space through these "antennae," your arms and legs become metaphorically endless.

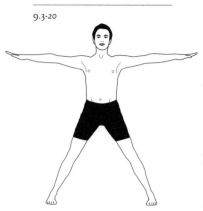

9.3-20

a feeling of lightness in this area. Connect the two gravity points so that, even in this intricate end position, the active aspect of holding the end position does not become the goal. Allow yourself to carry the pose with lightness and relaxation so you can connect intuitively with the space around you.

· Remain in this end position for 20 to 60 seconds. Then bend your right leg, rotate back to center and place your hands in front of you on your mat, and move back to Adho Mukha Svanasana I or II. Repeat this pose to the other side.

From Tadasana

Read the earlier instructions for Adho Mukha Svanasana.

· From Tadasana, jump with your feet approximately 3 feet apart. Extend your arms sideways at shoulder-height (figure 9.3-20).
· Pivot your right foot on your heel, turning it out 90 degrees, then turn your left foot in 45 degrees.

> **Note:** Try to keep your pelvis level when turning your feet. If it is misaligned in this phase, it can substantially limit the possibility of free movement. To prevent this problem, it is best to lift the front of your right foot and rotate it outward on the heel before turning the left foot in. When placing your right foot on the ground, move the left side of your pelvis inward to prevent misalignment. See the difference in figures 9.3-21a and 9.3-21b. Distribute your balance evenly between both hips.

· Keep your lower back stable in its extension and feel how your inner tube transfers weight to your tailbone. Place your left hand on the base of your sternum and rotate as far as you can to the right. The muscles of your back create the rotation. Make sure your right arm does not take over the initiative to twist, as this will disturb the free position of your shoulder blade.
· Place your right hand on your right buttock or sit bone, lift your left arm, and pivot around your hip as far as your hamstrings allow, without bending your lower back (figure 9.3-22).

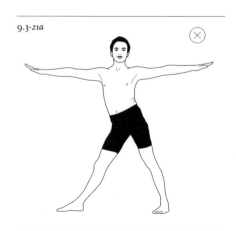

9.3-21a

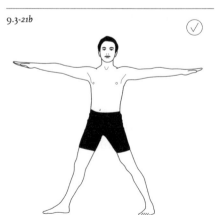

9.3-21b

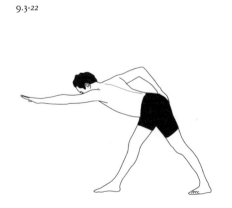

9.3-22

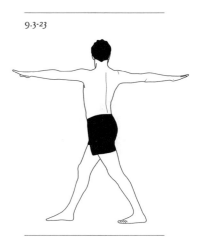

- Without bending your back, place your left hand against the outside of your right calf and feel the stable position of your lower back and the relaxation in both shoulders. Then rotate your chest farther up by pushing your left hand against the outside of your right leg (you can also place your right hand on your heart region instead of your right buttock to guide the extension of your neck and upper back from this point). Rotate the left side of your stomach and chest simultaneously toward the plane of the baseline between your feet, and extend your back to provide space to your heart region. Hold your right shoulder exactly above the left. Everything turns, except for your face which ends up above your right foot. Your right hip stretches farther back and your neck lengthens in order to connect with the heart region under your right hand.
- Lift your right arm and turn your face upward to look at your hand following the axis of your arm.

In regard to your legs and breathing, read the instructions in the description for "From Adho Mukha Svanasana."

- To come out, lift your left arm parallel to the floor. Pivot around your pelvis until you are standing as shown in figure 9.3-23.
- Turn your chest and feet to the front and repeat to the other side.

10. Utthita Parsvakonasana

***Utthita* means "erect"; *parsva* means "side"; and *kona* means "angle." (This is the extended side version of Virabhadrasana II.)**
This pose is similar to Utthita Trikonasana (see chapter 9.3, number 8) with respect to the position of the pelvis and the effect on the mobility of the SI joints, but it involves a bent front leg. Because of this, there is no constraint from the hamstrings in the bent leg's hip movement. This constraint makes the extension in the hip and lower back much more intense and makes the pose harder to maintain. This asana combines the benefits of Utthita Trikonasana and Virabhadrasana II.

This pose can be built up from Adho Mukha Svanasana (see chapter 9.2, number 4) or from Virabhadrasana II (see chapter 9.2, number 7).

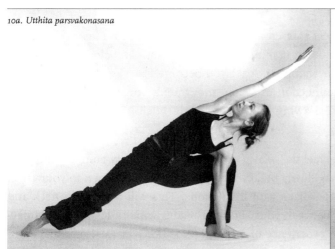

10a. Utthita parsvakonasana

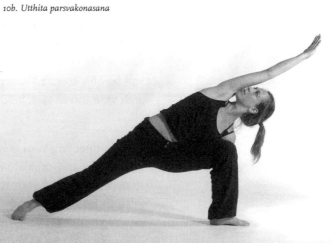

10b. Utthita parsvakonasana

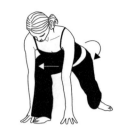

From Adho Mukha Svanasana I or II

- From Adho Mukha Svanasana, take a large step forward with your right foot so that your knee ends up in a 90-degree angle. Extend your lower back by pushing your abdomen into your thigh, allowing your shoulders to lower and your neck to rise and connect with your upper back and sternum.
- Feel how the extension of the upper part of your lower back pushes your right hip and the right side of your pelvis farther back. Increase the relaxation here by carrying your weight on your right heel and turning the left side of your pelvis forward.
- Keep the left side of your pelvis turning forward as far as possible as you position your back (left) foot on the floor. This will help to prevent your pelvis from ending in a diagonal. To make this easier, push your right knee against your upper arm (see the arrows in figure 9.3-24).
- Move the outside of your left foot toward the floor by turning your left leg outward and activating the inner arch of your foot.

From here, the end position can be done in various ways. A buildup in the sequence of movement is based on the use of the upper side engaged in combination with the front leg, which should remain at a 90-degree angle. This is often difficult to achieve, but it is easier to start with less of a bend in the front leg (meaning a less acute angle) and gradually move down to 90 degrees.

End position 1

- Place the upper part of your right arm against the inside of your knee, and put your hands together in front of your sternum. You are now free to change the height of your right thigh; use this freedom to position your straight leg correctly. From the inside of your left knee, turn your leg toward the outside of your left foot so the heel moves away from your body (see figure 9.2-31).
- As soon as you have established your straight leg, position your upper body over the baseline between your feet by moving your lower abdomen forward and extending your neck so that your face is above your right foot (figure 9.3-25).

> **Note:** To learn how to connect your core, always be certain that your lower back is arched. Arch it excessively at first, making it as hollow as you can before you bring your lower ribs toward your abdomen. After you become more experienced, you will be able to effect the connection in a fluid movement, but even then, always arch your lower back before drawing your ribs inward.

- After connecting your core, feel the relaxation in your hara gravity point during your inhalations and exhalations. Slowly breathe from your lower abdomen to your chest in order to extend your upper back with inhalations. This will bring your neck and head in line with the area between your shoulder blades without losing the connection to your core. With the experience of relaxation in your core, a strong feeling of lightness will spread through your entire body.

- In this end position, allow your knee to return slowly to 90 degrees and be mindful that the movement comes from the relaxation of your hamstrings and hip. This allows your sit bone to move farther back. It will produce more pressure and therefore more relaxation in your hip. It will also produce more strength at the front of your thigh. When this becomes a habit after sustained practice, your end position will become lighter. Use gravity to bend your leg; go with it instead of fighting it.

> **Note:** The release of your hamstrings and the aforementioned effects are very intense. Some people describe it as hard labor. I do not think that is the case. Rather, it is a strong release that produces intense feeling that is comparable to hard work. It is interesting to examine whether the release in your hip or the working part of your leg is what bothers you in the end position. When your strength comes to an end, your leg will start to shake involuntarily. But you will observe relaxation at the same time from the experience of open awareness produced by breathing.

- The contact of your upper arm with your knee is important. When you use your upper right side to place your body weight over your right hip, this part of your arm lifts the inside of your knee slightly higher, which should be your intention. Your shoulder should not carry your weight, as this will cause your upper arm and shoulder to sink toward the ground. Your weight should be carried by the left side of your core, which should end in a contracted position as it does in Utthita Trikonasana.

End position 2

- Place your fingers or the palm of your right hand on the inside of your right foot without leaning on it. When you have positioned your hand, release your hamstrings and hip by carrying your weight on your right heel. Lift your upper body toward your right hip. Your left side will feel hollow, active, and strong. Move your pelvis forward, and keep your face above your right foot.

> **Note:** Your arm can keep your knee in the correct position when you place it on the inside of your knee. A meaningful stretch will develop in your right groin when you move your pelvis forward.

- Rotate your chest upward and stretch your left arm up alongside your head. Make sure you keep your diaphragm relaxed in this position so that your lower ribs remain connected to your stomach. Your right hip and buttock keep moving backward in relation to your lower back. The left side of your pelvis moves forward (figure 9.3-26).
- The same rules apply here as in Utthita Trikonasana: your left (upper) side brings your body weight over your right hip, which allows the muscles around the hip to relax. The correct extension of your lower back makes it possible to rotate your upper back freely.
- The ribs on the left side of your chest should remain low when your arm moves over your head connected with your left side. Do not

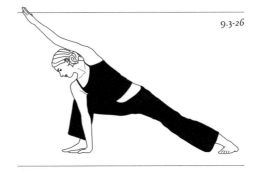

9.3-26

loosen the grip in the muscles in your left side when your arm moves over your head, but rather keep them active and engaged. The ribs on the left side of your chest should remain low.

- Remain in this end position for 20 to 30 seconds, then move back to Adho Mukha Svanasana or go immediately into the following position.

End position 3

- From end position 2, move your right arm to the outside of your knee without losing the strength in your left side. Push your thigh against your upper arm (figure 9.3-27). Now all the strength to stretch your groin must come from your leg.
- Position your face above your right foot. Without collapsing your neck, turn your face to the ceiling.
- This is the classic end position. Maintain it for 20 to 30 seconds. Then move back into Adho Mukha Svanasana I or II, or go directly into the following variation.

Variation

- Bring your right arm under your right thigh and your left arm down behind your back; clasp your hands together (figure 9.3-28). Place your right wrist on your right buttock to feel that your buttock is still moving away from your lower back.
- Constantly pay attention to the position of your lower ribs because they have a tendency to move too far up in this pose. Develop this movement by relaxing your buttock and allowing relaxation and mobility to develop around your SI joints.

From Virabhadrasana II

- From Virabhadrasana II (see chapter 9.2, number 7), with your right foot turned outward, lift your right arm and place your left hand on the left side of your pelvis. Contract the muscles in your left side and bend forward slowly without losing the control of that side. When the hamstrings of your right leg relax during the movement of your trunk, it will produce more pressure in your hip joint. This makes it possible to relax the movement muscles of your right hip even more.
- Turn the left part of your pelvis forward slightly so that your right lower back can relax.
- Observe and maintain the pressure on the outside of your left foot, and keep your inside arch active.

9.3-27   9.3-28

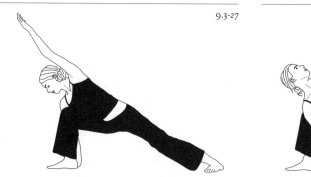
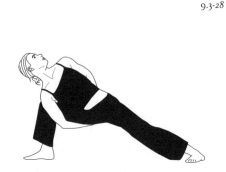

Note: The release of tension in your right hip will have an immediate effect on the release of the quadratus lumborum muscles on the right side of your lower back. Make sure that when your right lower back relaxes, you do not lose the rotation in your chest. If your chest falls inward when your lower back relaxes, it means you have not only lost the tension in your left side but also the extension and strength in the center line of your lower back (which will bend). Then the higher part of your lower back will no longer be in a position to carry your weight. When you notice this has happened, arch your lower back by pulling your shoulders backward. Then bring your lower ribs down to connect your diaphragm with the extension of your lower back. This will stabilize your core in this pose.

You should now be able to increase your rotation without using force. If you cannot lower your trunk completely, place your hands in front of your chest so that you can push against your knee with your arm or elbow to recover the rotation of your chest. You will end in position 1 (see figure 9.3-25). Remain in this position to increase the strength in your lower back.

Note: When your right hip, lower back, and buttock have relaxed, keep your left heel turned slightly outward. If your lower back contracts on the right side, then your left ankle will collapse inward. Thus, the position of your foot tells you what is happening in your lower back.

- Without losing the contraction in your left side, choose which of the three end positions you want to move to, or do all three sequentially.
- Remain in the end position for 20 to 30 seconds, then lift your right arm and feel your weight falling back toward your left side. This action transports weight to your pelvis, allowing you to move from your pelvis into Virabhadrasana II. If you have enough strength, end with your knee at a 90-degree angle, with a well-placed left hip and your arms extended.
- To come out, straighten your right leg and turn your feet forward. Repeat on the other side.

11. Parivrtta Parsvakonasana

Parivrtta means "rotated"; *parsva* means "side"; *kona* means "angle."
(This is the rotated version of Utthita Parsvakonasana.)
Just as in Parivrtta Trikonasana, the hip is extended backward so that both hips can be brought into line to complete the rotation of the upper body. Together with the extension of the lower back, the hips are extended as much as possible, allowing the deep muscles to stabilize the joints.

This powerful rotation is built up in phases. Every step is, in itself, a complete end position. For this reason, seek the one that is most effective for you. Note that your lower back is central to the development of the pose (also see chapter 10.2, coordination exercise 1). By elevating your body, you will be able to apply connection 6 (see chapter 6.3), which allows you to use your arms to increase the stretch in your lower

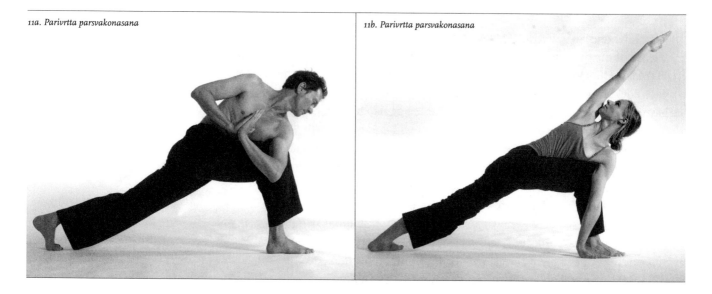

back. Do this by pushing your elbow or upper arm against your thigh rather than by pulling on your feet.

The pose can be built from Adho Mukha Svanasana (see chapter 9.2, number 4) or Virabhadrasana II (see chapter 9.2, number 7). For beginners, I recommend starting from Adho Mukha Svanasana, because you can place your back knee on the ground, avoiding balance problems, and the asana can be built more slowly and with more precision.

End position 1

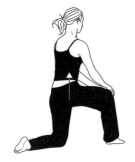

- Kneel on your mat and move your right foot forward so that your knee is above your ankle. Feel the difference between contracting your lower back and hip muscles by rotating your right outer thigh and hip upward (figure 9.3-29a) and then allowing them to lower and relax (figure 9.3-29b). Imagine there is a weight hanging off your upper thigh. Ensure that your knee does not turn outward during this movement. Carefully observe and maintain this relaxation, because your hip can develop tension easily, especially in the later position when your back leg is elevated.
- Extend your abdomen toward your thigh, keeping your shoulders low. Breathe in and out a few times, and accept the pressure around your hip by carrying your weight on your right heel.

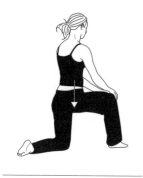

Note: Observe your breathing in the area below your navel very carefully. Read the instructions in chapter 6.3, connection 1 (the balance between the two centers of gravity). In this pose, this connection means that the end of every exhalation should produce a movement toward your leg at the hara level of your abdomen. This should happen throughout the whole exercise. When your lower abdomen starts to contract at the end of your exhalations, it tells you there is no proper support from your lower back.

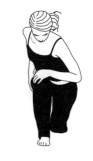

9.3-30

- Place your right hand against your right thigh, and hold your right knee with your left hand. Lift your trunk slightly higher, and feel the space and relaxation in your abdomen. Breathe into your abdomen. Pulling on your knee, start to rotate your chest to the right. This rotation extends into your abdomen, causing the left side of your abdomen to rotate toward your thigh. Your face should remain in the same position you started with, exactly above the floor just to the inside of your right foot (figure 9.3.30).
- When your abdomen can rotate no farther, press your right hand firmly against your thigh. This keeps your abdomen relaxed, while you place your left elbow against the outside of your right knee. Keep carrying your weight with your lower back, and increase the pressure of your left elbow against your knee to connect your arm with your shoulder blade. This allows your chest to turn farther toward your leg.
- Your upper arm connects with your shoulder blade and also with your lower back. Try to move in such a way that the pressure of your arm helps you extend your lower back. This will provide more space in your abdomen, chest, shoulders, and neck, and you will feel more pressure on your right hip (figure 9.3-31).
- When you have worked out the rotation and extension, place your palms together with your thumbs against the base of your sternum.

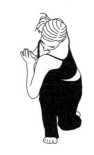

9.3-31

> **Note:** If you have not adequately developed the *rotation,* your thumbs will end on the right side of your chest (figure 9.3-32a). If the *extension* is not adequately developed, your hands will be too close to your chin (figure 9.3-32b). A combination of the two is also possible (hands too high on the right side of the chest and too close to the chin). In this situation, your back will bend under your right shoulder blade (see the arrows in figure 9.3-32c). The movement of your neck and right arm will not converge there to allow your back to extend. For all of these examples, the solution lies in working out the extension to your lower back so that you can develop both the extension and the rotation needed.

- When you use your lower back correctly, the skin of your knee will be lifted where your upper arm touches the outside of it. This lift also has consequences for your groin, to which much of your body weight will now be directed. When the outside of your knee lifts slightly, your groin moves down, and this—together with pressure from your right heel—ensures that your groin and hip can relax.

9.3-32a

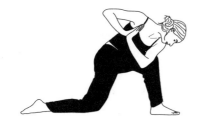

9.3-32b

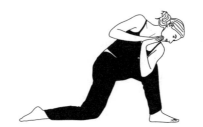

9.3-32c

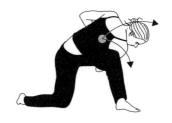

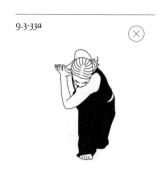

9.3-33a

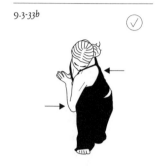

9.3-33b

- This is end position 1. Breathe regularly from your hara gravity point to your heart gravity point. If necessary, breathe slightly faster, which may encourage a freer movement in your back. Remain in this position for 20 to 30 seconds. Come out of the pose slowly and repeat on the other side.

End position 2

- The buildup of the pose is the same here as for end position 1, except for the positioning of your left arm. This should now slide further alongside your right knee toward the floor. In figure 9.3-33a, the elbow points diagonally downward. In this position, the upper arm cannot work effectively as a lever with the shoulder blade to turn the chest toward the leg. In figure 9.3-33b, the arrows show how this leverage should take place. Placing your arm lower in this way makes it difficult to extend your lower back, but it does have the following advantage.

The significance for the diaphragm when placing the arm lower

The advantage of sliding your arm along your knee from elbow to shoulder is that this movement prevents you from lifting your diaphragm. In twists such as in Parivrtta Parsvakonasana, as well as in seated twists (see chapters 12.3 and 12.4), the extension of your lower back often causes your diaphragm to "lift" erroneously. This is the same as the compensatory movement discussed for Utkatasana (see figure 9.2-9b), and it has two undesirable effects: the lower back loses its extension toward the pelvis, and the upper back contracts under the shoulder blades. This can also occur when your chest is stretched. Because of this, the extension of your back must be a subtle movement done with full attention. You must consider the different connections, such as your inner tube (see chapter 6.3, number 1) and the connection between your neck and your sternum (see chapter 6.3, number 3). They must be positioned correctly in relation to each other. These connections can only be worked out effectively when the position of your diaphragm is stable, which occurs in this pose when your arm slides below your knee. Then inhalations can isolate the extension of your upper back, producing more stability in your neck extension.

In this pose, the power to work out the extension of your back is created by the collaboration of your arm and lower back, through which the movement is brought strongly into your upper back. Many people have difficulty stretching this area (see chapter 6.3, numbers 2 and 3). Although your ribs should remain connected to your abdomen in the end pose, they must not feel blocked, because this causes you to lock up in the chest and abdomen. That, in turn, makes the pose unworkable, and your breath will no longer have an open passage from your abdomen to your chest.

- In the beginning, your face moves with whichever arm you place over your knee. But when you develop the extension in your back, your neck will be able to direct the weight of your head between your shoulder blades more and more. Then your face will return to its place above the inside of your foot.
- Breathe regularly—if necessary, a little faster—from gravity point to gravity point. Remain in this position for 20 to 30 seconds. Come out of the pose slowly and repeat on the other side, or carry on to end position 3.

End position 3

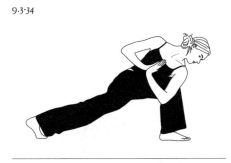

9.3.34

- From end position 2, lift the knee of your left leg (figure 9.3-34) without allowing your right thigh to rise (see the comments for end position 1). Lifting your back knee will allow your lower back to stretch deeply, causing your groin to move farther back. The effect is similar to that of the raised leg in Adho Mukha Svanasana II (see chapter 9.2, number 5).
- Make sure the weight of your body does not fall into your shoulders. Keep your upper body high enough that you can lift the outside of your right knee with your left upper arm. It is important that you keep your hamstrings, groin, and hip relaxed at this moment.

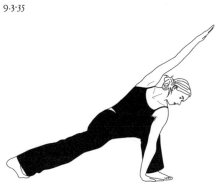

9.3.35

- Because of the new impetus to your lower back, you can now stretch your upper body farther toward your crown. This stronger extension provides more room for the rotation of your back. Rotate your chest farther, and lower your shoulders.
- Keep looking down in this end position, as this is better for balance and orientation. Keep your gaze on the floor just to the inside of your foot. This will provide awareness for the direction of your stretch.
- Keep breathing freely and, if necessary, slightly faster than normal. If you can keep your breathing free, you will become more relaxed and be able to extend and rotate more. Remain in this pose for 20 to 30 seconds. Return slowly and repeat on the other side, or carry on to end position 4.

End Position 4

- Place your left hand or fingertips on the floor against the outside of your right foot, rotate your chest upward, and place your right hand on your left thigh. Turn your right palm upward and stretch your arm over your head. This allows your entire trunk to stretch farther from your right groin (figure 9.3-35).
- Keep looking down, and breathe as freely as possible.

> **Note:** If you relax your abdomen, you will be able to extend your arm even farther. This can happen when you maintain your right knee at 90 degrees and keep your groin in the same position. It is the hip rather than the abdomen that tends to follow the movement of the arm. This is incorrect: when the hip is raised, tension develops.

- Breathe as freely as possible; if necessary, breathe somewhat faster than normal. If you can keep your breathing free, you will become more relaxed, as well as increase your extension and rotation. Remain in this pose for 20 to 30 seconds. Return slowly and repeat on the other side, or carry on to end position 5.

End position 5

- Turn your back (left) heel slowly to the floor without allowing your body to fall into a diagonal. Keep your abdominal muscles relaxed.

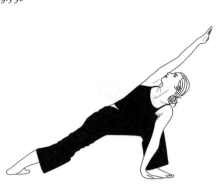

- Keep your face over the same area on the inside of your foot as in end position 4. Once you have positioned your heel, turn your head and gaze along the inside of your raised arm (figure 9.3-36). This is the end position.
- When you are able to connect your neck to your upper back in this position (or in the previous positions), your upper thoracic vertebrae get more space because of the strong extension of your neck. This can lead to faster and deeper breathing. Go with this reflex and ensure that your chest does not collapse when you exhale. Try to keep your chest open and broad with each exhalation.
- Stay in this position for 20 to 30 seconds. Return slowly and repeat on the other side.

9.4 Standing poses: leg stretches

Dandasana (standing), Virabhadrasana III, Utthita Trikonasana, Parivrtta Trikonasana, Parsvottanasana, Adho Mukha Svanasana II, and Ardha Chandrasana form the subgroup of standing poses also directed toward stretching the legs. Ardha Chandrasana and Parsvottanasana are described in this chapter; the others were described in the previous chapters. All of these asanas develop the lower back strength necessary for seated forward bends and are particularly important if you experience difficulty stretching in those poses.

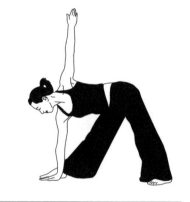

12. Ardha Chandrasana

Ardha means "half"; *chandra* means "moon."
In this pose, the body looks like a half moon—hence, the name. Ardha Chandrasana is a balance pose in which extension is developed in the standing leg. Correct balance is essential for developing relaxation around the large muscles of the hip, and weight is conducted through the muscles on the upper side of the body toward the hip of the standing leg. Relaxing the supporting foot helps to stabilize the postural muscles in the ankle. It is best to develop Ardha Chandrasana from Utthita Trikonasana.

Instructions

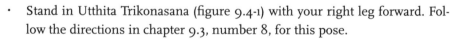
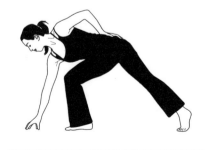

- Stand in Utthita Trikonasana (figure 9.4-1) with your right leg forward. Follow the directions in chapter 9.3, number 8, for this pose.
- Bend your right leg and place the fingertips of your right hand about 8 inches in front of your right foot. Extend your neck and look at your hand (figure 9.4-2). Bring your left hand down to your left hip, per the figure. Maintain the extension to your lower back, and observe it by directing your attention to your left shoulder. If your shoulder bends forward, your lower back has collapsed. To prevent this, keep your shoulder in the correct position during the movement and maintain the extension in the higher part of your lower back. Relax your right hip and the right side of your lower back; stretch both

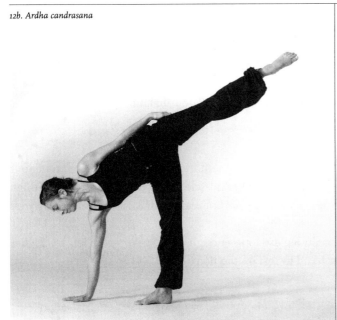

12b. Ardha candrasana

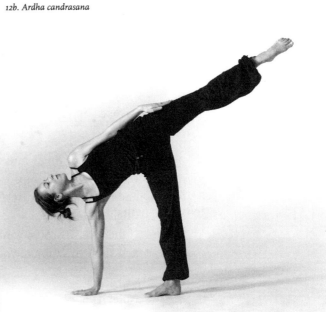

12b. Ardha candrasana

of these areas toward your left heel. The pressure developed in your hip transfers your body weight toward the upper part of your right thigh, which is then activated. This movement is developed later, but it is important to take the time to allow your thigh to accept the pressure, as this decides whether or not your hip can relax in the subsequent development of the movement.

· Push your right heel firmly into the ground to stimulate further relaxation in your right hip and lift your left heel (see figure 9.4-2).

· Keep your balance on the front of your right heel and lift your left leg sideways until you feel the muscles in your left side contract. The contraction of these muscles increases the pressure on your right hip, which accepts the pressure with relaxation when you remain correctly balanced on your right heel and keep your hamstrings relaxed. During this movement, keep your left shoulder high and your face positioned over your right hand (figure 9.4-3).

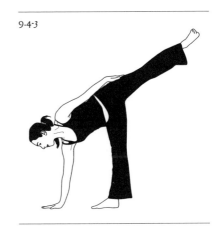

9.4-3

Note: Be aware of your left leg, as it often moves out of the frontal plane, causing tension to develop in your lower back. This will disturb the extension of your lower back, the control of your inner tube, and the relaxation in your hara gravity point.

You can do the following exercise to test how far your left (back) leg should move:

1. Lie supine on a block or yoga mat, with your knees bent.
2. Push your lower abdomen slowly against the floor; breathe into your lower abdomen, allowing it to expand.
3. Extend your knees and elevate your legs from the pressure on your lower abdomen.   *(continued)*

4. Because your pelvis remains in its neutral position, you will feel an end to the lifting movement of your legs. This is the same end you can feel in your left leg in Ardha Chandrasana when you imagine pushing your lower abdomen into the block. The push can be simulated by your inhalation, filling the space of your lower abdomen and moving it forward. The inhalation pulls your lower back into its neutral arch.

- Activate your thigh muscles so you can feel them transferring the extension of your right knee to your hip. To do this, activate the muscles from the hip end of your thigh and not from the muscles directly above your kneecap. Your kneecap is lifted by your thigh muscles.
- If the hamstrings of your right leg are long enough, you can lift your left leg higher and allow the palm of your hand to rest on the floor.

Note: If your leg muscles are not long enough, do not bend your side. Instead, use a block to elevate your hand, or bend your leg slightly in the beginning.

- Once your balance is secure, turn your head to the left and look upward.
- Remain in this position for 20 to 30 seconds, connecting your two gravity points with your breathing.
- Give your full attention to returning to Utthita Trikonasana.
  1. Slowly bend your right leg while keeping your right shoulder in position. Feel the pressure in your right hip, and place your left foot on the floor without losing the control in your left side.
  2. Place your right hand against the inside of your ankle and extend your right leg. Maintain the feeling that the extension of your right knee is passed on to your right hip without losing the strength in your left side.
- Follow the instructions for Utthita Trikonasana, then repeat Ardha Chandrasana on the other side.

13. Parsvottanasana

Parsva means "side"; *uttana* means "stretched out."
This pose is built up from Adho Mukha Svanasana I or II, with the legs alternately stretched forward. It is an intense stretch for the hamstrings of the front leg; for this reason, it is an ideal preparation for the seated forward bends described in chapter 10.5.

Instructions

- From Adho Mukha Svanasana I or II (see chapter 9.2, numbers 4 and 5), with your right leg about 3 feet forward, push your abdomen against your thigh to activate your lower back. After this, with your fingertips on the floor, you will be able to broaden your shoulders and extend your neck.
- Through the extension of your lower back and the release of your hamstrings, pressure is developed in your right hip. When you allow the front of your right heel to

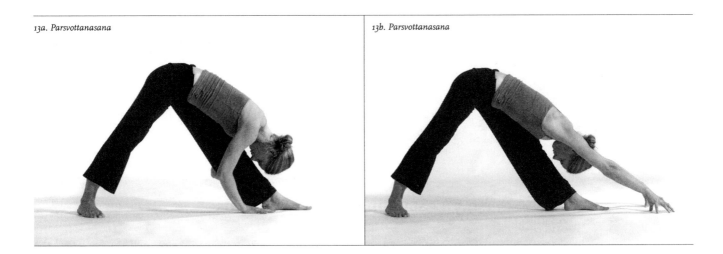

13a. Parsvottanasana

13b. Parsvottanasana

carry the weight of your body , the muscles in the fold between your abdomen and thigh are able to relax. This allows your hip to move farther back.

- Take hold of your right ankle and pull your lower abdomen toward your upper thigh. The traction created from pulling on your ankle allows your back to straighten. Use the connection between your hand and lower back while slowly straightening your right leg (photo 13a).

Note: The strength you need to straighten your leg comes from the upper thigh, close to your lower abdomen. Your abdomen moves in the opposite direction from your hip. This happens when you are able to keep your hamstrings relaxed during the straightening movement of your knee. Take your time when stretching your leg. If you move too fast, you may unconsciously tighten your hamstrings. Move slowly into the end position, and keep your attention on your hamstrings; allow your breath to circulate freely there.

- At the end of the stretch, pull your kneecap up by contracting the upper part of your thigh muscle (not the muscles just above your knee), with the image that the extension of your leg transfers the movement through your knee to your hip. (For more information about this, read chapter 6.3, connections 10 and 11.) Also read about the extension of the back versus the leg in the description of coordination exercise 2 in chapter 10.2.
- You can move into two variations from this end position.
  1. Move your fingers forward as far as possible while maintaining the feeling that the extension in your arms lengthens your abdomen. This happen when you do not lose the upward pull of your hara toward your navel and when you keep your lower ribs down.
  2. From this position, move as if you are going to lift your fingertips from the ground. This movement is initiated from your lower back and will make the extension in your hip and legs more intense.
- Relaxation in your hamstrings and hip will allow the weight of your body to move toward your right (back) heel. Initially, you may feel top-heavy over your left leg

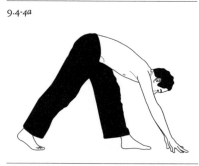

9.4-4a

9.4-4b

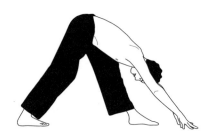

with hardly any pressure to your right heel. As the extension in your hamstrings increases and the pressure intensifies to your right heel, the stretch to your right calf will also increase (figures 9.4-4a and 9.4-4b).

· Breathe freely in your abdomen and chest, and remain in the end position for 30 to 60 seconds. Then bend your left leg, place your hands on your mat, and step back into Adho Mukha Svanasana I or II. Repeat the movement on the other side.

9.5 Standing poses: backbends

Here, the inner tube depends on the strength of the stomach muscles and the free movement of the hips and thighs. With this strength, the backbending movement does not become stuck in the lower back but is transferred to the legs. This is different from backbend (chapter 11), where the emphasis is also placed on the back and shoulders, because they are often stiff and demand all of our attention. Virabhadrasana I belongs to this subgroup.

14. Virabhadrasana I

This is the first variation from the Warrior series. It introduces the basic principle of backward bending of the lower back and will be discussed extensively from that perspective.

The free position of the lower back is intimately related to the free movement of the hips. For example, if the hips in both Trikonasanas (see chapter 9.3, numbers 8 and 9) cannot move freely, the movement will not be transferred through the back to the hips. That will cause tension to develop in the lower back and SI joints. For a free movement of the lower back in Virabhadrasana I, the movement must be transferred through the back to the hips, but now the free position of the pelvis and lower back also depends on the free movement of the *front* of the hips. When movement there is liberated, the gravity point can be placed in the pelvic floor, allowing the inner tube to stabilize the strength in the deep postural muscles of the lower back. When this occurs, relaxation can develop through respiration to the lower abdomen in this difficult pose.

When developing this asana, keep a careful eye on what your lower ribs are doing. Ensure that they push the movement through the arch of your lower back into your pelvic floor (figure 9.5-1). Then the movement will pass through your SI joints, stimulating their mobility.

This pose is important for people with discopathy (distortion of the intervertebral discs) in the (lower) back. This pose can positively influence the discs through the positioning of the back leg in combination with the positioning of the lower ribs. This allows the affected lower back vertebrae to

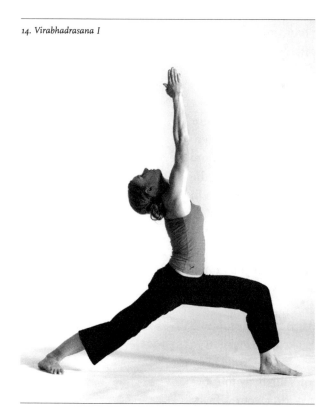

14. Virabhadrasana I

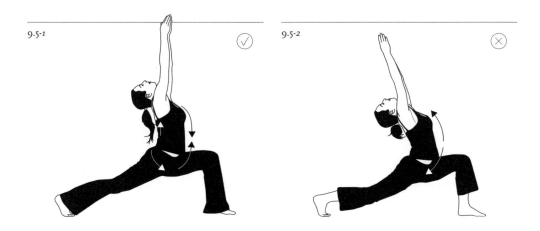

9.5-1 ✓

9.5-2 ✗

be stretched in combination with traction. Then they can fall back into their correct position, allowing the weight of the body to be transferred through the arch of the lower back into the pelvic floor (see the arrows in figure 9.5-1). The position of the front leg can stimulate the backward tilt of the pelvis, while the position of the back leg can stimulate the lumbar curve in the lower back. This is a formidable combination of movements, because although a back-tilted pelvis is often advised when standing (mostly in combination with abdominal exercises), it is detrimental to a stable lumbar curve. In this asana, you must use your stomach muscles — the upper stomach muscles pull your lower ribs toward your abdomen, and the lower stomach muscles allow your pelvis to tilt backward. If you do not use your abdominal muscles properly, they will lengthen, causing your lower back to collapse and lose its stability (figure 9.5-2).

Contracting the stomach muscles is also called the "air bag effect."

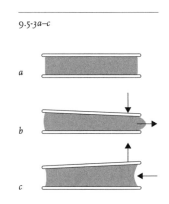

9.5-3a–c

a

b

c

The air bag effect

This effect is produced during Virabhadrasana I by maintaining the inner tube. Imagine two waffles filled with whipped cream with the cream evenly divided across the waffles (figure 9.5-3a). If pressure is applied to one side of the top waffle, the cream will be pushed out (figure 9.5-3b). This also happens to the intervertebral discs when the stomach muscles are flaccid.

Good-quality whipped cream will move back inside the waffles once they move apart (figure 9.5-3c). The same will happen to the intervertebral discs when the vertebrae are pulled apart, just like an accordion that is pulled open. The organs that lie between the abdominal wall and the vertebrae of the lower back push the vertebrae apart. Look carefully at the differences between figures 9.5-4a and 9.5-4b.

The buildup to the end pose is accomplished in two phases: one with the back knee on the floor, and one with the back leg straight. If you are not strong enough to hold the end position, use this buildup to increase your strength and endurance.

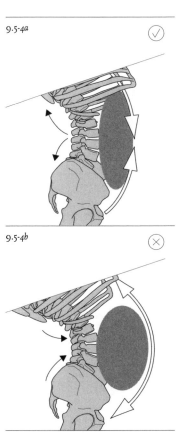

9.5-4a ✓

9.5-4b ✗

Phase 1

With your front leg bent beyond 90 degrees:

· Kneel on your felt mat and move your right foot forward; your foot should be slightly in front of your knee. Your left foot should be directly behind your left knee, and the top of your foot rests on the floor. Place your hands against your right knee, or push with both fists against your tailbone (figure 9.5-5). Move your lower ribs slightly back and feel how your tailbone moves away from your lower back when you contract the lower abdominal muscles 1 inch under your navel. The activation of your abdominal muscles should be light and should not obstruct free breathing.

- Keep your tailbone heavy, and breathe deeply into your lower abdomen. Bend your right leg until you feel an intense stretch in the front of your left hip. Breathing into this area will help you to dissolve the tension.

Note: Your upper body can react in various ways to this movement, and it is important to investigate why that happens.

First compensation

Your entire body leans forward over your front leg (figure 9.5-6), because the entire lumbar curve of your lower back has developed a preference for flexion. Lying on the thin lower back roll can increase the mobility to this area of your back (see chapter 6.3, connection 7).

Second compensation

Your diaphragm shifts forward and your pelvis remains (correctly) tilted forward (figure 9.5-7), because of the rounding of the vertebra(e) in your lower lower back. Your upper lower back is in its correct lordotic curve but the bottom vertebrae are rounded. Lying on the thick lower back roll and moving your pelvis up and down will help to mobilize these vertebrae.

Third compensation

Your body hangs back and puts pressure on the lower vertebra(e) of your lower back (figure 9.5-8), while your upper chest collapses. The cause of this is mostly stiffness in the higher upper back, as in the case of the person with a swayback, as shown in figure 9.5-8. Lying on the thin lower back roll, together with strengthening the lower abdominals, can assist your lower back in recovering its natural lumbar curve. Then your upper chest will be able to move forward.

Fourth compensation

Your pelvis gets pulled up toward your lower back, causing your entire lower back to become excessively hollow (figure 9.5-9). This can be caused by a hyperlordosis that pre-

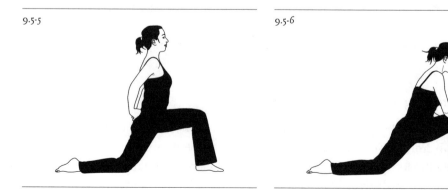

9.5-5

9.5-6

vents the transfer of movement into your legs. This hyperlordosis, caused when the air bag effect has been lost, holds on to the movement. The lower vertebrae are often stiff, but the overall posture is usually caused by weak abdominals. Abdominal exercises with your lower back on the rubber strip are the solution and make your stomach support the natural curve of your lower back.

Fifth compensation

This one is similar to the third compensation; the difference is that your body weight does not fall into the lower vertebrae of your lower back but into your left hip. This happens when the muscles at the front of your hip are too long and allow your body to lean back from your pelvis. To correct this, first lean forward with your upper body and then position your diaphragm directly above your pelvis. With a deep inhalation, position your neck above your upper back. It is especially important to complete the movement with these two steps:

- Slowly start to push the instep of your left foot into the floor. Use that pressure to lower your pelvis toward the floor as soon as the activity of your left leg starts to push your tailbone farther down. During this variation, your right leg may lower below 90 degrees.
- Keep your lower ribs secure by your abdomen so your weight can pass through the arch of your lower back and your SI joints and move freely down into your pelvic floor.
- To increase the extension in the curve of your lower back (see figure 9.5-4a), bring your arms overhead with the feeling that the floating ribs are lifted out of your lower back. (Read the instructions under phase 3 for more information.)
- Remain in this end position for 20 to 60 seconds. Use your breathing to develop relaxation in your lower abdomen. Repeat the movement on the other side.

Phase 2

With your front leg bent to 90 degrees:

- Kneel on your felt mat and move your right foot forward so your heel is directly under your knee. Your left leg should be at a 45-degree angle in relation to your trunk; turn the toes of your left foot under.
- Ensure that your inner tube—the connection between your diaphragm, lower back, and pelvic floor (see chapter 6.3, number 1)—is correctly positioned. Breathe slowly into your abdomen to develop a relaxed feeling throughout your body. Without losing

9.5-7

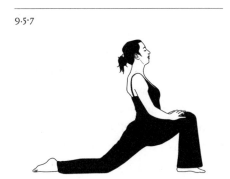

9.5-8

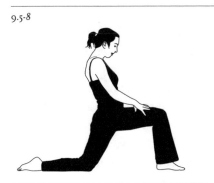

9.5-9

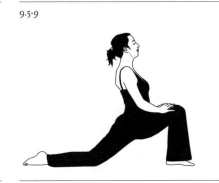

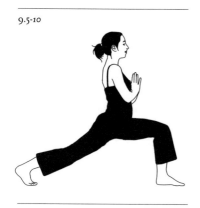

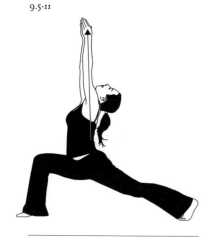

awareness of your breathing and the associated relaxation, lift your knee and stretch your left leg without changing the position of your lower back and pelvis. Place your hands in front of your chest, as shown in figure 9.5-10. Keep your diaphragm, lower back, and pelvis in position with your abdominal muscles.

· The upper part of your right thigh should be low, as if a weight is hanging from it. The pressure to your right heel and the relaxation in your right hip and lower back make this possible by reducing the exertion required from your right leg, especially to the hip and knee. You can hang on to a stool in this phase if you have difficulty maintaining your balance.

· Remain here for 20 to 60 seconds, relaxing your lower abdomen with the rhythm of your breath. Repeat the movement on the other side.

Phase 3
With your arms overhead:

· From the end position of phase 2 (with either a bent or straight back leg), first determine the effect that moving your front ribs backward has on the floating ribs (the bottom ribs on the back of your body, at the level of your kidneys) in your back. By moving your lower ribs backward, you should get the feeling that they are floating above your lower back. When you lift your arms overhead, direct this lift toward your floating ribs. If these ribs shift inward and become stuck, your lower back will immediately lose its free position. Then you can lift your arms all you like, but no space will develop in the curve of your lower back. But if your floating ribs keep floating, then your lumbar curve will remain free, allowing your lower back to react to the lifting action of your arms and the downward movement of your pelvis. This will allow space to be pulled into the curve of the lower back: the accordion is pulled open.

· Pull your hara area up toward your navel.

> **Note:** When your hips are stiff in the beginning, the upward movement below your navel originates from the movement muscles in your abdomen, but when your hips become freer and more open, you do not need that strength anymore. Then you are able to stabilize your core by using your transverse abdominals, the postural muscles of the abdomen.

· Bring your hands down next to your pelvis and turn the palms of your hands out. Place your upper arms in such a position that you can feel the connection with your shoulder blades. Slowly lift your arms without losing the support of your abdominal muscles and without your breath getting stuck in your chest. If your breath does get stuck, it indicates that your diaphragm has constricted and your floating ribs have become trapped in your back. Notice that your exhalations, which push your lower abdomen forward at the end, are able to maintain the coordination.

· Place the palms of your hands together, hook your thumbs, and stretch your arms toward the ceiling. As you do, visualize that your arms are lifting the top of your sternum and your floating ribs—but not the lower ribs above your abdomen (see the arrow in figure 9.5-11).

- Connect both gravity points through your breathing, and remain in this end position for 20 to 60 seconds.
- Try to keep your front leg at a 90-degree angle. If this is too difficult, build it up slowly, allowing your leg to start slightly higher.
- Repeat on the other side.

The end pose
With the back heel on the floor:

Lower backs are often rotated, causing one side of the spine to lie deeper inside than the other, which can result in a difference in muscle development between the left and right sides. If this has occurred in your back, one side of your lower back will be easier to stretch than the other. You can expect big differences in the end position between the left and right sides.

Do the following exercise if you want to research this problem in your lower back. Lie down on the thick lower back roll and follow the instructions described in chapter 6.3, connection 6, for stretching the entire lower back.

When your lower back starts to feel relaxed, you can do the following:

- Slowly move your pelvis up and down to feel whether one side of your pelvis is touching the floor earlier then the other. When the right side of your *pelvis* is moving down faster then the left side, it means the opposite side of your *lower back* is stiff, and vice versa.
- Try to balance your pelvis evenly between the right and left sides the next time you move it down. Then you can become aware of any uneven pressure between the left and right sides of your lower back. There will be more strain on the musculature on the stiff side. Allow the muscles here to relax while you move up and down slowly. When the musculature starts to release its tension, that side of your vertebrae can start to move properly again. This can produce unpleasant cracking sounds in the beginning.

Basic rule
If your lower back feels tight on one side, try to relax your back as much as possible and move your (front) lower ribs toward the contraction. Then use your arms to develop length and shift the gravity point toward the area of your back just *under* the area of stiffness or pain. This will allow the vertebrae to move into the correct position.

- Kneel on your felt mat and move your right foot forward. Place the toes of your left foot on the floor and lift your left knee as described above for phase 3. Place your hands on your right knee or thigh, without leaning on them.
- Keep your weight above your pelvis and turn your left heel toward the floor. Your pelvis will tilt diagonally, changing the pressure on your lower back. Keep turning the left side of your pelvis forward, stretch your left knee, and extend your arms toward the ceiling.

9.5-12

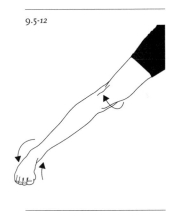

Note: Your back leg now becomes a "carrying" leg. Make sure you push your heel to the floor with the inner arch high and active. This movement is guided by the inside of your knee (see the arrows in figure 9.5-12). If your inner   *(continued)*

9.5-13

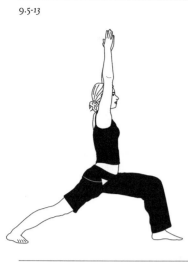

9.5-14

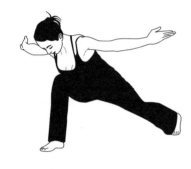

arch collapses, the inside of your knee will also collapse. This can overload the knee and cause the gravity point to shift from your pelvis to your knee. If this movement is difficult with your front leg at 90 degrees, increase the angle slightly. When your back leg is correctly positioned, you can try to lower the front leg to 90 degrees.

When you have positioned your back leg, turning it outward to position your foot, then turn your left hip forward (see the arrow in figure 9.5-13).

- From this position, turn the palms of your hands outward and lift your arms. When you extend your arms toward the ceiling, they lift your rib cage. By keeping your inner tube active and your pelvis stable, this movement of your arms pulls length into the contracted area of your lower back.
- You can keep looking forward or, at the end of an inhalation, lift your head and look at your hands. If your neck feels compressed during this variation, inhale toward the top of your sternum, keeping in mind the image that your inhalations are pulling the vertebrae under your neck farther inward. When your spine starts to respond well to this, its extension will lessen the pressure in your neck, because the weight of your head will then pass your neck and move into your spine.
- Use your breath, as already described, and remain in this end pose for 20 to 60 seconds.
- Bring your head back, bend your back leg, and repeat to the other side.

There are, aside from kneeling, two other possibilities for moving into the end of this pose—from Adho Mukha Svanasana and from Tadasana.

From Adho Mukha Svanasana

- From Adho Mukha Svanasana I or II (see chapter 9.2, numbers 4 and 5), move your right foot between your hands and activate your upper body by pushing your abdomen against your thigh while keeping your fingertips on the floor. Keep your shoulders low.
- Lift your left knee, stretching your leg and spreading your arms out to the sides (figure 9.5-14).
- Breathe deeply into your lower abdomen and develop a feeling of relaxation there. Keep observing your breath in this area. Slowly lift your upper body, following the upward pull of your lower abdomen to your navel at the front of your body until the back of your spine directs your weight to your tailbone.
- Fill your lungs, lift your arms, and stretch your rib cage away from your lower back. Lift your head at the end of an inhalation and look up toward your hands.
- Remain in this position for 20 to 60 seconds. Use your breath first to develop relaxation in your lower abdomen and lightness in your chest, then to connect you with the space around you.
- Keep your shoulders low as you spread your arms and lower your abdomen back to your thigh to come back. Place your hands next to your foot and step back into Adho Mukha Svanasana I or II. Repeat the movement to the other side.

From Tadasana

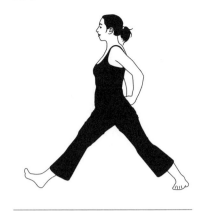

- From Tadasana (see chapter 9.2, number 1), jump with your feet approximately 4 feet apart. Place your hands on your hips; turn your left foot halfway in and your right foot 90 degrees out, but keep your right foot and toes pointing up. Allow your pelvis to turn with your right leg, and look forward over your right foot. Anchor the outside of your left foot to the floor.
- Keep your abdominal muscles firm to keep your weight in your pelvic floor, and push your fists against your tailbone. From this pressure, start to bend your right leg. Begin by placing the sole of your foot carefully on the floor without releasing the pressure on your right heel (figures 9.5-15a and 9.5-15b). Breathe in and out a couple of times.
- Place your arms besides your trunk and turn your hands out; lift your arms above your head in order to stretch your back. Relax the muscles in your shoulder girdle, breathe in deeply and lift your head, look upward, and breathe as described earlier.
- Remain here for 20 to 60 seconds, then straighten your right leg, and raise your head. Turn both feet to the front, and repeat on the other side.

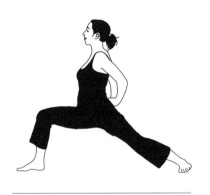

The steps for this asana are described so you can learn each step in the movement. Every time you go further in the process, it is important that you pause to oversee the movement you have already developed before moving to the next step.

After some time, when you are confident about the movement and what you are doing, you can start to move more fluidly. In the places where you originally paused, allow the movement to flow. However, do yourself a favor and take the time to develop the movement with the separate phases.

A personal story

I know how tempting it can be to attempt the most difficult poses you know. Often I felt uncomfortable when I was "wasting my time" on simpler exercises or easier phases of a pose. This goal-oriented manner of thinking ensured that I was often practicing at the limit of my ability. This immediately cut me off from any direct experience of relaxation and lightness. It was the source of an underlying tension in my poses that, after a time, began to dominate my practice. It caused a restlessness that kept me from being in the here and now. I even went through a period where I performed my practice with a sort of stressed haste.

When the time was right, the tide turned. I finally realized that I was trying to prove myself, even though there was nobody around for whom I had to do this. Still, it felt that way. I clearly remember the moment I realized this—it felt as if a heavy load dropped away. I immediately started to breathe more deeply, as if all the tension had disappeared. A totally different attention developed, one based on openness and relaxation. I realized the absurdity of the thoughts that measured my development by the poses I could do. Right away, the asanas developed a positive, intuitive meaning, and the feeling of dutiful compulsion fell away. The recovery of this intuition allowed me to consciously practice the more complicated phases of poses.

10

FORWARD BENDS

10.1 Introduction

The total movement of forward bending is initiated from the rotation of the pelvis on the hips. To achieve this, the spine must consistently transfer the weight of the body into the pelvis. This movement is initiated from the lower back and must be supported by the neck transferring the weight of the head through the upper back into the lower back. The lower back passes the movement on to the pelvis. Body weight is then passed to the hips, and when they relax, the pelvis rotates freely around the heads of the thighbones.

Many of our daily movements—sitting, bending and lifting—are essentially a form of forward bending, and we do them repeatedly. After many years of observation, I have concluded that these movements are nearly always done incorrectly. People often "break" in their back when bending or lifting, causing the functional relationship of the spine to be lost so that serious problems develop. If one point of the back has to make the same movement constantly, this will eventually lead to a loss of stability in that area. The back can become overloaded and develop all sorts of aspecific and specific problems (such as herniated discs). The question is then, how do we bend the back correctly? This question will be answered in this chapter.

During forward bending, the body moves from an upright to a bent position. The coordinated movement of the legs, hips, and spine is essential during this transition. In addition to this, the spine must not lose its connections, meaning the movement of neighboring vertebrae must be passed on and not stop in the break. Forward bends strengthen the postural muscles of the legs, hips, and spine.

How can the spine retain its functional relationship when bending forward?

The lower back plays a crucial role here. It must remain extended. This means that you must actively guide it while still relaxed. To understand this properly, you have to distinguish the different uses of the movement and postural muscles of the lower back. The movement muscles at the sides, such as the quadratus lumborum (see figure 6.3-53b), are able to create stability at the level of the L1, L2, and L3 vertebrae (the upper lower back). The postural muscles, however, can create strength in the complete arch of the lower back, including L4 and L5 and into the sacrum.

After contraction, a muscle is able to release its strength slowly. This is its only possible action. Because of this slow release, you are able to keep your spine stable in a forward bending position. It keeps your spine "together." This is not the case when there is a sudden and complete release of the muscles. Then the movement will break at its weakest spot over and over again. This unconscious habit increases instability in the spine. You have to be careful not to act accordingly when performing these asanas. Indeed, this group of asanas must be able to protect your lower back under these circumstances. You need to learn how to stabilize your lower back by using your muscles properly.

For instance, when you arch your lower back by rotating your pelvis, you generally use the movement muscles at the sides of your lower back. This means there is no strength provided to your lower lower back (L4 and L5). When you bend forward from this situation, you are able to release the strength in the movement muscles slowly, which gives support to your upper lower back but not to your lower lower back, because the muscles there were never activated.

Therefore, you need to create a contraction in the complete midline of your lower back first (see chapter 6.3, connections 8 and 9). Only then are you able to release your strength with control, including in L4 and L5. Then your *whole* lower back remains stable, even when there is no longer support from the quadratus lumborum muscles at the sides. This should always be the situation at the end of the movement in a forward bend asana.

The strength in the midline of the spine is always provided by the neck, which transports the weight of the head through the whole spine to the lower back and toward the sacrum. When the forward bend ends in this stable position, you are able to provide more extension to your lower back by using your hands as described in chapter 6.3, connection 6.

The pull of your hands develops more extension to the front of the spine and activates your hara gravity point, giving you the opportunity to experience relaxation. The pull of your hands transfers your body weight to your SI joints and pelvis. Subsequently, the movement is passed on from your pelvis through your legs and into your feet, which are held by your hands.

These complex movements allow space to develop in various parts of the body:

1. In the area *under* the lower back; specifically the pelvis, hips, and legs
2. In the area *above* the lower back; specifically the chest, heart gravity point, and the shoulders and neck
3. In the area to the *front* of the lower back; specifically, the abdomen and hara gravity point

Forward bends can be divided into four subgroups that have a logical progression in complexity of movement, going from relatively simple poses that form the groundwork to complex balance poses that are difficult to perform and require a high degree of flexibility.

1. Leg and back stretches

The groundwork for these asanas was done during the standing poses. That basic work can be developed with Navasana, Prasarita Padottanasana I, and Dandasana.

2. Standing forward bends

During these exercises, the spine moves with the force of gravity, which makes these movements easier to guide. Specifically, more relaxation is possible here, and there is less danger of losing the connection to the hips. These poses can also be done with bent legs, allowing the stretch to the hamstrings to be increased gradually. Uttanasana and Prasarita Padottanasana II belong to this group.

3. Seated forward bends

In these exercises, all the elements of forward bending come together, and the spine, hips, and legs are mobilized. Paschimottanasana, Janu Sirsasana, Kraunchasana (Heron Pose), and Kurmasana (Tortoise Pose) belong to this group.

4. Balance poses

Simple balance poses are introduced at the end of this chapter. These are easier to learn once the body has become more flexible through forward bending. These balance poses are a good preparation for the more complex twists that follow in chapter 12. Eka Hasta Bhujasana (Elephant's Trunk Pose), Dvi Hasta Bhujasana (Two-Legged Sage Kaundinya's Pose), and Astavakrasana (Eight-Angle Pose) belong to this group.

Before starting with forward bends, I will introduce two coordination exercises. These give a good first impression of forward bending and the correct feeling your body should be experienced. The basic principles of these coordination exercises apply during forward bend asanas as well. Reread chapter 6.3, connections 6, 7, 9, 10, and 11.

10.2 Coordination exercises 1 and 2

Coordination exercise 1

Instructions

- Sit on your yoga mat with your legs bent. Place your heels on a felt mat or the floor. Keep the front of your feet raised. Hold the outside of your feet with your hands.
- Allow your lower back to collapse totally and observe the result of this. If you keep looking straight ahead, your neck and chest will collapse as well, and your shoulders will rise. As if this is not bad enough, your abdomen will fall inward, and all guidance from your lower back to your pelvis and hips will be lost. There is no traction from your hands. What should be spacious and balanced in the body is gone. When I do this exercise during class, people often say, "Nice!" spontaneously. Many people would actually prefer to sit in this collapsed manner (figure 10.2-1a).
- Carefully observe what happens in this pose when you actively extend your lower back. Be vigilant in making sure you do not elevate your lower ribs during this movement, as that will negate the strength in your lower back. In the area directly under your lower back, you will immediately feel a movement toward your pelvis and hips. In the front of your body, space will develop in your abdomen, your chest will rise, and your shoulders will lower. Even your neck will lengthen and stabilize correctly above your upper back (see the differences between figures 10.2-1a and 10.2-1b). Extending your lower back gives space to other areas of your body (shoulders, neck, and hips) and ensures that those areas can move freely. When you consistently apply this coordination during movement, you will be able to develop space in your gravity points in the end poses. One detail (discussed in chapter 6.3, connection 6) is missing here. In the preceding end position, the lower back is used actively. It cannot be avoided, because it needs to work against gravity. The use of the lower back in seated forward bends is discussed at the beginning of this chapter. The lower back in standing forward bends is passive. But even then, thanks to connection 6, you can maintain the correct action in your lower back with the help of your hands.
- In the previous end position, your lower back took the initiative to extend, resulting in your chest being lifted up and back and becoming spacious. Because of this, your hands started to pull on your ankles. You can increase this tractional force by pulling your abdomen closer to your thighs. Be careful here that only your abdomen moves forward and not your head. When you feel that your abdomen has moved closer to your thighs, relax your lower back and keep guiding the extension of your vertebrae with your hands and the postural muscles connected to your spine. *This is the most crucial transitional movement in all forward bends:* the transition from an active to a passive positioning of the lower back; it is only possible when the neck and head stay connected with the spine while pulling on your feet or lower legs with your hands.

> **Note:** The word *passive* means either completely passive during a standing forward bend or active only in the postural muscles during a seated forward bend. During this transition from active to passive, the position of the neck and head is crucial. When the neck is kept in line with the spine, it is able to pass the *(continued)*

10.2-1a ⊗

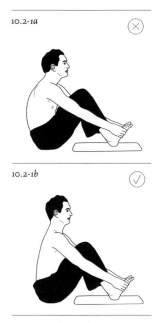

10.2-1b ✓

weight of the head toward the lower back. This is a movement through the center line of the spine. Therefore, it only affects the postural muscles of the back. When the head moves down toward the legs, the spine immediately loses its stability. Then the pull of the hands does not produce any extension in the lower back but increases tension in the shoulders and neck.

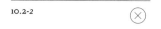

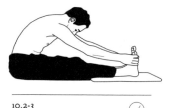

- Slowly push your feet out, sliding them forward gradually and straightening your legs. If your legs are stiff, the connection between your hands and lower back can be lost, as seen in figure 10.2-2. Therefore, it is important to stretch your legs daily, which makes it easier to control your lower back. When you maintain the correct connection (figure 10.2-3), your lower back can remain stable, ensuring the transfer of movement so the stretch can develop in your hamstrings. The feeling of stretching can be painful and, as such, have mental consequences (see chapter 3 for a detailed explanation).

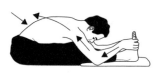

Note: The manner in which you pull on your feet changes during this movement. This change is designed to keep your lower back as flat as possible. In figure 10.2-4a, your hands pull your feet straight down toward your heels; in figure 10.2-4b, you pull your feet straight toward you; and in figure 10.2-4c, you pull your feet up, almost off the floor.

- Your entire spine can move with the extension of your crown when you maintain these connections. Then, when your hamstrings relax even more, your spine does not "break," and the front of your body lengthens. Your two gravity points become spacious and automatically move closer to your legs.

The coordination described here creates an end position where your legs, back, and arms work together harmoniously. This position should be tranquil, because every movement you make disturbs the balance. All movements should stimulate each other through the correct activity of the lower back, as described earlier. This tranquil end pose makes it possible to observe structure and possible tension. Then, through attention, breathing, and time, you can dissolve the stiffness.

This is completely different from end poses where restlessness and movement dominate. I often see the latter, and they are usually due to an incorrect buildup of the movement. Then the big picture (guidance from the lower back) is lost in the end position. Restlessness results, because the hands are still pulling—but not with traction guided

10.2-4a   10.2-4b   10.2-4c

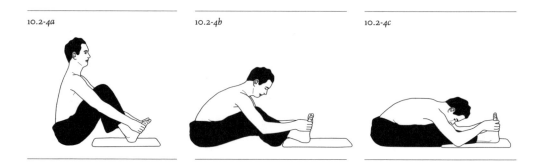

from the lower back. Senseless ambition has become predominant and causes tension in the shoulders and neck. This restlessness generally shows in two ways. Both reactions are described here using Paschimottanasana.

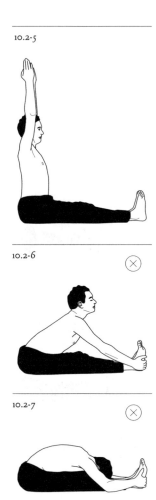

Problem 1: Your shoulders are placed in such a way that cramps develop under your shoulder blades.

Solution

Instead of your head and neck automatically connecting with your upper back as a result of the extension of your lower back (as described earlier), the action of your lower back has been lost. Then your shoulders take over the initiative to provide space to your chest. The result is that your shoulders and chest lift instead of your neck. This leads to tension in the middle of your back and a burning feeling under your shoulder blades. The free movement of your spine—a result of extending your neck—becomes blocked. In this case, you should start the movement again. Give more attention to the pull of your hands and ensure that this pull is connected to your lower back and not your midback.

10.2-6

The movement of your neck deserves a separate discussion. The following occurs frequently: In the beginning, the neck is often correctly extended in Dandasana (figure 10.2-5; see also chapter 10.3, number 3), the starting position for Paschimottanasana. Then it incorrectly becomes excessively concave about halfway through the movement, as the head is pulled back in an attempt to forcefully stretch the back (figure 10.2-6). To alleviate the tension in the head and neck, the face moves toward the legs in the end position (figure 10.2-7). This breaks the connection with the upper back and chest and is usually accompanied by mental restlessness.

10.2-7

To analyze the position of your neck, do the following:

- Sit in Dandasana (see chapter 10.3, number 3) and hold your legs or feet with your hands. Move back as far as possible by contracting your lower back muscles so that traction develops from your hands, as shown in figure 10.2-8.
- Breathe in deeply and place your chin on your chest (figure 10.2-9). Relax your shoulders as you exhale. Remain in this position for a few breaths.
- Slowly pull your abdomen forward as described for Paschimottanasana (see chapter 10.5, number 6), and start relaxing your hamstrings. As your body lowers, your chin will move away from your chest, and your neck will automatically elevate and connect with your upper back (figure 10.2-10). Once your leg muscles lengthen and your upper body moves closer to your legs, your neck will move higher.
- Keep your neck and head motionless in the end position and allow the pose to develop further. This will keep your neck open and extended, allowing your spine to extend in

10.2-8

10.2-9

10.2-10

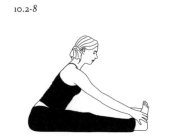
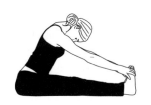
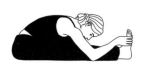

three ways. First, as mentioned earlier in this chapter, your neck provides stability to your lower back, because it transports the weight of your head through the midline of your spine to your lower back. Second, the constant extension of your neck pulls the tension out of your upper back. Third, it allows mental repose. Then mental awareness can move easily to the back of your head (see chapter 5.2).

Problem 2: You lose awareness in your lower back because your hamstrings are too long.

This is a problem that can happen to people who have been practicing yoga for many years or people who have overstretched their muscles in other disciplines. Here, the upper body can lie on the legs easily, but there is no resistance feeding awareness into the pose. The gravity point is not in the pelvis. The body hangs from the chest, and the head lies on the legs (figure 10.2-11). This is often followed by a sort of "waking up and stretching" feeling, where the head and the chest are elevated as the lower ribs shift forward (figure 10.2-12). This movement *removes* the strength from the lower back. Subsequently, the previous position is adopted: the head lies flat on the legs without any sort of awareness. This is like a cat that stretches and then continues to doze.

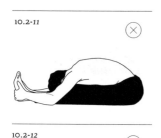

10.2-11

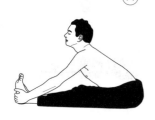

10.2-12

Solution

Focus on the connections. The strength of the pull from your hands is important and is only effective when your neck is in line with your spine. Do not relax completely; keep the center line of your back active by transporting the weight of your head to your lower back. This keeps your neck alert and your attention in the here and now. Try to keep the strength of the pull constant, just as you keep a part of your attention on the extension of your neck during meditation. This will help you maintain awareness. Concentrate on positioning your neck so you can develop an awareness that guides and opens your heart region, similar to when you lie on the block (see chapter 6.3, connection 3). Your hamstrings may have sufficient length, but that has nothing to do with the form and structure of your upper back. Keep in mind that Critical Alignment always tries to develop relaxation in an active structure. Otherwise, relaxation merely leads to exhaustion and sleep. In this pose, you must use your neck to keep extending and relaxing your upper back. Do not disregard the principles of alertness, being present in the here and now, and relaxation within an active structure just because you think you "know" the pose.

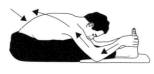

10.2-13

Coordination exercise 2: Sitting on the backbender

This exercise is subtle and effective, and everyone will understand its purpose instantly. First, it is important to investigate anatomically how the large movements within Paschimottanasana develop. These principles apply to all forward bends.

If you look at the arrows in figure 10.2-13, you can see that the correct guidance for your lower back (see coordination exercise 1) comes from your neck, over your back, and into your pelvis. I am not talking about activity to the entire pelvis—only to the sacrum (see the darker-shaded section of figure 10.2-14).

Afterward, the pull of your hands and extension of your neck develops a forward movement in the front of your body that begins in your lower abdomen. This is a softening of the hip flexors and the psoas major muscle, which lengthens your lower abdomen. The stretch of your legs is directed into both sides of your pelvis (the ilia, or hip bones). This is the part of your pelvis to which your legs are connected by the hip joints (see the

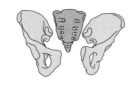

10.2-14

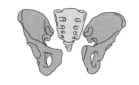

10.2-15

darker-shaded section of figure 10.2-15). These two halves of your pelvis can move backward in relation to your sacrum. The sacrum itself, together with the front of the pelvis (or lower abdomen), moves forward in relation to the two pelvic halves (see the arrows in figure 10.2-16). Keep this image in mind when you are doing this exercise. Think of the sacrum as a sword being pulled from its scabbard (the pelvis, or SI joints).

10.2-16

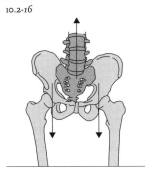

Instructions

- Place the backbender on your yoga mat and cover it with a felt mat.
- Place your sit bones on the highest point of the backbender, extend your legs, and loop a belt around the broadest part of your calves. This will keep your legs turned inward. Allow your feet to point forward (figure 10.2-17).
- Make sure you keep your heels in exactly the same place during the following movement!
- Take hold of your feet or lower legs, use your back to extend forward, and make your exhalations as long as possible. You will feel as if your back is moving forward from your pelvis.
- Pull on your feet or lower legs so that your heels remain in exactly the same place but your hips and pelvis move *backward* over the backbender. During this movement, your spine, beginning in your lower abdomen, simultaneously follows your crown *forward*, mobilizing the muscles around your SI joints. A lot of people actually feel movement in that area of their pelvis.

10.2-17

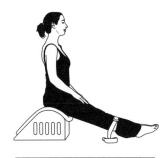

Applying this coordination exercise to forward bends ensures that they become total movements requiring consistent, total attention. This should not be a tense attention obsessed with technique but one that is directed toward releasing tension within your body. What is so beautiful about this technique is that you start to feel accurately how the movements and connections complete the picture and how relaxation within the structure generates increasing space and tranquillity.

Coordination exercise 3

The following powerful exercises are excellent for lengthening your hamstrings and preparing your hips for forward bends. They provide insight into the coordinated use of your abdominals and back muscles during forward bends.

Preparation
Begin by stretching the upper part of your lower back as described in chapter 6.3, connection 7. Have a belt next to your mat.

Instructions with the pelvis on the floor
Your lower back is constantly extended during this phase so the movement can be isolated in your hips and legs.

10.2-18

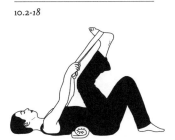

- Pull your right leg in toward your chest and loop the belt over your right foot. Keep your knee bent (figure 10.2-18). Keep your thigh in this position, diagonally above your trunk. This allows you to clearly feel your hip joint. Pull on your foot to increase the pressure to your hip while keeping your pelvis on the floor. If, after 1 minute, the roll feels too thick, make it smaller.

- Extend your right leg as far as possible while maintaining pressure on your hip joint and keeping your pelvis on the floor. Keep your thigh diagonally above the trunk; otherwise, the pressure to your hip will be lost. Maintain the pressure in your hip, even if you are not able to extend your leg fully.
- Remain in this end position as long as you want while breathing into your abdomen. Use the feeling of relaxation that develops there to help your hamstrings relax.
- Repeat on the left side.

Instructions with the pelvis lifted off the floor

During this phase, you lift your pelvis off the floor. This places your lower back in a position similar to the one that occurs when you bend forward. Bending the lower back can occur in two ways. In the first instance, contact with the pelvis and hips is lost, and in the second, the lower back passes movement on to the pelvis and hips even while bending. The abdominal muscles play an important role in this movement. The description in the first part of the ensuing exercise will clarify this.

- Still lying on the roll, lift both feet from the floor and take hold of your knees (figure 10.2-19) or place the belt over your knees. Forcibly contract your abdominal muscles and pull your knees as close as you can to your chest. Maintain the contraction of your abdominals and feel how these muscles push your lower back into the roll. This causes your lower back to bend in such a way that the connection to your pelvis is lost. In this position, you feel no pressure in your hips.
- Keeping your legs in the same position, slowly relax the contraction of your abdominals. This relaxation causes your pelvis to lower slightly. The pressure of the roll extends your lower back slightly, providing space to your abdomen and recovering the connection with your pelvis and hips. Your lower back is now in a position, albeit bent, to pass movement on.
- To activate your inner core (or inner tube), you only need to pull your hara point up toward your navel. This activates your transverse abdominals, which pull your stomach in and up. This is a subtle contraction and should not lift your pelvis.
- Your abdomen can now receive your breath and support feelings of relaxation. These, in turn, can be used to neutralize the discomfort of stretching your legs during the next phase of the exercise.

With the legs extended

Your pelvis does not touch the floor during this phase of the exercise. Your legs are extended and pulled toward your body, forming a reverse Paschimottanasana (see chapter 10.5, exercise 6). Subsequently, you move your legs up and down to analyze the action of your abdominals more precisely.

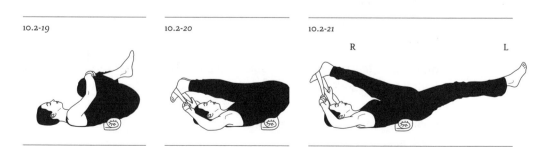

10.2-19   10.2-20   10.2-21

                                                   R   L

- Loop the belt around both feet and extend your legs slowly. Pull your legs as close as possible to your chest while keeping your pelvis on the roll (figure 10.2-20). Keep a firm grip on the belt to maintain pressure to your hips. Relax the muscles of your posterior pelvis and lower back.

- It is important to realize that your back is now in an ideal forward bending position. The back of your head and your upper back rest on the floor, allowing movement to be passed on. The area of your upper back between the shoulder blades is connected to the area of your lower back where it makes contact with the roll. This area, in turn, is connected to your pelvis. This cohesion of the back of your body creates space for the two gravity points in the front of your body.

- Remove your left foot from the belt while keeping your right leg in the exact same position. Slowly lower your extended left leg toward the floor (figure 10.2-21). Observe the action of your abdominals: are they starting to contract forcibly? If this happens, keep your right leg in position and relax your abdominals slowly. Then the reason for contraction will become clear — relaxing your abdominals causes your pelvis to lower slightly, resulting in a marked increase of pressure in your right hip and stretch to your hamstrings. This can be very uncomfortable, and the body never chooses discomfort. Contraction of your abdominals can therefore be seen as a compensation, and your body has (unconsciously) resisted relaxation.

Note: This situation of relaxation causes pain and discomfort, which in turn creates feelings of restlessness. When relaxing your abdominals and increasing the stretch to your hamstrings, watch for feelings of agitation. The advantage of this exercise is that the transition from contraction to relaxation is very slow and can therefore be done with conscious attention. Precisely at the moment when feelings of agitation take over, you can ask yourself what exactly is causing this. You can often choose between the following two reactions:

1. The pain is intense, and the reaction is justified. In such a situation, it is impossible to relax, and you must slowly release the stretch to your hamstrings. At a certain point, you will find the sweet spot where pain can be tolerated and neutralized through your breath.

2. A feeling of discomfort arises, and this causes a steadily increasing restlessness in the thinking mind. This can, consciously or unconsciously, have numerous consequences for your behavior. Very often, people become physically restless and their facial expressions become tense. Attention to the breath is lost. One solution is to look at the cause of this response and to question whether the discomfort in your hip and leg justifies such a strong emotional reaction. Observe your leg rationally. Which muscles are causing this unbearable pain that has so disturbed your emotional state? Try to feel exactly where these muscles are located and whether the painful sensations are moving and changing or constant. This scrutiny often shows that the pain is actually not that bad; then the stress reaction lessens and, with that, the pain.

- Remain in this end position as long as you want, then return both legs to the reversed Paschimottanasana position and repeat on the other side.

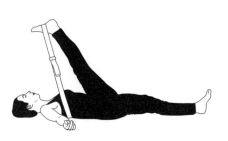

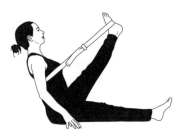

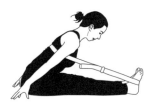

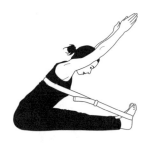

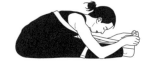

You can repeat this exercise until the reaction of your abdominals lessens or disappears completely. This means your body is starting to accept the stretch in your legs and the pressure in your hips.

Using a belt without the roll

This phase goes further than the previous one. Up until now, traction has been provided by your hands, which allowed you to vary the intensity. Now, with the belt looped around your body, the intensity remains the same or is increased by tightening the belt.

Apart from the fact that this pose can feel intense, it can also provide a profound sense of relaxation. Pulling with your hands often means you do the exercise ambitiously, and ambition can cause restlessness. Your hands do not have to pull during this phase, and this creates more scope for attention to be directed to physical relaxation and mental tranquillity and for the breath to soften the pain.

Preparation

You will need a long belt for this variation or two belts strung together so you can make the loop shown in figure 10.2-22. The exercises that follow can be divided into two series. The first provides support under your shoulder blades and clearly shows the connection between your neck and midback. During the second series, the belt is placed against your lower back so you can closely monitor the connection between your neck and lower back.

First series

- Place the belt under your shoulder blades and lie down. Place your right foot in the loop and extend your leg. Tighten the belt so that your leg is firmly supported. Keep your left leg extended on the floor.
- With both hands, push against your upper right thigh and feel the space that is created in your lower back and hip. Contract your thigh muscles under your hands, lifting the kneecap. Remain in this position; until relaxation occurs and you feel more space in your hamstrings, you can tighten the belt a little more.
- Pull your left leg in and lean against your elbows to come to the position shown in figure 10.2-23. Pull your left leg in and lean against your elbows to come off the floor with your trunk and take the position shown in figure 10.2-23. Keep your neck connected to the place where the belt is positioned in your midback. Remain in this position for 30 to 60 seconds.
- Keeping your neck connected to your midback, move forward into the position shown in figure 10.2-24. Remain in this position for 30 to 60 seconds and then return to the position shown in figure 10.2-23.
- Repeat the same forward movement with your arms lifted. Keep your arms and neck connected with your midback, and move slowly to the position shown in figure 10.2-25. Keep your arms lifted for a couple of breaths before slowly lowering them to take hold of your foot or calf, without losing the connection between your neck and midback.
- During the entire exercise, your midback supports your heart region and provides space there. Without losing the connection between your neck and midback, move into Paschimottanasana, as shown in figure 10.2-26.

Second series

- Place the belt against your lower back at the position where most movement occurs when you bend forward, then lie down. Follow the instructions from the first series, but keep connecting your neck with your lower back at the position of the belt.
- During the final position, Paschimottanasana, the emphasis is on maintaining space in your lower abdomen.

10.3 Leg and back stretches

Navasana, Prasarita Padottanasana I, and Dandasana form the subgroup of forward bends where emphasis is placed on stretching the legs and back.

1. Navasana

Nava means "boat."

This is an important exercise for preparing your lower back for Dandasana, the following pose. It is a difficult pose in which all the connections necessary for providing space (see coordination exercise 1) are in danger of being lost. If they are, habitual patterns such as a bent upper back, collapsed chest, head too far forward, and collapsed lower back will take over, as seen in figure 10.3-1. The upward strength of your lower back is the crucial point on which everything depends: strength (or lack of it) in this area makes the pose either a floating yacht or a sinking ship. For this reason, it is important to prepare with the exercises in chapter 6.3, connection 6, before asking your lower back to carry the pose independently, and the pose is explained from this connection.

Instructions

- Sit on your yoga mat with your legs bent, and take hold of the backs of your thighs. Pull your thighs toward your hips so the extension in your lower back is strengthened, as in coordination exercise 1.
- Lean your upper body farther back so that your lower back becomes stronger and more active. This allows your shoulders to lower and your neck to connect with the erect position of your upper back.
- Lift your feet a little way off the floor and find your balance (figure 10.3-2). Use the pull of your hands on your thighs to support your lower back and begin to straighten your legs without collapsing your chest.
- Slowly start to lessen the pull from your hands on your thighs; feel how your legs, lower back, midback, and abdominal muscles have to take over.

Note: The reduction of pull does not have to happen all at once. To start with, share the work between your arms and the rest of your body. It is much more important that you maintain the correct position of your upper body.

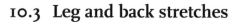
1. Navasana

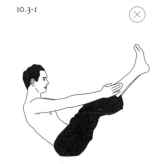

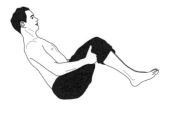
10.3-1

10.3-2

Cramp in the hips

Letting go of your legs can be difficult in this pose. It reveals what happens when your lower back and legs are not working together optimally. Your legs have a tendency to turn outward. To prevent this, use your hands to rotate them inward, and push your ankles and knees together firmly before releasing your legs. The increasing support required from your lower back can cause cramps to develop in your hips. This can be unpleasant, but it does show that you are maintaining the movement in your pelvis, that your lower back is strengthening, and that you are on track. Cramps often develop on the outsides of your hips and cause your lower back to collapse slightly and your legs to turn outward. This pulls the movement out of your hips. When your lower back strengthens, your hips gain flexibility, and your adductors get stronger, the cramps will lessen and eventually disappear altogether.

· If you are able to let go of your legs and maintain the position, then place your finger-tips on the ground to keep your balance. Next, lift your arms parallel to the floor, alongside your knees.

· Keep breathing into your abdomen and chest, and remain in this position for 20 to 30 seconds.

This pose is partially an abdominal exercise. During such exercises, it is important that your heart gravity point remains flexible and your lower back stays active. (Read chapter 13.4 for more information about abdominal exercises.)

The following variation of Navasana is useful for those with short hamstrings, and it can help if you have difficulty with balance because you visually fix on a single point.

· Sit on a felt mat with your legs bent. Let your knees fall slightly apart and take hold of the insides of your feet, ankles, or lower legs. Lift your feet off the floor, and keep looking at one point on the floor to maintain your balance.

· Slowly spread and stretch your legs.

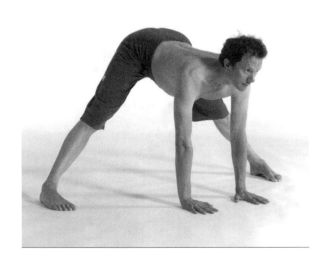

2. Prasarita padottanasana I

2. Prasarita Padottanasana I

***Prasarita* means "extended apart" or "stretched out"; *pada* means "foot."**

Prasarita Padottanasana comprises two variations: Prasarita Padottanasana I and II. In the first variation, the upper body is parallel with the floor; in the second, the upper body is stretched toward the floor. Because the back is bent in the second variation, it will be discussed in chapter 10.4, number 5.

Instructions

You can move into this asana in two ways: from a wide-legged stance or by jumping with your feet wide apart from Adho Mukha Svanasana (see chapter 9.2, number 4).

· Standing in a wide-legged stance with bent knees, place your hands on the floor under your shoulders. Keep your upper body parallel with the floor. Your lower back and legs should bear your weight.

- Feel the pressure of your weight falling into the front of your heels and how your hips are "suspended" directly above. When your hips start to relax, allow your sit bones to move up by consciously releasing your hamstrings. This will change the position of your pelvis and extend your lower back.
- Without losing the full extension in your lower back, slowly pull your lower ribs toward your abdomen until you become aware of the stop in the movement of your ribs. Pull the area below your navel up. Your abdomen should now feel like a firm column, an inner tube that supports the neutral arch of your lower back. After stabilizing your core this way, slowly stretch your legs.
- It is relatively easy in this pose to feel how your legs transfer the action from your heels through your knees and into your hips, which — through the correct balance on your feet and extension of your lower back — move backward.

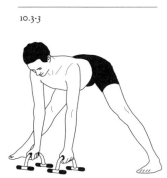

10.3-3

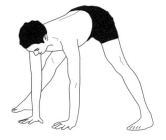

10.3-4

> **Note:** If your hamstrings are of sufficient length, you can place your fingertips or your palms on the floor. If this is not possible, elevate your hands as in figure 10.3-3.

- As your thighs, hips, and both halves of the pelvis move posteriorly, the front of your spine extends forward (coordination exercise 2) toward your crown, as shown in figure 10.3-4. This movement depends on the inner tube. If your lower back is bent, as in figure 10.3-5, your diaphragm will move too low to compensate for the lack of extension in your lower back. Thus, the cohesion of the spine, which makes the extension possible, will be lost. In this situation, elevate your hands to ensure that your lower back is correctly positioned, or keep your knees bent for a longer time to allow your hips to relax more fully. This will help you to extend your lower back farther. If you find it difficult to tell whether or not your lower back is extended, use a mirror or ask someone to observe your back. When your neck is correctly placed in relation to your upper back, look forward and feel how the movement of your head straightens your upper back even more.
- Divide the pressure evenly over the inside and outside of your feet.
- Breathe freely and remain in this end pose for 30 to 60 seconds.

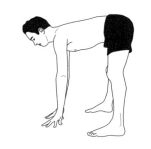

10.3-5

3. Dandasana (seated)

Danda **means "stick."**
The arms, legs, and back are as straight as a stick in this pose, hence the name. The lower back is extended, with the (lack of) length in the hamstrings being the constraining factor. I used to think the pelvis had to tilt for the lower back to extend in Dandasana. I'm afraid many people from the yoga and medical worlds still believe this; however, I have changed my opinion.

As stated earlier, normal daily movements like sitting or standing erect start from the eyes. The eyes send movement to the spine, and the spine transfers it to the pelvis.

Tilting the pelvis in forward bends causes the upper lower back — the part that lies above the pelvic rim — to move actively inward with the support of the movement muscles in the lower back. But this action has no effect on the lowest segment of the lower back, the vertebrae below the pelvic rim (L4, L5, and S1; figures 10.3-6a and 10.3-6b).

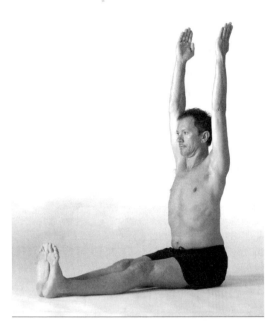

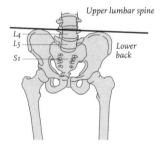

10.3-6a

Upper lumbar spine

L4
L5
S1

Lower
back

10.3-6b

The diaphragm pulls the upper part of the lumbar spine forward, and the lower back moves backward (see arrows).

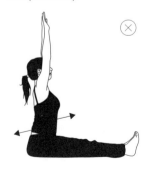

Therefore, the activity of arching the lower back is actually directed toward the diaphragm. In that position, pressure is most likely to be felt in the front of the hips. But this pressure is caused by the superficial movement muscles transferring the body weight into the groin. The pressure is not created by the transfer of movement through the entire lower back, as only the upper lower back is involved in this movement. In fact, the movement is away from the pelvis instead of toward it. The lower back shown in figure 10.3-6b has an S shape. The strength developed in the upper lower back (by tilting the pelvis) will be unusable in the forward bend that follows Dandasana, because the back must be able to relax the superficial muscles in that movement. This tilt breaks the connection between the back and the pelvis and hips, and the lower vertebrae of the lower back (L4, L5, and S1) will not get the opportunity to strengthen. This connection, described in coordination exercise 2, has the leading role in forward bending, because the movement of the spine and the legs meet there.

If the postural muscles of the entire lower back are active from the start of Dandasana, then the lower back is able to transfer the movement to the pelvis during the ensuing forward bend. Even then, the vertebrae of the lower back pass the movement on to the hips. The quality of the forward bend strongly depends on the buildup of strength in Dandasana. If this does not happen in the correct manner, the lower segment of the lower back becomes lazy, and the intervertebral discs start to deform. This is why many yoga practitioners and dancers develop lower back and hip problems after many years of incorrect practice.

Therefore, it is very important to include the lower vertebrae of the lower back in the movement chain. You should ascertain that they are passing the movement on to your pelvis. Only then can you begin to develop the movement.

The way to do this (without extension in your legs) was described in chapter 6.3, connection 9. This is an important starting point for using your lower back in Critical Alignment.

Do not worry if you cannot position your back correctly yet. It is more important that you realize how to develop correct control. From that, you will gain body awareness and increased mobility. It is important, certainly to start with, that you pay a lot of attention to correct positioning so you can make proper connections that allow you to develop strength, as in Utkatasana (see chapter 9.2, number 2) and standing Dandasana (see chapter 9.2, number 3).

In the instructions that follow, a number of methods are introduced so that people with a bent lower back and stiff hamstrings will be able to activate their lower back. With practice, the 90-degree angle between the legs and trunk and the lordotic curve of the lower back will become possible.

Instructions

Method 1

· Sit on your mat with your legs extended. If you have a lot of difficulty with this, sit on one or two shoulderstand blocks; the angle between your upper body and legs will be greater, and tight hamstrings will not interfere (figure 10.3-7).

- Lean your upper body forward so that you feel your body weight moving into your groin.

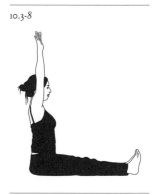

> **Note:** You can lean forward from any part of your spine, but you need to imagine that the movement starts from the release of your hamstrings. Then your sit bones move away from your legs, and the position of your pelvis changes, not through the force of contraction of your lower back muscles, but through the release of the muscles on the backs of your legs.

- When you feel pressure in your groin, you know that your pelvis is correctly positioned. This makes it possible to press your upper thighs into the floor when stretching your legs. Unlike in Navasana, cramps do not usually occur, because the weight of the upper body helps the hips relax. Contracting your thigh muscles will help you keep your pelvis in position prior to extending your lower back. Your lower back is bent, but your pelvis is straight.
- Place the back of your left hand against your lower back and the palm of your right hand against your lower ribs in front. Without changing the position of your pelvis, shift your diaphragm back over the lower vertebrae of your lower back so they slide down deeper and your back straightens. (This was described in chapter 6.3, connection 9.) The movement is transferred to your groin and hips by the extension of your lower back. All of the vertebrae in your lower back are now involved in the movement, and the strength of your lower back can be stabilized by the deep postural muscles. Your pelvic floor, lower back, midback, and abdomen have now formed your inner tube, which can guide the process of bending forward into the end position.

> **Note:** You need mobility in your lower vertebrae to complete this movement effortlessly. If such mobility is lacking, improve it by practicing regularly with the lower back rolls (see chapter 6.3, number 7).

- Mobility is also required in your upper back to position it without disturbing your inner tube. If your back can move easily between your shoulder blades, then one deep inhalation is enough to place your neck over your upper back. Your ribs spread and your sternum is elevated through the movement of your diaphragm and the air entering your lungs. Your sternum, in turn, pulls your upper back straighter with your ribs so that your neck automatically places the weight of your head above your spine.
- Connect your arms with your shoulder blades and lift them above your head (figure 10.3-8).

- Rotate your legs inward so that your ankles are parallel with each other and your toes point directly upward.
- Hold this asana only briefly (but a minimum of 20 seconds) before moving into the forward bend. Use this time to work it through properly.

This is the traditional end position of Dandasana. The following two methods are both excellent ways to start the forward bend. They are a good preparation and excellent for increasing strength in the arch of your lower back. Use them regularly as a preparation for forward bends.

Method 2

- Sit on the floor with your legs extended; if necessary, sit on a shoulderstand block as described in method 1. Place your hands diagonally behind you and lean on your hands. The angle between your legs and lower back has now changed, and consequently the movement of your lower back is not as restricted by tight hamstrings.
- Arch your lower back as much as you can. An increasing amount of weight will be transferred into the front of your pelvis, building pressure to your upper thighs. Push the back of your pelvis into the floor; this gives the same effect as lying on the thick lower back roll described in chapter 6.3, connections 7 and 8. This movement develops strength in the lower segment of your lower back. From this, you will get the feeling that you are sitting on your pelvis instead of leaning on your hands.
- Keeping your face forward, direct your breath to the middle and upper parts of your chest. Feel how these areas move upward with inhalations; ensure that your lower ribs do not follow this movement. Tip your head toward your back (figure 10.3-9a).
- After overarching your lower back for a while, move your lower ribs toward your abdomen. When your lower back is well arched, this movement will come to a stop. This break in your movement means your diaphragm is connected to your pelvic floor. Your extended lower back transports your body weight to your pelvis.
- Move your lower abdomen forward. Keep your lower back strong, and lift your arms up, ending in Dandasana.
- Alternatively, lift your head, and lean your upper body forward diagonally, leaving your fingertips on the floor behind you. Maintain the strength in your lower back (figure 10.3-9b).

Method 3

- Sit on the floor with your legs extended. Place more height under you, if necessary.
- Lift your arms overhead and lean back as far as you can (figure 10.3-10), as if you are trying to touch your fingertips to the wall behind you. Keep your lower back in a deep arch. Keep your breathing regular, and remain in this end position for as long as you can. Ensure that your lower ribs remain low and well connected to the arch of your lower back.

You will realize quickly that this movement is an excellent abdominal exercise that strengthens your lower back.

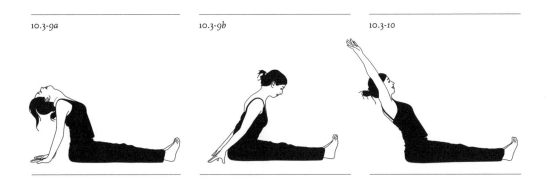

10.3-9a   10.3-9b   10.3-10

> **Note:** You can also move into this position from Navasana by slowly lowering your legs to the ground without collapsing your lower back. You can start this movement with your fingertips on the floor. Lift your arms, one at a time, to increase the difficulty.

- Move back into the 90-degree angle as if someone is pushing you forward from your lower back without losing the strength you have developed.

10.4 Standing forward bends

Uttanasana and Prasarita Padottanasana II belong to this subgroup. The spine moves with the force of gravity in these asanas. The knees do not have to be extended immediately; the spine can guide the movement more easily with bent knees.

4. Uttanasana

Ut means "out"; tan means "stretch."

This asana is an intense stretch to the entire back of your body. It is particularly appropriate if you do not feel that your hamstrings are stretching adequately during seated forward bends (see chapter 10.5) because your back is bending instead of your pelvis (figure 10.4-1).

It is important to realize that you bend your back *as little as possible* when bending forward (contrary to what the name implies). To maintain the cohesion of your spine, you have to move so that each vertebra passes the movement on equally. These connections ensure that your back does not "break" consistently in the same place. Such a break occurs constantly in daily life when you bend forward from the back — usually an automatic movement. You can imagine how such singular use of your lower back can lead to overload. Learning to use your back correctly during this exercise is important, because you can use what you learn in your daily life when lifting and bending. The correct balance of your spine ensures that your two gravity points (see chapter 6.3, connection 1) can remain relaxed and open as the movement progresses toward the end position. The art of Uttanasana and the ensuing forward bends is to give correct guidance to both gravity points; they must remain spacious. The heart gravity point maintains its space under the guidance of your neck, and the hara gravity point from the activity of your lower back. This ensures that both areas are lowered simultaneously toward your legs when the length and relaxation of your hamstrings increases.

You should feel relaxed and light in the end position. This occurs through the hierarchy of movement in your spine. The strength of your lower back generates free movement to your shoulders, neck, and upper back. Without the active support of your lower back, you will lose the spaciousness in your chest. *The activity of your lower back always has priority.*

4. Uttanasana

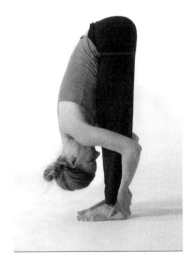

10.4-1

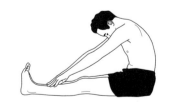

Instructions

- From Utkatasana (figure 10.4-2), place your hands lightly on your knees—do not lean on them. Your weight is borne by your lower back and legs. Make sure your hamstrings do not contract, and pull your sit bones toward your legs. Allow your sit bones to move back as far as possible, away from the backs of your knees (see the difference between figures 10.4-3a and 10.4-3b). When you do this correctly, your lower back will be concave. Move your lower ribs toward your abdomen. This will place the power line (midline) in your lower back all the way down to L4 and L5. Then, when you bend your back, you can maintain strength in the midline and bend your lower back gradually.

> **Note:** When your lower back moves from concave to convex, slowly release the lower back muscles that attach to your pelvis. If you have not made your lower back strong by activating the midline when your lower back is concave and moving your lower ribs toward your abdomen, then your lower back will always break during bending once the muscles on the sides of the lower back lose their control (read the introduction to Utthita Trikonasana page for more information about this).

- Keep your balance on the front of your heels and slowly move your abdomen toward your upper thighs. Keep your back as straight as possible, and when you bend forward, feel your lower back keep transferring movement to your pelvis. When you do this correctly, you will feel pressure on your hips. This is the first condition for maintaining relaxation in your hips and lower back. The second condition is contingent on the position of your knees. They must move inward slightly so that your hip flexors are released. The third condition for relaxation around the hips is contingent on the position of your thighs. They must rotate inward slightly so that your groin can relax. If you have difficulty with these movements, you can use your hands to push your knees slightly closer and rotate your thighs inward. Then try to take over the movement actively with your leg muscles.
- Your shoulders should be low and your neck extended to provide space to the base of your sternum (figure 10.4-4). This is the ideal position for your back and is comparable to the end position of the forward bend.

10.4-2

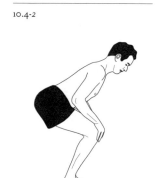

10.4-3a

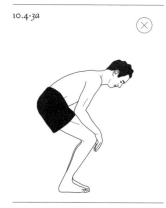

10.4-3b

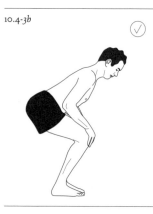

10.4-4

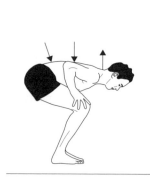

10.4-5

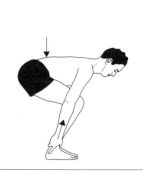

- Take hold of your ankles, push your abdomen firmly against your upper thighs, and elevate your upper body and neck as far as possible. This should create a feeling that you are about to lift yourself off the floor (figure 10.4-5). The movement of your lower back creates the pull of your hands; keep your arms straight.
- Turn the activity around. Instead of your lower back taking the initiative to pull on your ankles, pull with your hands, relax your lower back at the sides, and allow your pelvic rim to move away from your back. Then pull your abdomen firmly against your legs, without lowering your face and chest.
- When your neck is in line with your spine at this stage of your movement, it indicates that the center line of your back is still active.
- *The strength of the pull of your hands makes your lower back flatter.* Remember that your arms and lower back can work in this manner whenever you lift something heavy. Maintain this connection as you develop the movement. Once you start to extend your legs, your lower back can take advantage of the pull of gravity and start to relax. You can then control the bending of your lower back from your arm pull.
- Slowly straighten your legs. Maintain your balance on the front of your heels. Bring your attention to your hamstrings, and try to consciously guide the release of tension in this area. Let your breathing circulate freely in the areas where you feel tension. Bend forward as far as your legs allow. If the pain of stretching gets so acute that your breathing becomes irregular, stop stretching. Regulate your breathing and wait until your legs relax before moving farther. Toward the end of the movement, your legs should extend as described in Dandasana, where your legs transfer the movement through your knees to your hips (figures 10.4-6 and 10.4-7).
- In the end position, observe the placement of your neck in relation to your chest. Position it in line with your upper back. Keep pulling actively with your hands. You can vary the amount of strength you use, but remember that this pull provides structure. Try to find relaxation within the structure, not by letting go of the structure. Through that structure we are able to isolate the areas which we want to relax and which are specific for that asana: hips and hamstrings. People tend to lose their structure or "frame" when they start to relax (for instance when they lose control over the spine) and therefore they are not able to relax the areas that are essential for this posture. When the structure collapses we are not able to isolate the areas in which we want to relax. Instead we move into our preferences. When your legs relax more fully, your back lengthens immediately, allowing your two gravity points to move closer to your legs.

> **Note:** Do not push your head toward your legs. This will disturb the balance in your gravity points immediately and annihilate the positive feelings you have developed in the pose (figure 10.4-8). A stable neck is one of the goals of forward bends. If you do not keep this in mind, your habitual postures will only be strengthened.

- You can remain in this pose for 1 to 5 minutes. Come out either with straight arms and legs into Tadasana or with bent knees into Utkatasana.

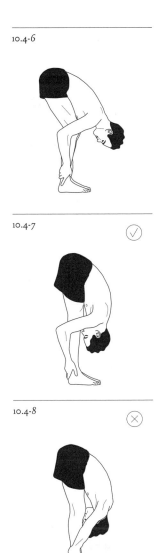

10.4-6

10.4-7

10.4-8

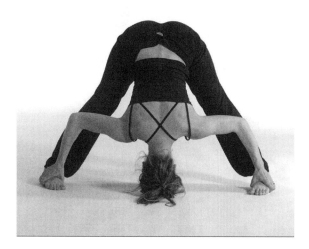

5. Prasarita Padottanasana II

When moving from Prasarita Padottanasana I (see chapter 10.3, number 2) into Prasarita Padottanasana II, it is wise to give attention to the cohesion of your spine first. Work on this connection initially with bent legs. You will be able to mobilize your hips easily and determine exactly how much they thwart the movement. If the extension of your legs does not disturb the position of your lower back too much, then you can do the movement with straight legs. The following description remains the same.

Instructions

· From Prasarita Padottansana I, bend your legs while keeping your balance on the front of your heels, which are turned outward slightly. Take hold of your ankles and direct the pull of your hands to the extension of your lower back so that pressure on your hips increases. Do not lower your head and shoulders when you pull, but elevate your upper body slightly to arch your lower back completely. Pull your lower ribs inward without losing the extension in your lower back to stabilize the arch of your lower back. Now your diaphragm is firmly connected to your pelvis and hips. If it did not happen automatically, pull your hara area up to your navel to establish complete stability of your core.

· Bend around your hips when bending forward maintaining control in your core.

· Move as far as your leg muscles allow; extend your crown and neck toward the floor. Keep your breathing relaxed, and slowly begin to straighten your legs without losing your balance. If you do lose your balance, your hips and hamstrings will probably contract. Therefore, pay attention to these areas and move slowly toward the end position without decreasing the pull of your hands.

· Breathe from your abdomen to your chest, and move with both gravity points engaged slowly toward the plane of your legs (if your hamstrings allow it).

· Remain in this position for 30 to 60 seconds. Use the strength of your legs and lower back to return to a standing position. Do this by first stretching your arms sideways like a pair of wings (figures 10.4-9a through 10.4-9c).

10.4-9a

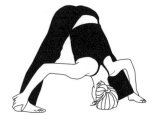

10.4-9b

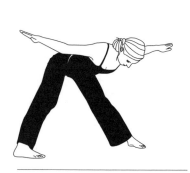

10.4-9c

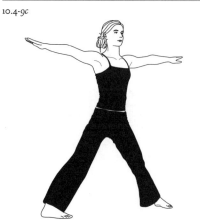

10.4-10

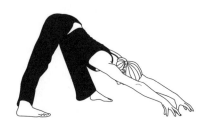

- Figure 10.4-10 shows a variation that can be done from Prasarita Padottansana II. From the end position, walk forward with your hands as far as possible without losing the pressure balance on the front of your heels. You can stop at this point or continue using your lower back to lift your fingertips from the floor. This immediately activates the entire cycle of movements that was described in the coordination exercises. The lordotic curve of your lower back will be enhanced, creating more space (flexibility) in your hips, legs, abdomen, chest, shoulders, and neck.
- Remain in this position for 30 seconds and then walk back into Prasarita Padottansana I with your fingers.

10.5 Seated forward bends

Paschimottanasana, Janu Sirsasana, Kraunchasana, Kurmasana, Dvi Hasta Bhujasana, and Titibhasana belong to this group. All of the elements of forward bending come together in these asanas, with the result that the spine, hips, and legs are mobilized.

6. Paschimottanasana

6. Paschimottanasana

Paschima refers to "back (of the body)"; *uttana* means "stretched out."

Paschimottanasana was described in the introduction to this chapter. The two coordination exercises gave important information about this pose. Earlier in this book, attention was given to the psychological and meditative aspects of this exercise (see chapters 3.3 and 5.6). Re-read these chapters together with the description that follows.

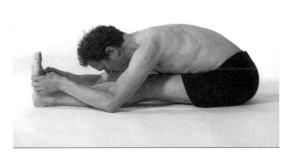

In this chapter, after the seated Paschimottanasana has been described, a number of other variations will be introduced that illuminate particular aspects of this asana. These concern the extension of the midback, the calves, and the back of the pelvis.

Instructions

- Sit in Dandasana.
- Slowly bend forward from your hips by releasing your hamstrings. Keep your arms well connected to your lower back. If your lower back loses its strength, your back will end up in the situation discussed under coordination exercise 1 (see page 245). The first sign of this failure is tight shoulders and a concave neck. Then your abdominal muscles will contract, your chest will collapse, and your breath will get stuck in your

Note: When it is difficult to straighten your lower back in this seated position, read the instructions given in chapter 10.3, exercise 3, and use the different methods to extend your lower back. Leaning backward first helps to extend your lower back and creates more stability in your core before you move forward.

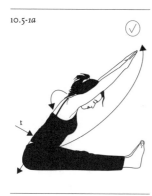

10.5-1a

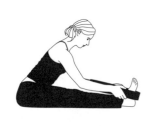

10.5-1b

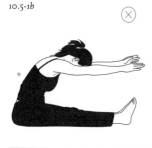

10.5-2

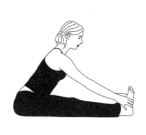

10.5-3

chest. These are all signs that your lower back is no longer bearing the weight of your upper body.

- When you notice one of these signs, stop immediately. Do not think that your lower back is straight in this position. The natural lordotic curve will be lost, but your lower back must retain its cohesion even when it is bent. The arrows in figure 10.5-1a show the effect of the proper use of your lower back. Keeping it strong maintains its cohesion thanks to the direction of the strength developed, which is toward your abdomen (see arrow 1). Through this strength, or cohesion, activity develops in the direction indicated by the arrows placed at each end of the arch: the lowest arrow points toward the pelvis and hip region, indicating that activity should be directed there, while the the upper arrow indicates activity in the upper body space above the diaphragm. In this position, the bend of the lower back is kept as flat as possible. Because of that, it stays connected. The flatter the arch, the better. The arch in figure 10.5-1b has lost its cohesion and broken, causing a loss of activity to the extremities. The space in the pelvis and upper body is no longer supported, and the abdominal muscles will harden.

- In this situation, *without bending your back any farther*, lower your hands and take hold of your feet or lower legs, or place a rubber strip around your feet and hang on to the ends (figure 10.5-2).

Note: This is a crucial point in the movement. Many people make the mistake of taking hold of their feet and bending their backs too far. Take hold of what you can (legs, ankles, or strip) while maintaining the correct active position of your back, and don't go any farther. Take the time necessary to perform this movement correctly.

- When you grasp your legs or feet, relax your shoulders immediately to create a strong feeling of relaxation before you continue the movement. Breathe deeply into your abdomen to transfer the physical feeling of relaxation produced by your shoulders to your breath. Then elevate your upper body slightly so that your lower back extends a little more (figure 10.5-3). This movement, which is more like a backbend than a forward bend, creates a resistance pull in your hands. You can turn this action around, as described in Uttanasana. Pull with your hands to control your lower back and keep it as flat as possible. Slowly move forward, keeping your neck aligned with your lower back. Imagine that your hands are pulling your abdomen forward, and allow your spine to bend—vertebra by vertebra—until your hamstrings are in a strong stretch. Stop moving and remain in this end position, breathing slowly in and out.

Note: Remember that, during this movement, the *lengthening* of the front of your body always precedes the *bending* of your back. This sequence is very important to prevent your back from "breaking."

- Once in this position, the nature of the pose changes dramatically. If you have followed the technique correctly, there is structural integrity in the end position. You should feel that the front of your body is lengthening from your lower abdomen due to the pull of your hands. The art lies in not wanting too much too soon. All you have to do is wait for your hamstrings to relax. Sometimes this occurs quickly; sometimes it takes a long time. The speed can vary from day to day. Use your breath to stimulate the release of tension. Send your breath to the places where you feel resistance and allow it to circulate freely, as if you are massaging the stiffness out of your muscles with your breath.

· When your hamstrings do relax, it is seldom a slow and gradual movement. Usually, it occurs abruptly. Then your two gravity points (the hara and heart regions) will automatically move closer to your legs. This is not a movement that you *do;* relaxation is not something that your willpower can create. In the end position, the movement occurs automatically as soon as your hamstrings relax. Your head does not lower, because your neck remains connected to your upper back in order to provide space to your heart region.

· Stay in this position for 1 to 5 minutes. Sometimes it is good to hold the pose for a long time; then you can work out the psychological aspects of this asana, reflecting on how you can deal with tension (see chapter 3.3). Long holds (in my lessons, I often maintain this pose for 15 to 20 minutes) have a positive effect on the length of the muscles by penetrating the stiffness there. Sometimes it is more pleasant to hold the pose for shorter periods with more repetitions.

· To return, stretch your arms forward and use your lower back to elevate your fingertips. Your fingertips lead the movement back to Dandasana, ensuring that your back is erect and strong. Relax your arms. If your lower back protests at this stage because the vertebrae have been in a bent position for a long time, keep your arms extended overhead and follow your arms until you are leaning farther back, as shown in figure 10.5-4. This movement will stretch and strengthen your lower back.

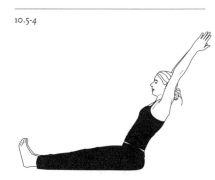

10.5-4

You can also move from the position described in coordination exercise 1 (see chapter 10.2) to the end position. The difference of this buildup from the one described here is that the length of your back, not the stretching of your legs, is the focal point. You can alternate between both methods. Your hips and lower back get more benefit from the pose with bent legs.

Two variations of Paschimottanasana

1. Paschimottanasana with your back on the floor (figure 10.5-5)
Do not confuse this pose with Halasana, in which the weight of your body is borne by your shoulders; in this variation of Paschimottanasana, your weight is borne by your midback. Many backs have a preference for "breaking" at this point instead at the lower back. When this happens, you immediately lose the connection to the space in the front of your heart region. Paschimottanasana is a challenging pose in which to develop feelings like lightness and space. Try to develop this feeling when you lie in this position and stay connected to it when you move to the seated variation at the end of the exercise. That variation provides a beneficial stretch to the area around your SI joints for a stiff lower back.

10.5-5

· Lie on your back on a felt mat with your head about 1 foot from the wall. The distance differs from person to person and will become clear after a few attempts.
· Lift your legs and take hold of your ankles with your hands. Bring your feet over your head and place them against the wall; slowly start to bring your hands and feet closer

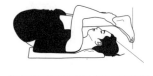

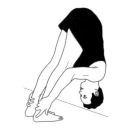

to the floor. Ultimately, they will reach the floor. Be careful to maintain your weight under your shoulders in your midback. Do not roll farther onto your shoulders.

· Remain in this position, straightening your legs. The pressure that the floor exerts on your midback allows it to stretch. (In the seated variation of Paschimottanasana, it is your neck that initiates the stretching of your midback.)

· During exhalations, relax this part of your back so that your entire spine can lengthen.

· Push with your toes against the wall and move your heels away from the wall. Feel the length and space that arises in L4 and L5 and your SI joints. This is an intense stretch in an area that is difficult to feel.

· Remain in this end position for 30 to 60 seconds. Take your feet off the wall, and in a fluid movement, roll back into Paschimottanasana. Bend forward and take hold of your lower legs or feet, using the image of the connection between your neck and midback. Your neck will immediately move up to connect to your midback when you start to bend forward.

2. Paschimottanasana with the back against the wall (figure 10.5-6)

· Stand with your feet at hip-width, about 15 or 16 inches from the wall. Bend forward and allow your back to slide down the wall as far as you can, without letting your head touch the ground. Ensure that your midback is against the wall. Breathe in and out slowly a couple of times.

· Keep your head at the same height above the floor and slowly straighten your legs. This movement pushes your pelvis higher. Turn your heels outward slightly by turning your thighs inward, and place your heels on the floor. You will notice that the stretch to your calf muscles is more intense.

· The extension in your legs has probably ensured that your lower back has moved closer to the wall. During exhalations, release the tension from your entire trunk, starting with your pelvic area. Your back and head will move progressively closer to the floor.

· Remain in this position for 30 to 60 seconds. Bend your legs to return, and with a fluid movement, move back into Paschimottanasana, without losing the connection between your neck and midback (from the previous variation). Try to apply the same feeling of release starting at your pelvis so that your entire back can *lengthen*—make sure that it does not *bend*. Since the wall does not provide any support to your back in the seated position, the release is made possible through the pull of your hands, which controls the bending of the lower and middle parts of your back.

These two variations teach you how to actively guide and maintain spaciousness in both gravity points effortlessly. These points are less likely to become obstructed than in the seated version. Therefore, you can easily develop the feeling of breathing freely.

7. Janu Sirsasana

Janu means "knee"; *sirsa* means "head."
In this pose, one leg is bent while the head is brought over the knee of the extended leg.

7. Janu sirsasana

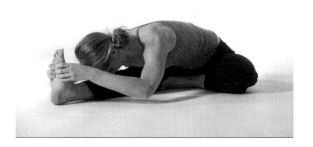

Instructions

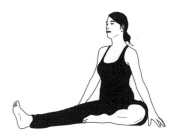

- Sit on your yoga mat with your legs extended in front of you. If your lower back has difficulty extending, sit on a shoulderstand block.
- Keep your pelvis straight and bend your left leg, placing the sole of your foot as high as possible against your inner right thigh (figure 10.5-7). If your knees are stiff, slowly move your foot higher up your thigh. Ultimately, your heel should be against your perineum.
- Place your lower back in the Dandasana position by allowing your weight to move forward so that you feel pressure on your knees and in your groin. Press your right thigh and your left knee toward the floor, then extend your back and lift your arms overhead. Remain in this position for 10 seconds, breathing from your abdomen to your chest to connect the two gravity points.
- Lean your torso forward, and from this point, follow the instructions for Paschimottanasana.
- Remember that the middle of your body should not be aligned over the middle of your extended leg but to the inside. This way, your nose will end up above the floor, not above your shin.
- Relax your abdominal muscles in the end pose by breathing into your abdomen. This will help to relax your lower back and hamstrings; when this occurs, use your hands to lengthen and develop the stretch of your spine further.
- Stay in this end position for 30 seconds to 2 minutes. Then stretch your arms forward and use your lower back to lift them, returning to the seated position with an extended back.
- Repeat the movement on the other side.

Note: Do not follow the movement of your arms when you raise back up; instead, think about placing your pelvis, lower back, and diaphragm in the right position. Try to organize the connection of your core quickly but pay attention to the correct sequence:

1. When you maintain the extension of your right leg and the downward pressure of your left knee, it helps you keep your pelvis straight.
2. When you raise up with a straight pelvis, the upward movement of your body produces more extension in your lower back.
3. Once your lower back feels properly arched, finish the movement with the inward pull of your lower ribs.

Regarding the hamstrings, Janu Sirsasana is more beneficial than Paschimottanasana, because only one leg is stretched out instead of two. Restricting the movement of one leg is more intensive for the hamstrings than when two legs are resisting the movement.

8. Upavista konasana

Upavista **means "seated";** *kona* **means "angle."**
During Paschimottanasana and Janu Sirsasana, the free movement of the hips and lower back is achieved by lengthening the hamstrings. In Upavista Konasana, you stretch not only your hamstrings but also your adductors.

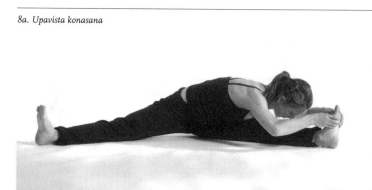

8a. Upavista konasana

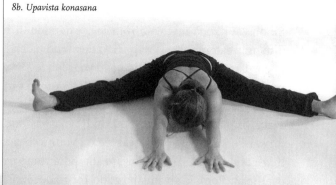

8b. Upavista konasana

Upavista konasana to the side

- Sit on your yoga mat and spread your legs as wide as possible. Lean your trunk forward, allowing your hamstrings to relax. Your body weight will shift to the front of your pelvis and exert pressure on your groin. Relax your groin. If this is difficult, sit on a shoulderstand block. Press the backs of your thighs into the floor to keep your feet straight and perpendicular to the floor. Contract your quadriceps. Do not lift the back of your pelvis; keep that part of your back passive. It is the release in your hamstrings, not the tilting of your pelvis, that transfers the movement to your groin.

- Place your left hand against the inside of your left knee and your right hand on the floor behind your right leg; use the pressure of your right hand to keep your groin low. This will keep your pelvis straight when you extend your upper body. Shift your diaphragm back as described for Dandasana until your body weight allows your lower back to extend toward your pelvis. Rotate your body to the right (figure 10.5-8) and feel how the left side of your abdomen turns from your groin toward your right leg. This rotation will increase when your abdominal and lower back muscles are relaxed, which will occur when your lower back is extended. Make sure that your upper back is extended in this position and that your neck and head are in line with your back. Feel how your body weight is supported by your lower back and pelvis rather than by your arms and tense shoulders. Take some time to become aware of the release in your shoulders and the relaxation of your breath in your lower abdomen.

- Keep pressing your left hand against the inside of your knee to maintain the rotation in your abdomen, and bend forward over your right leg. Notice whether your lower back is adequately carrying your weight (figure 10.5-9) by observing the position of your shoulders (low), chest, and abdomen (spacious).

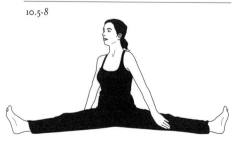

10.5-8

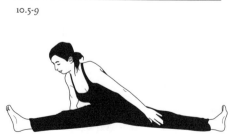

10.5-9

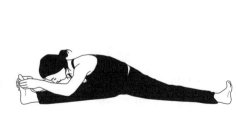

10.5-10

- Without bending your lower back any more, take hold of your lower right leg or foot and pull your lower abdomen farther forward. Only now should your back continue its bend from your pelvis, vertebra by vertebra, until an intensive stretch to your hamstrings restricts further movement. Do not attempt to keep moving deeper, but wait here until your hamstrings allow you to move farther (figure 10.5-10).

Note: To make the forward bend easier, you can lift the left side of your pelvis slightly, but keep your hip heavy. This creates space around your left SI joint.

10.5-11

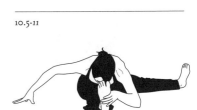

- Keep your right leg aligned, as described in chapter 6.3, connection 11. Rotate your thigh inward, maintain the pressure to the right side of your groin, and ensure that your foot stays straight. If you still have the feeling that you are rolling your leg out, use your right hand on the floor to apply counterpressure (figure 10.5-11).
- Remain in this end position for 30 to 60 seconds and breathe freely. Move your hands back, and repeat the movement on the other side.

10.5-12

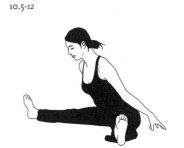

Upavista konasana to the middle

- Once you have completed both sides, move back to the middle and lean forward so that pressure can develop in your groin. Then sit up straight with an erect lower back, as in Dandasana.
- Bend forward from your hips without losing the weight-bearing action of your lower back (figure 10.5-12).
- Move your hands forward and remember that lengthening the front of your body precedes the bending of your back. Observe this sequence of movement carefully so that your back remains connected, meaning that your neck is able to transport the weight of your head toward your lower back continually. Stretch your hands forward as far as you can (figure 10.5-13), and pay attention to your heels, as described in coordination exercise 2 (see chapter 10.2). If you keep your heels in the same position on the mat while flexing your feet toward you, you will feel your hips moving backward. Your upper body moves forward in relation to the movement of your hips.

10.5-13

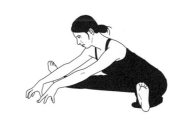

Note: If it is difficult for you to get your body weight to move forward over your hips because your hamstrings are too tight, sit on one or two shoulderstand blocks. If that does not help, spend more time in the standing variation of this pose—Prasarita Padottanasana II (see chapter 10.4, number 5).

9. Kraunchasana

Krauncha means "heron."

This is also the name of a mountain pass in the Himalayas that was, according to Indian mythology, made by Parasurama's arrow. Parasurama, also known as Rama with the Ax, was the sixth incarnation of Vishnu.

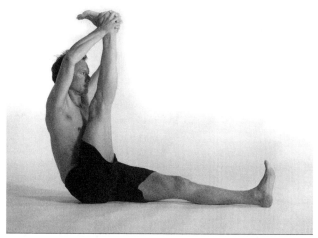

9. Kraunchasana

10.5-14   10.5-15

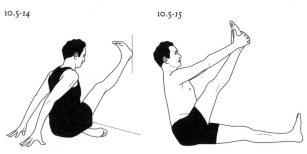

Instructions

- Sit on your yoga mat with your legs extended in front of you. Bend your right leg and take hold of your foot. Pull your thigh toward your abdomen, and extend your lower back so that your abdomen moves actively toward your thigh. The strength in your lower back helps with the positioning and release of strain in your neck, head, and shoulders. This movement is similar to that in coordination exercise 1 (see chapter 10.2).
- Slowly straighten your knee by lifting your foot and maintaining the upward extension of your lower back. Stretch your leg and use your hands to pull your abdomen and heart region toward the leg. If this combination of movements is too difficult, then the variation shown in figure 10.5-14 is a good alternative.
- Lean your elevated leg against the wall and support your lower back with your arms by pushing your hands into the floor behind you. Or try the variation where you move your upper body as far away from your elevated leg as possible. Then your body takes on a Navasana position (figure 10.5-15).
- Keep breathing freely and hold the pose for 30 to 60 seconds, then repeat on the other side.

> **Note:** You can also exchange the extended leg on the ground for the leg position from the seated pose, Virasana (Hero Pose; see chapter 13.2, number 2), or Baddha Konasana (Bound Angle Pose; see chapter 13.2, number 3).

10. Kurmasana

Kurma means "tortoise."

Many of the asanas are named after animals. By taking its form, the belief is that you appropriate the powers of the animal.

There are various variations of this asana: a standing, or "suspended," variation, in which your body is balanced on your arms (this pose is described here, but it also belongs in the balance poses in chapter 10.6), and two supine variations. They can be completed in the following order.

Standing variation

- Stand with your feet against the sides of your yoga mat and bend your knees. Slide your arms as far as you can under your knees, until your shoulders and knees meet.
- Take hold of your ankles and maintain the contact of your knees with your shoulders while you straighten your legs as much as you can (figure 10.5-16).

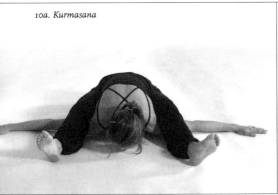

10a. Kurmasana

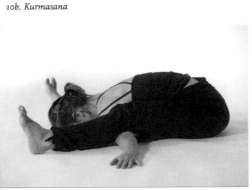

10b. Kurmasana

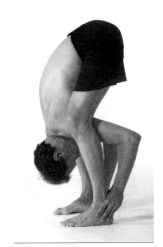

10c. Kurmasana

10.5-16

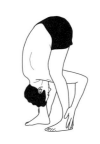

- The stretch of your legs produces pressure against your upper arms and shoulders. Try to coordinate this pressure so that your arms stay connected with your shoulder blades. Then the pressure of your knees will improve the extension of your lower back. Otherwise, your knees will push your arms away from your shoulder blades, and you will lose the connection with your lower back.
- Remain in this pose for 10 to 20 seconds, breathing as freely as possible. Return to standing or move into the following pose.

11. Dvi hasta bhujasana

Dvi means "two"; *hasta* means "hand"; *bhuja* means "arm."
This pose also belongs to the balance poses described in chapter 10.6.

11. Dvi hasta bhujasana

Instructions

- From the preceding position, bend your knees and place your palms flat on the floor. Your hands and arms will now be able to carry your body weight so that you can lift your feet off the floor. Keep your shoulders low and your abdominal muscles relaxed.

> **Note:** You can also cross your feet (figure 10.5-17). This pose is called Bhujapidasana (Shoulder-Pressing Pose). *Bhuja* means "shoulder" or "arm"; *pida* means "pressure."

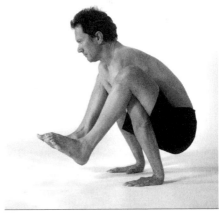

- Remain in this pose for 10 to 20 seconds. Allow the space and tranquillity of your breathing to become central.
- Now you can complete the two variations of Titibhasana.

10.5-17

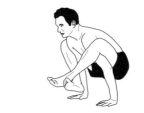

12. Titibhasana

Titibha means "firefly."
This pose also belongs to the balance poses described in chapter 10.6.

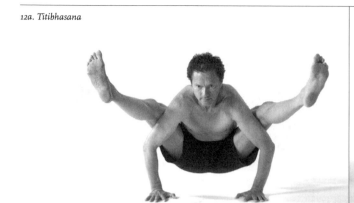

12a. Titibhasana

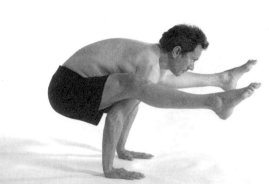

12b. Titibhasana

Variation 1

· Slide your pelvis forward and extend your legs, lifting them as high as you can.
· Hold this position for 10 to 20 seconds, then return or move into the following pose.

Variation 2

· From variation 1, with your pelvis high, look straight ahead, and extend your legs parallel to the floor.
· Remain in this end pose for 10 to 20 seconds, breathing as freely as possible. Return or move into the following pose.

Kurmasana end pose 1

· When taking the pose from variation 2, bend your arms so that you can sit on the floor.
· Stretch your arms sideways under your knees, and push your knees against your upper arms without loosening the connection between your upper arms and shoulder blades. This extends your back, and your abdomen moves closer to the floor. Keep pushing back with your upper arms, or your legs will push your arms into the ground.
· Remain in this asana for 10 to 12 seconds, and breathe as freely as possible from your abdomen to your chest. Return or move into the following pose.

Kurmasana end pose 2

· From end pose 1, bend your legs and place your left foot on top of your right. If necessary, use your hands to do this. Rest your forehead on the floor between your ankles. Take hold of your hands behind your back (figure 10.5-18). This pose resembles a tortoise that has pulled its head and feet into its shell.
· Reverse the crossing of your feet after 10 to 20 seconds.
· Release your feet and arms to come out of the pose.

10.5-18

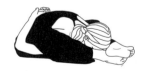

All of these variations are more intense than Paschimottanasana for stretching L4, L5, and your hips. Therefore, it is important to position your lower back correctly. If your back protests after these asanas and you feel that you cannot stand up straight for a long time, this says something about the preference position of your lower vertebrae. Allow them to extend by lying on your back or on a thick lower back roll, or jump up into Adho Mukha Vrksasana.

10.6 Balance poses

13. Eka Hasta Bhujasana

Eka means "one"; *hasta* means "hand"; *bhuja* means "arm."
You can do this pose after Kraunchasana (see chapter 10.5, number 9).

Instructions

- Complete Kraunchasana with your right leg high and your left leg extended. Bend your right leg and slide your right arm under your knee until your shoulder meets your knee. Place your right hand flat on the floor, just in front of your pelvis.
- Take hold of your right foot with your left hand and pull your foot toward your left shoulder so that your leg does not slide down your right arm. Lean forward and shift your weight toward your right hand, increasing the contact of your right leg with your right upper arm.
- Push your right thigh firmly against your arm and slowly release your right foot. Your foot moves outward, but your leg stays in the same place.
- Place your left hand approximately 20 to 24 inches to the side of your right hand along the same plane and push your body away from the floor. In phase 1, you can keep your left foot on the floor to maintain your balance. In phase 2, place your left foot on top of your right and then extend your left leg forward. This end pose works your abdominal muscles.
- Keep your shoulders low and breathe freely, keeping your neck and face relaxed.
- Remain in this end pose for 10 to 20 seconds, and repeat on the other side or move into the following pose.

13a. Eka hasta bhujasana   13b. Eka hasta bhujasana

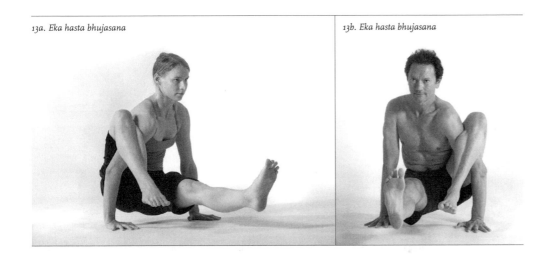

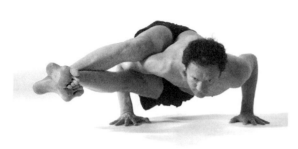

10.6-1a   10.6-1b

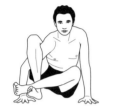 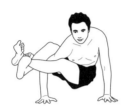

14. Astavakrasana

Astavakra is the name of a Brahman.

The story of Astavakra, the son of Kahoda, is told in the *Maha-bharata*—the longest epic poem in the world. It recounts the war of the Bharata family.* Kahoda married Uddalaka but was so dedicated to his study that he neglected his wife. When Uddalaka was in the last weeks of her pregnancy, her unborn child commented on the behavior of his father. His father was furious and cursed his son, who was born misshapen (*vakra*) in eight (*asta*) places. Only after twelve years did his father remove the curse, and Astavakra's limbs became straight.

Instructions

- From Eka Hasta Bhujasana, place your left foot on top of your right. Push your right leg firmly against your right upper arm and extend your right knee, keep your leg high by bending your right arm slightly (figures 10.6-1a and 10.6-1b).
- Lift your pelvis off the floor and lean forward. Bear in mind that your left shoulder will be carrying most of your weight. Push your left hand firmly into the floor.

Note: The strength must come from your left arm and not from pulling up your left shoulder. As soon as you pull your shoulder up, your arm will twist, and you will end up with your chest on the floor. Here, your arm must remain connected to your shoulder blade (see chapter 6.3, connection 4).

- Remain in this pose for as long as you can, remembering that you need to reserve some strength for returning to the pose in figure 10.6-1b.
- Relax and repeat on the other side.

---

* Bharata was a legendary hero and monarch of India, and the word *Bharata* was originally understood to mean his sons and family. From that, it has come to mean "India, the land of the Bharatas."

II

BACKBENDS

11.1 Introduction

When you bend backward, your head, sometimes together with your arms, initiates the movement toward your upper back and chest. Then the movement is passed on to your inner tube, which transfers the movement through the midline of your lower back and into your pelvis and legs. Many back problems stem from sitting for long periods with a bent back, from incorrect bending and lifting, and from stress. All of these cause areas of your spine to become progressively stiffer so that eventually the areas are unable to extend and stretch adequately. Stiffness makes it difficult to move with ease and that, in turn, diminishes your desire to move. Children have difficulty sitting still; adults have difficulty moving.

In the changing room of my studio in Amsterdam, differences in behavior after a backbend lesson are immediately obvious: students are physically more active and talk more than after other lessons. The atmosphere is full of energy.

Backbends are invaluable for the spine. They help prevent malformations of the vertebrae, and they increase the mobility of the intervertebral discs. They develop feelings of lightness in the upper back and chest and feelings of alertness, quickness, and strength in the lower back.

Backbends can be divided into three subgroups that work on the upper back, lower back, and entire body.

1. Backbends for the upper body

Salabhasana (Locust Pose), Urdhva Mukha Svanasana, and Bhujangasana—as well as a passive coordination exercise (lying on the backbender) in which your upper back, arms, and shoulders are prepared for the asanas—belong to this subgroup.

The coordination exercise and the asanas target the connections between your head, upper back, and sternum, as well as between your arms and shoulder blades. You need to pay attention to the location of your breath and how it guides movement in your chest.

2. Backbends for the lower body

The coordination exercises in this subgroup focus on how movement from your spine is transferred through your pelvis to your hips and legs without overloading your lower back. In these asanas, I emphasize the role of the inner tube, or air bag, during backbends. (For this, reread the discussion of Virabhadrasana I in chapter 9.5, number 14.) Ustrasana, Dhanurasana, and Parsva Dhanurasana (Side Bow Pose) belong to this subgroup.

3. Backbends for the entire body

The characteristics of the previous subgroups are combined in these asanas, with emphasis on the total movement of backbending. In Bhekasana (Frog Pose), the emphasis is on actual spinal strength. In the other poses, your arms and the legs become the pillars of strength that carry the movement, allowing your spine to move freely and easily. Bhekasana, Urdhva Dhanurasana, and Viparita Chakrasana belong to this subgroup.

11.2 Backbends for the upper body

The exercises in this subgroup are directed toward the connections between your head, upper back, and chest, as well as between your arms and shoulder blades. Again, you need to pay attention to the correct use of breathing during movement.

A passive coordination exercise, Salabhasana, Urdhva Mukha Svanasana, and Bhujangasana belong to this group.

Coordination and preparation exercise 1

In this exercise, your upper back lies on the backbender, and your arms are stretched over your head. I always use it in my lessons as a preparation for advanced backbends; I use it regularly in my beginner lessons and almost always during therapeutic lessons. Because the stretch is held for long periods, you can gain insight into the basic movement of backbending—that is, the backward bending of your upper back. During actual backbends, this insight is more difficult to realize, because you can hold poses for only short periods (compare with Urdhva Dhanurasana and Viparita Chakrasana, for example).

During this coordination exercise, you learn how to stretch your arms over your head without tensing your back muscles, how to connect your neck with your upper back, and how to use your breathing to release tension so that energy can flow freely through your body. In addition, this exercise has a strong effect on the position of your vertebrae and the shape of your intervertebral discs as they are pushed back into a balanced, even position. This gives the exercise a distinct therapeutic value.

Lie on a rubber strip with one end folded double to prepare for this exercise. Move your pelvis up and down, as described in chapter 6.3, connection 2.

Coordination exercise 1: upper back on the backbender

Phase 1

- Place the backbender on the front of your yoga mat, with the sloping edge facing forward. Lay the rubber strip on top, with the majority of the strip hanging over the sloping edge. Sit down and lean against the backbender. The rubber strip should press against your spine between your shoulder blades. Take hold of the back of your head with your hands (figure 11.2-1).
- Raise your pelvis until it is even with the top of the backbender. Push with your feet toward the place where the strip and your back meet. Feel the movement in your skin. With one hand, make sure the last neck vertebra (C7) is free, just above the strip. Place both hands behind your head again, and from the place where your back meets the strip, lift your head so that your neck lengthens; move your elbows toward each other until they are about shoulder-width apart. When you relax your neck muscles, your head will become heavy in your hands; keep holding your head up with your hands.
- Feel the pressure of the strip against your back (see the shaded area for phase 1 in figure 11.2-2) and relax that area with exhalations. At the same time, with every exhalation, lower your head *without losing length in your neck*. Imagine that your neck originates at the place where your back and the strip meet. Move slowly; divide the movement into three or four parts with a pause between each. Do not move according to the speed and force of your will as you do in ordinary movements. Here, the movement should contribute to relaxation. Visualize that the pull of your hands not only lengthens your neck but also creates a little space between the vertebrae that are in contact with the strip. Let your hands pull your vertebrae apart to improve the extension.

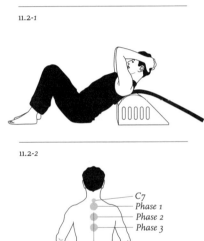

11.2-1

11.2-2

C7
Phase 1
Phase 2
Phase 3

Note: If you notice at the end of the movement that your neck starts to arch and you are not able to correct that tension, double the rubber strip under your head. Then you do not have to lower your head as much.

- Place the palms of your hands against your forehead while keeping your elbows together. Push the back of your head firmly against the strip. This point becomes your "anchor." Move your diaphragm and pelvis gently up and down to mobilize your upper back.

Note: If your neck moves with the movement of your pelvis (that is, becomes more concave when you lower your pelvis), then the effect of the exercise will be compromised. When you notice your neck beginning to shorten, do not move farther with your pelvis. Instead, make sure that you keep pushing with your feet to direct pressure toward the place where the strip and your back meet.

- After a couple of minutes, hook your thumbs together and extend your arms over your head. Your arms also move toward the place where your back and the strip meet. When your arms are in their end position (see chapter 6.3, connection 4), you can create length in your upper back by extending them away from your back. Imagine that your arms are pulling your vertebrae apart, creating space.
- Remain in this position for 1 to 2 minutes.

> **Note:** Instead of hooking your thumbs together, you can place the headstand bench or a chair behind the backbender, then take hold of the horizontal bar of the bench or the chair legs so that you do not have to bear all the weight of your arms. This is a good variation for lengthening your back. If you want to stretch your back even more, move your hands down the headstand/chair legs toward the floor.

> **Note:** This exercise can create a tender feeling in your upper back that can linger for a couple of days. Do not worry if this occurs; it is a sign of positive change. In fact, it means you have entered the deeper layers of tension and are releasing them. One of the characterizations of structural tension is our lack of awareness of it in daily activities. We carry it with us unconsciously day after day. Exercises like this make us conscious of it and give us the opportunity to free ourselves from it. Nevertheless, if you have the feeling that it is overwhelming, shorten the length of time you spend doing the exercise.

Phases 2 and 3

- Lift your pelvis until it is even with the top of the backbender, and hold the back of your head with your hands. Lift your head and slide over the backbender until your back is lying on the place indicated for phase 2 in figure 11.2-2. Do not be in a hurry to lower your head. Keep it high and feel the precise spot where your back meets the strip. Guide your breath toward that spot and let yourself become heavy. Lower your head and move your arms in the same manner as described for phase 1.
- After phase 2, move your back to the place shown for phase 3 in figure 11.2-2 and repeat the exercise.
- Remain in each phase for 1 to 2 minutes. To return, lift your pelvis, hold the back of your head with your hands, and during exhalations, slowly lower your pelvis to the floor.

If the following exercise is too stressful, keep practicing with the upper back roll (see chapter 6.3, connection 2).

11.2-3

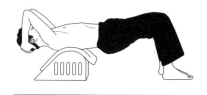

With the midback on the backbender

- Place a felt mat over the backbender with the sloping edge facing away from you. Sit with approximately 4 inches of space between your buttocks and the backbender so that you can lift yourself up and lie on top of it. Hold the back of your head with your hands. Lift your pelvis so that your midback, just under your shoulder blades, is resting on the backbender. Your body should be level from head to knees (figure 11.2-3).

- Guide your breath toward the spot where your back is resting on the backbender and release the tension there while *simultaneously* lowering your head and pelvis. If your head cannot reach the backbender, place a doubled-up rubber strip under your head so that you can extend your arms over your head without tension in your neck.
- Remain in this position for 1 to 3 minutes. Return slowly.

1. *Salabhasana*

1. Salabhasana

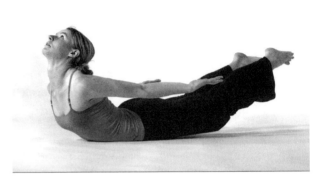

Salabha **means "locust."**

Instructions

- Lie on your stomach on a felt mat or a shoulderstand block. Rest your forehead on your hands and relax your upper back, shoulders, and arms so that the weight of your body descends to your chest. Gently push your hara area just below your navel toward the floor; feel the inward movement of the arch of your lower back. This correctly positions your lower back and pelvis.
- Breathe in toward your sternum. The inhalation pulls the vertebrae between your shoulder blades inward, which allows your neck to rise so that your forehead moves away from your hands. Raise your neck until it is in line with your upper back; this movement can be compared to an elevator (see page 103) moving straight up, and it produces pressure in your heart gravity point.
- Distribute the pressure between your two gravity points evenly and extend your arms back alongside your body. At the end of an inhalation, elevate your chest, and move your head toward your upper back during exhalations. In the beginning, this may cause some strain in your neck. Try to solve this problem by directing your inhalations to the top of your lungs. This produces an upward movement in the top of your sternum and your first ribs. This movement, in turn, helps you extend the vertebrae just below your neck. When this starts to happen, you can release your upper back more, allowing it to sink deeper between your shoulder blades during exhalations. Then your neck is able to transport the weight of your head into your spine, and the pressure in your neck is released. Take your time and analyze this movement precisely. Coordination exercise 1 is an important preparation for this.

Note: The movement of your head may remain "hanging" in your neck if your upper back is not properly extended. Alternatively, the movement may go straight into your lower back. If this happens, your upper body has lifted, and your weight is being carried by your abdomen. There will be no pressure on your heart gravity point because the movement is not initiated from your breath, as described earlier, but from the activity of your lower back.

This movement of the head is also used in the standing variations of backbends. Many people find it scary to let their head drop back. The advantage of this prone variation is that your head moves against the force of gravity.   *(continued)*

- Feel how your inhalations fill your lungs right up to your collarbones; allow every inhalation to elevate you farther until you carry your body weight with your lower abdomen.
- When you cannot move any farther, lift your arms as far as you can without tightening your shoulders. Your arms push against your shoulder blades, the weight of your head is transferred to your upper back, and your inhalations fill your lungs completely—everything is directed toward the upward force of your upper chest. This force, which can be isolated well in this pose, plays an important role in backbends.
- Elevate your stretched legs with your heels turned out, which keeps your sacrum and buttocks relaxed.

All of the strength for this end position must come from your back. For this reason, it is a powerful antidote to habitual movements that tend to encourage a stiff posture and a bent back. Backbends increase the flexibility of your back.

11.2-4

Note: A second variation is aimed at increasing strength in the lowest vertebrae of your back. In this version, the palms of your hands are placed on the ground and your knees are bent (figure 11.2-4). Ensure that you keep your knees together, even though you will be able to go higher if you allow them to spread apart.

- Remain in this position as long possible, breathing freely from your abdomen to the top of your chest. Return and relax with your forehead on your hands, or move immediately into the following pose.

2. Urdhva Mukha Svanasana

Urdhva mukha means "face upward"; *sva* means "dog."
The difference between this pose and Salabhasana is that strength is replaced with relaxation of the back in Urdhva Mukha Svanasana. This relaxation does wonders for the vertebrae and intervertebral discs. Read the instructions carefully (even if your back is flexible) to learn how to transfer the movement of your lower back into your pelvis and hips.

You can move into this pose in two ways. The first is from Salabhasana; the second is from standing on your hands and knees. Both ways are discussed here. If your lower back or wrists are very sensitive, you can do this pose with your hands on a chair (figure 11.2-5).

Instructions

From Salabhasana

- Return your feet to the floor and keep pressing your lower abdomen into the floor.
- Feel the connection between your arms and shoulder blades by lifting your arms as high as you can. Feel the end of the movement exerting pressure on your back,

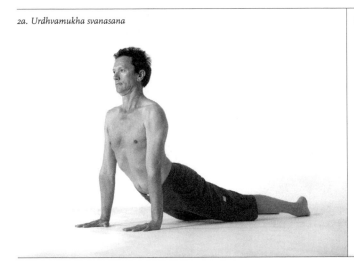

2a. Urdhvamukha svanasana

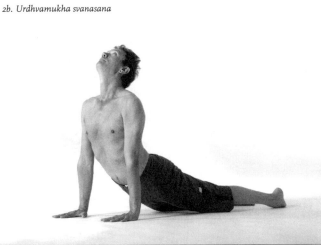

2b. Urdhvamukha svanasana

not creating tension in your shoulder girdle or neck. Place your hands on the floor next to your diaphragm without tensing your shoulders; keep your upper arms pushing against your shoulder blades (visualize this), as shown in figure 11.2-6.

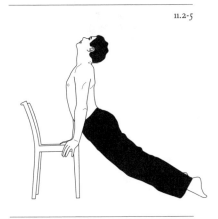

11.2-5

- Be very conscious about the pressure of your abdomen on the floor. This pressure ensures the air bag effect, which your abdominal muscles must take over as soon as your abdomen lifts off the floor.
- Breathe in deeply and feel the space that is created in your upper chest. Push this area up using your arms with their connection to your shoulder blades intact and the weight of your head extending your upper back. Relax your lower back as soon as your arms become active.

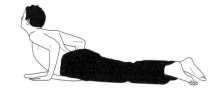

11.2-6

Note: Make sure to relax your back and not your abdominal muscles. Your abdominal muscles keep your diaphragm and pelvis in the correct position and guide the movement toward your SI joints, tailbone, and hips. From this perspective, it is helpful to experience the effects of coordination exercise 3 before performing this asana. Coordinate your breathing so that your abdominal muscles remain active when you breathe deeply—right up to the top of your lungs. Rotate your arms inward so that you can push with the inside of your hands. Your shoulders broaden in relation to your collarbones (see the arrows in figure 11.2-7). Initially, this may feel like an obstructive movement, but it maintains the correct connection to your shoulder blades so that they, in turn, can support the space in your chest. Press your fingertips lightly into the floor to strengthen the cohesion in your wrists.

Feel where the movement "lands" in your back. If you have the feeling that you are hanging in your lower back, use your exhalations to move your lower ribs back toward your abdomen and contract your lower abdominals (just below your navel) until you feel that your tailbone is becoming heavier. Experiment with this movement; try bending your knees so *(continued)*

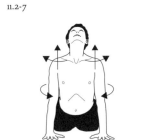

11.2-7

that your pelvis can move more easily. If you do not feel that your weight is moving into your tailbone but remains hanging in your lower back, you should use Virabhadrasana I (see chapter 9.5, number 14) to prepare. That will release your hips so that you can use your lower abdominals to tilt your pelvis backward. When your tailbone finally lengthens your lower back, the vertebrae and intervertebral discs (the cream inside the waffles, as described with Virabhadrasana I) will be pulled apart, allowing the discs to move back to a balanced position.

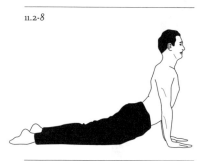

11.2-8

Note: If your neck is painful when your head is elevated, look straight ahead (figure 11.2-8). Develop the head–spine connection as described for Salabhasana.

· When you feel that your tailbone is moving downward, start to push your feet into the floor while slowly stretching your knees. Do not lose the upward grip of your lower abdomen toward your navel at this stage of the movement. The arch of your lower back will extend even more, and when your lower back stays relaxed, your tailbone will move farther down. Ensure that you keep your shoulders down. The additional weight of your legs makes your pelvis heavier.

Note: During this phase of the movement, you may develop certain reflexes that disturb the relaxation. If your lower back experiences pain, then it will (unconsciously) start to resist the movement. Your body never chooses to move into pain. The question is, what is causing the pain? It may be that your body is resisting the movement, but it also may be due to the recovery of mobility in your back. Lying on the lower back roll can also be painful initially, but that pain diminishes with relaxation or after longer practice. If the pain begins to dominate, move more slowly. Learn to recognize the moment when your body starts to resist. Holding your breath or irregular breathing and muscle contraction are the first signs of resistance. This reaction starts *before* you experience pain and blocks movement.

The source of this reflex can also be rooted in your thinking. Before the movement arrives in the sensitive area of your lower back, unconscious or automatic negative thoughts, or memories. The cause of the past experience could be, for example, an injury, or a strong manipulation by a teacher, or stiffness when you started to practice yoga. Even when the body is healed, it does not always means that the thinking patterns vanish. Often, these automatic thoughts dominate your behavior for years. The only way to break these thoughts is to develop a positive experience in another area of your body. When you are fully submerged in that experience, you may forget the original pain.

You can use this exercise to determine whether the theory works, because an experience of lightness is connected to the openness in your chest, which has been emphasized, from the beginning of the exercise. Do not break that experience. The tendency to do so comes at the moment when you stretch out your arms. This action can be done quickly and from willpower, which immediately breaks the experience and allows your negative thoughts to become active. This will happen when the movement arrives in your lower back. Therefore, stretch out your arms as slowly as possible and stay immersed in the experience of lightness, which is carried by your breath, when you push your chest upward. When this experience stays dominant, unconscious thoughts do not have a chance to become active, and I have experienced many instances when the pain seemed to be gone. To my unpleasant surprise, it seemed as if I had become attached to the pain. I felt disturbed when I noticed it was not there anymore; I had to focus on something else (the positive experience), which felt strange and uneasy in the beginning.

Pain in the lower back feels fearful, but when you are aware of the experience of space and feelings of lightness during the movement, you have a tool with which you can examine your pain and the fear connected with it, and possibly break the habit. It is only then that you are able to experience the exercise fully.

- Remain in this pose for 20 to 30 seconds. Bend your arms and relax, lying on your stomach with your forehead resting on your hands. Repeat the movement three times.

From hands and knees

- On your hands and knees, allow your upper back to sink deeply into the area between your shoulder blades so that your arms can connect to your shoulder blades. Allow your hamstrings to relax completely. All this produces an excessive arch in your lower back. Draw your lower ribs in without losing that arch, and pull your hara area up to your navel. Keep your abdominal muscles compact. Imitate the feeling of lying on the floor (where your lower ribs are pushed toward your abdomen, and your lower abdomen is pressed into the floor), as shown in figure 11.2-9.
- Connect your abdomen to your chest with your breath, and move the back of your head backward. Breathe deeply into your chest, and lower your pelvis toward the floor in the direction of your hands. Remain conscious of your breathing. Move slowly so that you can maintain the contraction of your abdominal muscles.
- Allow your tailbone to become heavy, and push your chest high. Slowly straighten your knees as described in the preceding variation, coming from Salabhasana.
- Remain in this pose for 20 to 30 seconds, then lift your pelvis and return to your hands and knees. Repeat the movement three times.

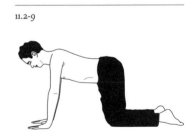

11.2-9

3. Bhujangasana

Bhuj means "bent"; *anga* means "body" (and secondarily "cobra," because the body rises up as in the asana).
The difference between Bhujangasana and Urdhva Mukha Svanasana is that the hanging of the lower back is central to the latter pose. The weight of the pelvis and legs is used to pull the accordion of the lower back open. This is possible because the legs are off

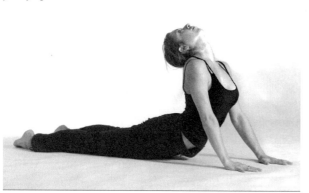

the floor. Contrary to this, in Bhujangasana, the lower back is extended through *pressure*. The arms push the upper body up against gravity, but the thighs remain on the floor — there is no hanging. The pressure to the lower back is supplied by the weight of the upper body. The pressure is less than that experienced in the standing variations of backbends like Viparita Chakrasana (see chapter 11.4, number 9). The pressure on the lowest vertebrae during that movement is much greater, because the weight of the body is guided there with the force of gravity.

Bhujangasana is a classic pose that is used in many physical therapies. Physiotherapists and the McKenzie Method apply it to treat lumbago, herniated discs, and other lower back problems. It is used therapeutically during yoga as well. It can be a rather advanced pose for practitioners with stiff backs. Therefore, it should not be done without preparation. The back should be prepared for this pose with the thick lower back roll (see chapter 6.3, connection 7), followed by Salabhasana and Urdva Mukha Svanasana.

Instructions

- Lie on the floor with your stomach on a felt mat or a shoulderstand block. Let your head rest on your hands. Relax your shoulders, arms, and upper back. Use exhalations to relax your lower back.
- Gently push your lower abdomen into the floor to position your pelvis and lower back. Turn your heels out slightly to keep your buttock muscles relaxed. Keep the lowest vertebrae in your back heavy and relaxed. Your exhalations should end with a push toward the floor at the level of your lower abdomen. This type of exhalation pulls the arch of your lower back farther in. It also makes it possible to start your next inhalation with a feeling of relaxation.
- With an inhalation directed to your sternum, allow the vertebrae between your shoulder blades to extend. Let your head rise. Your forehead moves away from your hands, and the weight of your head is transferred through your neck and upper back into the heart region.
- Place your hands next to your face and in front of your shoulders on the floor. Lift your head and sternum during the next inhalation, and let the weight of your head roll through your neck into your upper back and heart region. Balance on your lower ribs and breathe deeply toward your chest. Stay in this position for a few breaths.
- With every inhalation, allow yourself to rise toward your lower back without using the strength of your arms. When you cannot go any higher with the strength of your back, press your hands into the floor without moving farther up. Your arms take over the movement, making it possible to relax your back completely. Continue as far as you can, and allow the movement to move toward your tailbone. Every time your back resists the movement, stop and consciously use your exhalations to relax and release the tension. Move farther only when the muscles have eased. If stretching your arms is too difficult, lean on your elbows and wait until your lower back relaxes.

Note: Relax your back and buttock muscles but not your abdominals. Your abdominal muscles create the air bag effect, as described for Virabhadrasana I (see chapter 9.5, number 14), and they transfer the movement toward your pelvic floor.

- Keep your shoulders low and straighten your arms. Rotate your arms inward while keeping your shoulders low and broad, as described for Urdhva Mukha Svanasana, so that your arms remain connected to your shoulder blades. Your shoulder blades, in turn, elevate your chest.

Note: If this movement is painful for your lower back, remain aware of the space around you. Instead of becoming absorbed in the pain, feel how your body can open by breathing into the space around you. This difference in attention can increase your relaxation and lessen the pain (also see Urdhva Mukha Svanasana).

- In the end position, allow your lower abdomen to rise from the floor so that the movement can be transferred through to your hips and thighs (figure 11.2-10).

Note: It can be helpful to do this exercise with your toes against a wall, which prevents your legs from sliding farther back. Then your legs can offer resistance to your pelvis, making it easier to complete the movement.

- Keep breathing deeply, while maintaining control of your abdominal muscles. Allow your breathing to stimulate feelings of relaxation in your abdomen and lightness in your chest. Be especially vigilant about not relaxing your abdominals when breathing.
- Remain in this pose for 20 to 30 seconds. Return slowly, vertebra by vertebra, with your head last.

11.2-10

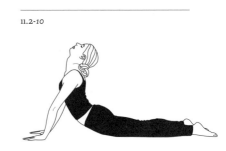

11.3 Backbends for the lower body

Two passive coordination exercises, Ustrasana, Dhanurasana, and Parsva Dhanurasana belong to this subgroup. All of these exercises are directed toward transferring movement through the spine to the pelvis and hips without overloading the lower back. The role of the inner tube is especially important here. Reread the instructions for Virabhadrasana I (see chapter 9.5, number 14).

Coordination and preparation exercises 2 and 3

Coordination exercise 2: hip stretch with the knee against the wall

This exercise stretches both your quadriceps and the muscles in the front of your hips. It releases both these areas, allowing the backbending movement to transfer from your

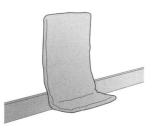

back through your pelvis and into your legs. When these areas are sufficiently mobile, a lot of pain and tension will disappear from your lower back.

The exercise is described in two phases. The first phase is directed toward your quadriceps, while the second phase is an intensive stretch for your quadriceps and the muscles in the front of your hips.

Phase 1

- Place a felt mat against the wall, as shown in figure 11.3-1.
- Place your right knee on the floor, hard against the wall; the front of your calf and top of your foot are also against the wall. Position your left foot in front of you. Place your hands on your left thigh, and use your left foot to push your pelvis toward the wall. (Ultimately, the back of your pelvis will meet the wall.) Make sure you keep your pelvis level so that your left hip does not rise.
- When your pelvis touches the wall, contract your abdominals so that the arch of your lower back is lengthened. This increases the stretch to your quadriceps. In this position, it is easy to feel how the weight of your body lands directly above your tailbone and how the contraction of your abdominal muscles lengthens the arch of your lower back. Once your muscles relax, your pelvis will move along the wall toward the floor. Hold this pose for 1 minute (figure 11.3-2).

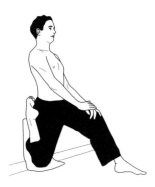

Note: You can move into a supine variation of this pose from Virasana (see chapter 13.2, number 2).

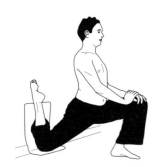

Phase 2

- Keep the upward pull of your abdominal muscles just below your navel active and start to bend your left leg until you have reached the maximum stretch in the front of your hip and thigh (figure 11.3-3).

Note: Reread the comments for Virabhadrasana I that explain the principle of the air bag effect during backbends. They apply here as well.

- If the tension in your thigh is excessive, push your right hand against your right calf. That almost always lessens the pain.
- If you are comfortable with the stretch, you can increase it by pushing your right foot into the wall. This pushes your tailbone down farther.
- Remain in this pose for 1 minute, then repeat on the other side.

Coordination exercise 3: lower back and tailbone on the backbender

Many people hang in their lower back in backbends. Some experience a lot of pain during this movement; others, none at all. To complete the movement in a natural way, it is important that the movement can leave the back. Many exercises are initiated from the head and move, vertebra by vertebra, down the spine toward the pelvis, SI joints, and hips. The exercises here are directed toward the last phase of this movement. If the muscles in the back of the pelvis are stiff, they will narrow the pelvis and block the free flow of movement into the hips. Because of this, the lower back can overload easily.

If your back is stiff, prepare it first by lying on the thick lower back roll. The following exercise is described in two phases. During the first phase, your lower back is placed on top of the backbender; during the second phase, your tailbone is on top. Critical Alignment applies phase 2 in the therapeutic treatment of a (beginning) herniated disc, because the spinal cord (on which the bulging disc often presses) receives traction in this position. This makes it possible for the disc to move back toward its correct position.

Phase 1

With the lower back on the backbender

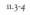

- Place a felt mat on the backbender so that the straight edge is toward your feet. Bend your legs and lie with your lower back on the backbender so that your shoulders are almost touching the ground (figure 11.3-4). You can vary the placement of your lower back—from the kidney area just below your ribs to the pelvic rim—so that you can relax the most painful parts of your back.
- Keep your knees together, and when the pain begins to lessen in your lower back, slowly extend your right leg and then the left. Make sure that the toes of your extended legs point straight up and that your legs are rotated inward, as described in chapter 6.3, connection 11.
- Remain in this pose for 1 to 2 minutes. Return or move into the following exercise.

If you are unfamiliar with this exercise, begin with shorter time spans—1 to 2 minutes—and see how your back reacts.

11.3-4

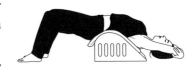

Phase 2

With your tailbone on the backbender

- From the previous exercise, move so that your tailbone is on top of the backbender. Do not go too far or you will slide past that point.
- Rest your shoulders on the floor and your feet firmly on the floor (see figure 11.3-5c). If your feet do not touch the floor easily, put a shoulderstand block under them. Place your hands on your lower ribs. Relax your ribs with exhalations so that additional space can develop in the vertebrae (and spinal cord) of your lower back. This traction has been described, together with the air bag effect, for Virabhadrasana I (see chapter 9.5, number 14).
- Observe the position of your knees, as they give you valuable information about stiffness in the back of your pelvis and your SI joints. If your knees move outward, the back of your pelvis will narrow, and that will be detrimental to the mobility of your SI joints. Then the transfer of the backbend from your back to your tailbone will be blocked: the sacral area of your lower back will hold on to the movement, which will overload your lower back. Try to move your knees toward each other. Make this an easy movement; do not force it. Imagine the back of your pelvis broadening, starting from the place where you feel your tailbone on the backbender.
- After 1 minute, take hold of the sides of the backbender and lift both knees. Keep them together, and move your feet up and down slowly, without relaxing your abdominal

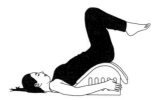
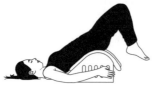
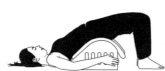
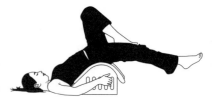

muscles (figures 11.3-5a through 11.3-5c). Keep bending from your hips rather than your lower back. Your abdominal muscles prevent the movement from shifting into your lower back.

· After 1 minute, lift your knees and extend your right leg (figure 11.3-6). Your bent leg should keep your pelvis in the correct position, while your extended leg stretches your hip on that side. Remember that the weight of your leg is 16 percent of your total body weight. Remain in this position for 30 to 60 seconds, and repeat on the other side.

· Extend your bent leg toward the ceiling and begin a sort of "cross-country skiing" movement with your legs. Once you feel that you have warmed up, you can begin to let the descending leg fall from an increasingly higher level without bending your knee. Finally, extend both legs together to a horizontal position without releasing your abdominal muscles. Your tailbone should always move away from your lower back in this exercise.

· Take 1 to 2 minutes to complete these variations, then bend your knees and place your feet on the floor.

· Take hold of the backbender and slide off backward toward your shoulders. You will end with your pelvis on the floor and the backs of your knees resting on the backbender. Stay here for a moment, feeling the space you have developed in the back of your pelvis.

4. Ustrasana

4. Ustrasana

Ustra means "camel."

The benefit of Ustrasana is that the knees are fixed on the ground. As seen from coordination exercise 3, this provides space to the pelvis so that the movement can be transferred from the back to the pelvic floor, hips, and thighs. For this reason, it is a safe exercise for those with lower back issues.

The movement can be initiated from the knees or from sitting on the feet.

Variation 1: from the knees

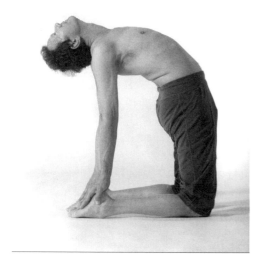

· Kneel with your knees hip-width apart on a felt mat. Push your fists against your tailbone, and position your pelvis as if you were lying facedown on a shoulderstand block and pushing your lower abdomen into the floor. Move your lower ribs toward the arch of your lower back to activate your inner tube. The area under your fists (your tailbone) moves away from your lower back.

- Breathe from your lower abdomen to the top of your lungs, and use the space created in the top of your chest to connect your neck to your upper back. Let your head drop down. Imagine your chin moving back from the top of your sternum and *not* from your throat. This will create pressure in your neck. Use the weight of your head and allow your head to hang, but do not stop the movement.

> **Note:** If this is too painful for your neck, keep your gaze straight ahead and move your chest farther back at the end of each inhalation. Practice placing your head in the prone position described for Salabhasana (see chapter 11.2, number 1). Make sure you direct your breathing toward the elevation of your sternum and not your lower ribs.

11.3-7

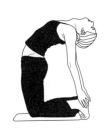

- Two movements are now occurring simultaneously: at the end of each inhalation, your chest moves farther up and back over your fists, while your thighs move forward. Relax your neck, shoulders, and upper back during exhalations. Maintain the height of your chest, and push your feet against the floor to keep your tailbone and thighs in position. This way, the arch of your back can develop with every inhalation without losing the air bag effect. Carry on until you feel that your upper body has stretched back fully from the front of your thighs.
- Keep your thighs in front of your knees and (if standing on your toes) try to take hold of your ankles (figure 11.3-7), or place the palms of your hands on the soles of your feet (figure 11.3-8).

11.3-8

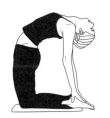

> **Note:** Observe the position of your thighs closely. If your pelvis moves back too far, your legs will build up tension. As usual, tension and stretch do not go well together. Using the headstand bench (see the following variation) can be very helpful in such circumstances.

- Breathing in and out deeply, remain in this position for 20 to 30 seconds. Push your feet firmly into the floor to move your pelvis forward. Move your fists back to your tailbone and return. Do not lead with your head when returning; use your abdominal muscles. Your head should be the last part to come out. When contracting your abdominals, keep pushing firmly against your tailbone. It is important to keep your tailbone in the correct position when returning. Alternatively, you can bend your knees and sit on your feet.

If your pelvis moves too far back when you take hold of your ankles, try using the headstand bench.

Variation 1: with the headstand bench

- Place the headstand bench against the wall and place your ankles against the insides of the bench legs (figure 11.3-9a).
- Start to bend backward as already described. When you can go no farther, take hold of the bench legs. Fill your lungs with inhalations, and with exhalations, allow your hands to slide down the bench legs toward the floor without losing the space in

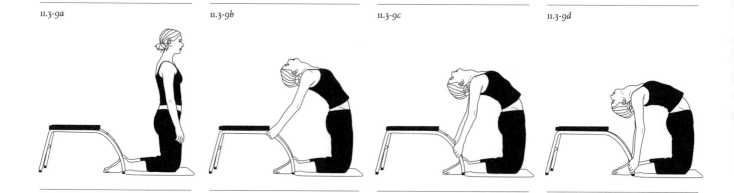

your chest. Your thighs will now remain easily in front of your knees (figures 11.3-9b through 11.3-9d). Ultimately, your hands and ankles will meet.

Variation 2: sitting on your feet

· Sit on your feet, and place your palms on your soles or take hold of your ankles.
· In a fluid total movement, on an inhalation, push your feet into the floor to lift your body up and forward. Use your hamstrings to push your pelvis and thighs forward powerfully. Your chest lifts with each inhalation.

5. Dhanurasana

Dhanur **means "bow."**

Your body forms a taut bow from your shoulders to your ankles in this pose. The knees often move apart in Dhanurasana. Keep them close together so that your leg muscles develop the correct strength. The air bag effect is strengthened and easy to maintain, as your abdomen carries the weight of your body. This is beneficial for opening the vertebrae and discs and makes this pose suitable if you have weak abdominal muscles. You can develop your breathing in the hara area well in this pose.

Instructions

5. Dhanurasana

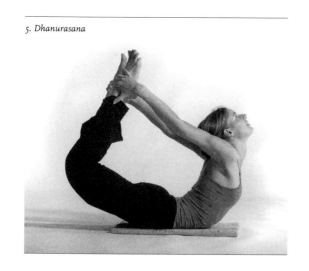

· Lie with your abdomen on a felt mat and take hold of your ankles. Position your lower back and pelvis by pushing the area just below your navel into the floor. This brings the weight of your body into your hara. Transfer the weight of your head into your upper back. Breathe deeply and feel how your exhalations, directed to the spot where your body is in contact with the floor, help you to relax your lower back. Every exhalation allows the arch of your lower back to move farther in. Maintain this type of breathing during the following steps.
· Lift your chest and knees during inhalations. Retain your body weight in the hara area of your abdomen. *Push* your feet into your hands, relax your shoulders, and simultaneously *lift* your knees and feet with your hands. Keep your knees at hip-width, even if this means that you cannot lift them as high.

- Breathe into your abdomen and chest. Relax your shoulders and back, and keep pushing your feet into your hands. Remember that relaxation clears the way for a new structure to emerge. Therefore, when your back relaxes, strength immediately develops in your legs.
- Remain in this pose for 20 to 30 seconds. Then return and rest your forehead on your hands or move directly into the following pose.

6. Parsva Dhanurasana

6. Parsva dhanurasana

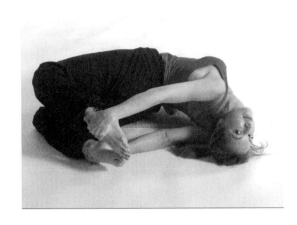

Parsva means "side"; *dhanur* means "bow."
Here, you complete Dhanurasana while lying on your side. Apart from the fact that your body weight is lying on one shoulder, which increases the stretch to your shoulders, the difference between Parsva Dhanurasana and Dhanurasana is mainly in the position of your knees, which move toward each other in Parsva Dhanurasana.

Instructions

- From Dhanurasana, roll onto your right side without losing the tautness of your bow. Keep pushing with your feet and lifting with your hands, even when you feel your knees moving closer together.
- Your right shoulder is pushed away from your right collarbone. Breathe into the top of your lungs to increase the space here from the inside out. Turn your head to the left and look over your shoulder toward your hands.
- Remain in this pose for 20 to 30 seconds. Roll back into Dhanurasana, maintaining your taut bow. Repeat the movement on the other side.

11.4 Total backbending movements

Bhekasana, Urdhva Dhanurasana, and Viparita Chakrasana form this subgroup. The focus here is on the total movement of backbends. In Bhekasana, the emphasis is on the strength of the spine itself. The other poses use the arms and legs to carry the movement, allowing the spine to move freely.

7. Bhekasana

7. Bhekasana

Bheka means "frog."
This pose stretches the front of the legs, freeing up the movement in the front of the pelvis for backbends. This makes it easier for the lower back to let go of tension.

Bhekasana is completed in two phases: initially with one leg, where the posture is held longer, and then with both legs together. Phase 2 is an intense stretch of the back and shoulders, and it emphasizes total movement from strength rather than suppleness.

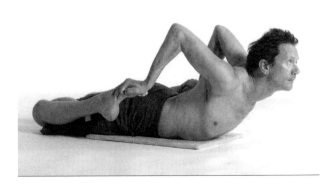

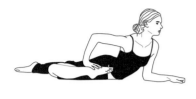

Phase 1: with one leg

- Lie on your abdomen on your yoga mat and lean on your elbows. Position your pelvis by pushing your lower abdomen into the floor.
- Bend your right leg and place the palm of your hand on the top of your foot. Push your foot down until it touches the floor next to your pelvis. Feel the pressure of your thigh on the floor, and visualize this pressure making the muscles of your leg relax and widen; this will help you release tension. Keep your pelvis balanced, and keep pushing your lower abdomen into the floor.
- Observe the position of your foot, and keep pushing your big toe and the ball of your foot down (figure 11.4-1). This keeps the stretch in the midline of your foot.
- Move slowly and ensure that your knee remains relaxed. This is an ideal stretch for athletes who use their legs a lot. The stretch takes the tension out of the muscles so that they do not stiffen. I have never felt that regularly stretching my leg muscles has diminished their strength. On the contrary, when running, my legs feel light and fast.
- Move the right side of your chest forward so that you can initiate the stretch to your shoulder. If you can complete this pose easily with your left elbow on the floor, try it with your arm stretched out as in Bhujangasana (see chapter 11.2, number 3). This will increase the stretch to your thigh immensely. The stretch to your leg in this pose can be compared with that in Virasana (see chapter 13.2, number 2).
- Remain in this pose for 1 minute, then repeat on the other side.

Phase 2: with both legs

- Lie on your abdomen and bend your knees. Place the palms of your hands on both feet.
- Raise your chest and head as high as you can, and push your feet toward the floor in the same way as for one leg. Share the action of pushing your feet down evenly with the elevation of your chest. Look up toward the ceiling and breathe regularly.
- This end pose strengthens your back muscles, relaxes your legs and knees, and creates a good stretch in your feet. Stay in the end position for as long as you can, return, and rest with your forehead on your hands.

8. Urdhva Dhanurasana

Urdhva means "up"; *dhanur* means "bow."

In contrast to many other asanas, this pose is well known in the West. Children often do this pose spontaneously, because it feels good to stretch the body this way. And many adults still associate this asana with feelings of freedom, youth, and joy. Unfortunately, time often wreaks havoc on the body, and many adults have adopted the exact opposite overall posture, bending or slumping forward.

The movement into Urdhva Dhanurasana often occurs impulsively and with haste, which means it may be performed in a sloppy manner. It is important to build it up slowly. It is much better to take your time and prepare yourself so that you can complete the pose with a good focus. Otherwise, you will return to habitual movements that may cause pain or exacerbate existing problems and bad posture.

Most of the problems that occur in this pose are related to the shoulders and/or lower back. Both areas will be addressed with extra exercises in the following description.

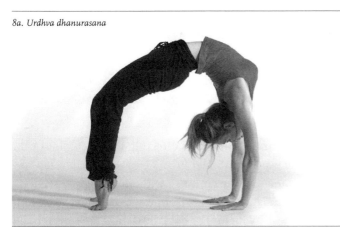

8a. Urdhva dhanurasana

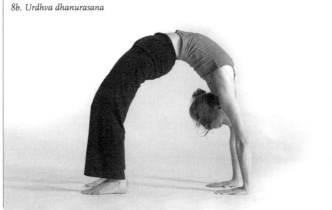

8b. Urdhva dhanurasana

Choose the appropriate exercises for your situation—the lower back rolls (see chapter 6.3, number 7) and/or coordination exercises 2 and 3 (earlier in this chapter). Prepare your shoulders with coordination exercise 1 combined with Adho Mukha Vrksasana variations and Pincha Mayurasana.

Urdhva Dhanurasana can be initiated from the floor or from Tadasana.

Variation 1: from the floor

· Lie on your back with your knees bent, and take hold of your ankles. Position your feet at hip-width on the floor and turn your heels slightly outward. Keep both knees at hip-width.

· Use the strength of your inner thighs and hamstrings to push your thighs and pelvis high. If you find it difficult to keep your knees at the right width, loop a belt around your knees and under your feet, as shown in figure 11.4-2. Then, by pushing your legs lightly against the belt, you will create more space around your SI joints and sacrum. For many people, using the belt greatly lessens their pain and increases the freedom of movement in their lower back.

· Lift your chest as high as possible, moving from your upper back between your shoulder blades, while keeping your neck and shoulders relaxed. Make sure your lower ribs stay low toward your abdomen. If your ribs move forward, movement will no longer be transferred to your lower vertebrae, and your pelvis will drop slightly. This can cause problems in your lower back.

11.4-2

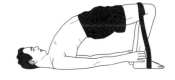

11.4-3

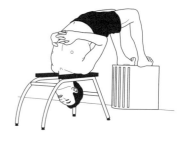

Note: To work out this coordination further, do the following exercise:

· Place the backbender or a chair on your mat against the wall. Place the headstand bench 20 inches in front or the backbender with the straight legs facing it.

· Place your shoulders on the middle of the rubber strips. Jump up into Sirsasana, and place your feet against the wall. Bring your feet down the wall until they reach the backbender. Keep your feet and knees hip-width apart.

· Place your hands on your lower ribs (figure 11.4-3), and move them toward your abdomen without losing the strength in your legs. The moment that your diaphragm relaxes, your legs will activate and be able to push your tailbone higher. If your ribs move away from your abdomen, your legs will not be able to push your tailbone

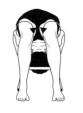

11.4-4

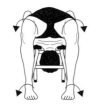

11.4-5

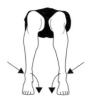

11.4-6

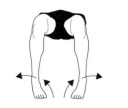

11.4-7

effectively. Then the activity of your legs lessens, and your midback gets overloaded. This also removes the extension and partial contraction from your lower back and has a detrimental effect in Viparita Chakrasana.

This sliding forward of the diaphragm is a serious mistake that is made repeatedly. Because the break constantly occurs in the midback, this area becomes weak, as does the lower back due to the loss of an effective lumbar curve.

· By moving your lower ribs toward your abdomen and directing the strength of your legs to your tailbone and hips, you activate your inner tube. Then you can develop spaciousness in your chest with your breath. Fill your lungs without losing the strength of your abdominals, and feel how your chest expands from the inside out. Relax your shoulders, and move your head toward your upper back. Feel how this movement pushes your vertebrae deeper between your shoulder blades. Movement is developed and transferred through your entire spine.

· The pose in figure 11.4-2 is similar to Dhanurasana (see chapter 11.3, number 5) and Ustrasana (see chapter 11.3, number 4). The difference is that the soles of your feet have contact with the floor (backbender) here. Try to position your feet so that you feel the strength being transferred to your pelvis and back through the midline. Rotate your legs slightly inward (see the arrows in figure 11.4-4). It is important to keep your outer ankles firmly in place and to activate your inner arches. When your feet lose their balance, their strength often "leaks out" through your ankles (figure 11.4-5). Then, you lose strength that should have reached your back.

· Place your hands next to your head on the floor. Push your body up and stand on the crown of your head and your toes.

Note: The movement of Urdhva Dhanurasana runs through the middle of your body, right through your spine. The arch it forms is supported by two pillars: your arms and your legs. They propel the movement through the midline, each in their own particular manner. When the movement is done correctly, the arch in your spine develops farther through relaxation. In this part of the movement, your legs are the guiding force.

Note: The purpose of standing on your toes is to give your upper back, shoulders, and chest more space in the movement. Keep your ankles in the correct position. As figure 11.4-6 illustrates, the feet must be placed correctly—when you lift your heels, the balls of your feet transfer movement through the insteps. In figure 11.4-7, the ankles fall outward, making it impossible to transfer movement through the midline of the body; accordingly, the lower back will not be able to relax. It is important to start the movement with the correct use of your feet. Later, in Viparita Chakrasana, this is the origin of the jump.

Keep your knees hip-width apart so that the insides and backs of your thighs can transfer the movement toward your tailbone. Your hamstrings should be active and your buttocks relaxed. Push your thighs, hips, and pelvis high; this will alleviate feelings of overload to your lower back.

- Breathe from your abdomen into your chest, and develop feelings of relaxation and lightness, which are very important during this stage of the movement. The activity of your arms pushing your body up often makes your body and breathing contract. Allow your breath, rather than your effort, to guide you during this phase of the movement. Become aware of the space around you, and imagine your body filling the space with your breath.
- Moving from this perspective, stretch both arms and, together with steady, deep breaths, use your legs to push your chest forward. On an exhalation, move your head backward to connect it to your upper back.

> **Note:** Two basic shoulder structures have different effects on the stretching of the arms:

1. The arms can immediately straighten fully.

In this case, the connection between your arms and shoulder blades (see chapter 6.3, connection 4) plays an important role. As described there, your arms connect to your shoulder blades when the upper arms transfer movement through your shoulders toward your back. This is the stable position required for your shoulders to be able to receive the movement of your chest and later, during Viparita Chakrasana, to organize the jump.

The connection can be broken by bending excessively at the shoulders. This often occurs when people have flexible shoulders. It causes the palms of the hands to lose their contact with the floor and the arms to lose contact with the shoulder blades (figure 11.4-8). This usually indicates a weak connection between the head and the upper back. When the head is connected properly to the back, it is easier for the arms to maintain their connection with the back and to remain perpendicular to the floor. The chin is often lifted toward the chest, causing the movement to hang in the unstable shoulder position. If the shoulders overextend, this does not mean that the upper back is flexible; on the contrary, it means the upper back is stiff and the shoulders need to compensate.

If you can do Adho Mukha Vrksasana (as described in chapter 8.4, number 18), then you can do the following exercise to facilitate the connection between your arms and shoulder blades:

- With your hands approximately 1 foot from the wall, jump into Adho Mukha Vrksasana and balance your weight between your shoulder blades. Place your feet against the wall; move your chest forward and your pelvis and diaphragm back toward the wall.

11.4-8

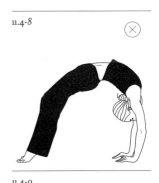

11.4-9

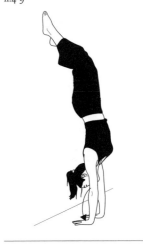

> **Note:** Keep your arms aligned (see the arrow in figure 11.4-9) so that the point just above your elbows keeps turning toward the back of your hand. This ensures that your hands remain stuck to the floor like barnacles. Push your fingertips lightly against the floor.

- When your chest moves into a free position in front of your arms, your shoulders must pass the power of your arms into your shoulder blades and back. Keep your head connected to your upper back.

- When the back of your pelvis moves toward the wall, keep your chest in a free position in front of your shoulders. If you cannot reach the wall with your pelvis, come down and move your hands closer to the wall. When your pelvis touches the wall, slowly slide it up and down the wall and feel how the arms–shoulder blades–upper back connection receives the movement of your pelvis. Maintain the connection between your head and your upper back, and keep pushing your fingertips lightly into the floor so that your arms remain extended. Then you will experience a resilient movement in your upper back but not in your shoulders. Compare figure 11.4-10a, where the chest has fallen back and the shoulders have contracted, with figure 11.4-10b, where the chest has moved too far forward, making the shoulders unstable so that the fingertips and hands lose contact with the floor and the shoulders overextend. Here, your back is not moving forward; your entire body is moving forward from your shoulders and wrists. This makes you feel top-heavy and disturbs your balance.

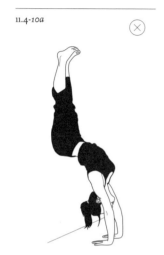

11.4-10a

2. The arms cannot extend completely.
This is often the situation with beginners and is painful for the wrists, because the arms cannot be positioned vertically above the hands; instead, the arms remain at an angle that causes excessive pressure on the wrists (figure 11.4-11). This can be corrected by placing the palms against the wall (figure 11.4-12) or by taking hold of the legs of the headstand bench (figure 11.4-13). Lying on the backbender (coordination exercise 1) will ultimately create more space in the upper back and shoulders.

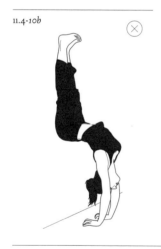

11.4-10b

Note: Students often say they do not have enough strength in their arms to straighten their elbows. This lack of strength is caused by tension in the upper back and shoulders. When the arms are lifted, the back and the shoulders often contract reflexively, creating a lot of tension in these areas, which can impinge on the nerves in the shoulder girdle. This causes the upper arms to lose strength. Regular practice on the backbender helps the upper back to relax. This reflex of the back and shoulder muscles can be broken by moving slowly with awareness. Then the arms will be able to regain their strength.

Using the support of a belt around the upper arms, as shown in figure 11.4-14, can also help break through these tension patterns.

- Remain in this position for 20 to 60 seconds. Bend your arms and return.

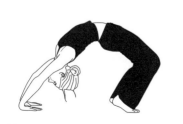

11.4-11

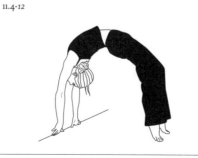

11.4-12

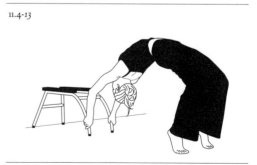

11.4-13

294   LEARNING THE EXERCISES

When I began practicing Urdhva Dhanurasana, it was clear to me that I was very stiff in this pose. The moment I pushed my head off the ground, my awareness narrowed, which caused me to cramp reflexively in my back and shoulders. It was a huge victory for me to dare to release this tension for a few seconds and focus on relaxing my breathing. In those short moments, I learned that the pain in my body diminished immediately. Evidently, it was caused by my cramped muscles. At first, I did not dare to extend these moments of relaxation, because it was too frightening. I was afraid of falling and ending up on the floor. I was afraid of losing control. I often remained caught in these cramped feelings.

Finally, I started to figure out where I needed to release tension and, particularly, where not to. This gave me something to hang on to. I could start experimenting with letting go of control, learning to trust the new structure (a posture not held together by tensed muscular patterns) that was supporting the pose with only a few muscles in my upper arms and legs. As my trust in my new structure grew, my fear of letting go lessened. At first, I was scared that letting go of the tension in my breathing, shoulders, and back would also take the strength out of my arms and elbows and cause me to fall. But then I began to focus clearly on the extension of my elbows and a few muscles in my upper arms. I realized that I could release the tension in the bigger muscle groups. Mentally, I constantly had to "go through" something. It reminded me of jumping over ditches as a child—every time I was in front of a broad ditch, I would hesitate: "Should I, or shouldn't I?" Ultimately, I would make myself mentally strong and breathe deeply a few times before jumping. Releasing my tension in Urdhva Dhanurasana felt like a victory, just like jumping over a ditch and ending up clean and dry on the other side.

In retrospect, I realize that my behavior in those years was dominated by fear, a feeling that was fed by thoughts of falling. The turning point came when I changed my thinking pattern by concentrating on how I could support my structure. By directing my attention to this, my feelings changed, the fear dissipated, and the pain in my shoulders and lower back—which had been present for years—began to lessen and finally disappear. Still, if I did not concentrate during practice, the pain and fear would return immediately.

With the tranquillity that came from my change in thinking, I started to concentrate on space and relaxation during this pose. That was the defining moment. It felt as if I was released from my body and absorbed in the space around me. To my surprise, I realized that, just by distancing myself, I was much more present in my body. This distance enabled me to observe precisely what I was doing. The need to control my body vanished, and relaxation emerged.

This is the image that this pose inspires: the hara gravity point, which is the abode of relaxation, is the highest point in Urdhva Dhanurasana; the head (control) is far below.

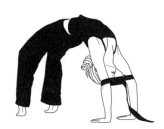

11.4-14

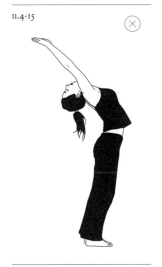

11.4-15

Variation 2: from Tadasana

Correct balance between the two gravity points is important in all asanas, but there is often a preference for one over the other: either the chest takes over the initiative and leads the movement at the expense of the space in the lower abdomen (figure 11.4-15), or the pelvis leads the movement, to the detriment of space in the chest and shoulders (figure 11.4-16).

Note: *Practice this variation with an experienced teacher.*

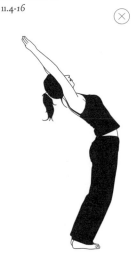

11.4-16

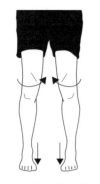

- From Tadasana (see chapter 9.2, number 1), lift your arms over your head while maintaining control of your inner tube. Your lower ribs should remain connected to your abdomen and transfer the weight of your upper body into your tailbone.
- Breathe deeply into the top of your lungs, feel the space in your chest, lift your head, and look upward.
- Keep your feet hip-width apart. Rotate your legs inward (see the arrows in figure 11.4-17).
- At the end of every inhalation, your arms lift your chest and back over your tailbone, while your pelvis and thighs simultaneously move forward (see figure 11.4-18c). When these two movements are synchronized, your weight is balanced precisely on the front of your heels. This balance is important, because it keeps your back and chest muscles relaxed so that your upper body can move in a free and relaxed way. Then your breath is truly able to provide space and movement to your chest, which you can then use to move farther into the pose. Move slowly during inhalations; with every inhalation, wait before you move and check that your breathing is free — that it is really elevating your sternum — before moving farther.

11.4-18a   11.4-18b   11.4-18c

11.4-19a   11.4-19b   11.4-19c   11.4-19d

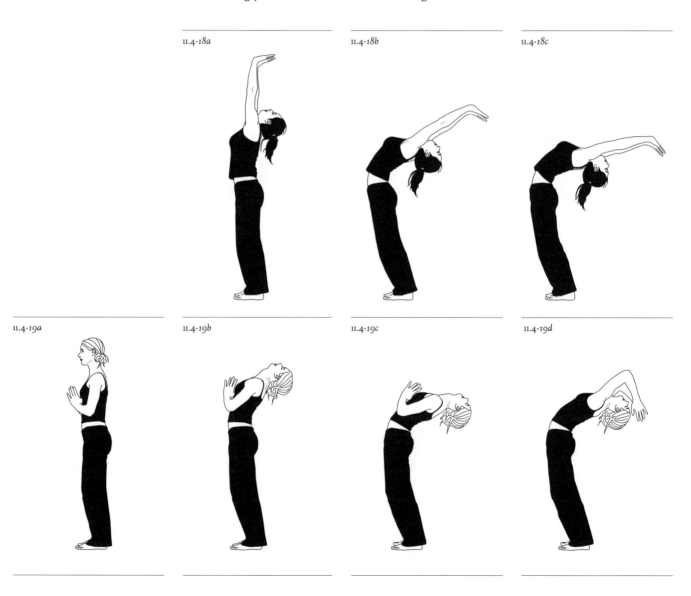

- In this way, you transfer the movement from your arms and head, vertebra by vertebra, through your mid- and lower back to end in your tailbone. Then the movement is transferred to the front of your thighs (figures 11.4-18a through 11.4-18c).

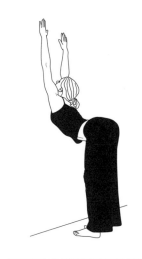
11.4-20

> **Note:** If leading with stretched arms overhead is too difficult, press your fists against your tailbone or start the movement with your hands in front of your chest in namaskar (figures 11.4-19a through 11.4-19c). Then, without collapsing your chest, stretch your arms over your head (figure 11.4-19d), keeping your hands in namaskar.
>
> If it is difficult for you to keep your chest high, try the following variation:

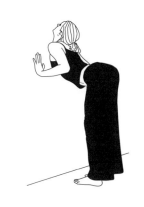
11.4-21

- Stand with your arms straight overhead and pressed against the wall, as shown in figure 11.4-20. Your chin touches the wall. Make sure that your pelvis moves backward, away from the wall. *Breathe* your chest closer to the wall by relaxing your shoulders and back. Remain in this pose for 30 seconds.
- When space has been developed in your chest, place your hands against the wall next to your chest (figure 11.4-21), and push yourself away from the wall. Keep your head connected to your upper back and your weight balanced on the front of your heels. Place your hands in front of your sternum and bend backward as far as you can (see figure 11.4-19c).
- Make sure that, when you relax around your lowest vertebrae, you keep your knees stretched and rotated inward. Relax your back, not your knees.

Once you can easily stretch your arms overhead, you can progress with this asana.

11.4-22

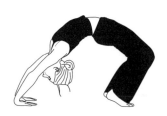

- When you have bent backward as far as you can, it is time for the scariest part of this asana—dropping back. Lift your heels, while keeping your knees together, and follow the movement of your hands as they pull your body, from your legs, to the floor. Drop back so that when your hands touch the ground, your chest immediately moves slightly forward (as described earlier for Urdhva Dhanurasana). Allow your head to move toward and connect to your upper back right away.

11.4-23

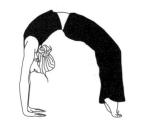

> **Note:** The moment that you lift your heels, your control over the movement is gone; there is no way back. Students frequently change their mind halfway through the movement and try to come back up, lifting their head and arms while they are falling. This is disastrous and can cause an ugly fall. The only thing you can do once you start to drop back is to keep your attention open and follow your arms. When you land on your hands, make sure your knees do not collapse (figure 11.4-22); keep your thighs and pelvis high so that your upper body drops back from the height of your pelvis (figure 11.4-23). When your hands touch the floor, the position of your arms allows your chest to move forward and your head to connect to your upper back. This can only occur when your arms are straight—do *not* bend your elbows.
>
> You can either lie down on the floor to come out, or jump over in the following asana.

9. Viparita Chakrasana

***Viparita* means "turned back"; *chakra* means "wheel."**

Most asanas have a static end position; however, Viparita Chakrasana comprises continuous movement. During this asana, your spine makes two opposing movements. First, it bends backward, vertebra by vertebra, from your head toward your pelvis. Then you jump up into Adho Mukha Vrksasana. After a moment of stillness, the opposite movement of your pelvis and legs toward the floor begins.

The pose originates from Western gymnastics and was introduced to yoga by B. K. S. Iyengar. Gymnasts complete this movement mainly from the strength of their movement muscles; in yoga, the movement is created from the breath, from balance, and from open attention. This makes it effortless, which is essential since the pose is traditionally repeated 108 times.

In India, the number 108 is holy. It is related to the concepts of space and time, and it is the result of adding the sun, the moon, and the seven planets (which makes nine) and multiplying by twelve (the waxing and waning moon through the twelve months of the year); this makes 108. The association with this asana is that time gets turned back, that the asana makes you younger and increases energy.

Viparita Chakrasana shows how movement is increasingly taken over by the superficial movement muscles when attention lapses; thoughts pass through and block the process of open movement. This asana, more than any other, teaches how meditative, quiet attention is the only way to create movement through the middle of your body. This process must be completed at a high speed that is closely related to the speed of your daily movements.

When open attention moves into thought, movement is blocked, effortlessness turns to exertion, and the movement muscles take over. If Sirsasana is the ultimate example of tranquillity, then Viparita Chakrasana is the ultimate example of free, effortless movement.

Obviously, this movement must be learned from an experienced teacher, but the pose can be practiced initially in the following way.

With the headstand bench

· Place your shoulders on the middle of the rubber strips and jump up. Bend your knees and lift your head. When moving your legs, remember coordination exercise 3 (see chapter 11.3). Keep your inner tube active, and move your knees back over your tailbone (follow the arrows in figure 11.4-24).

11.4-24

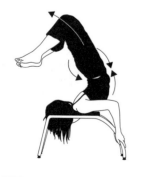

Note: There is a big difference for your lower back when you perform the dropback movement on the headstand bench as opposed to doing it from Tadasana (see chapter 9.2, number 1). The pressure to your lower back is much less in the headstand bench variation. Here, you can use your legs to effectively "pull" the arch of your lower back open. Do this by energetically activating your feet as described for Ustrasana (see chapter 11.3, number 4). This pose is excellent for freeing your lower back and preparing your back for dropping back from Tadasana.   *(continued)*

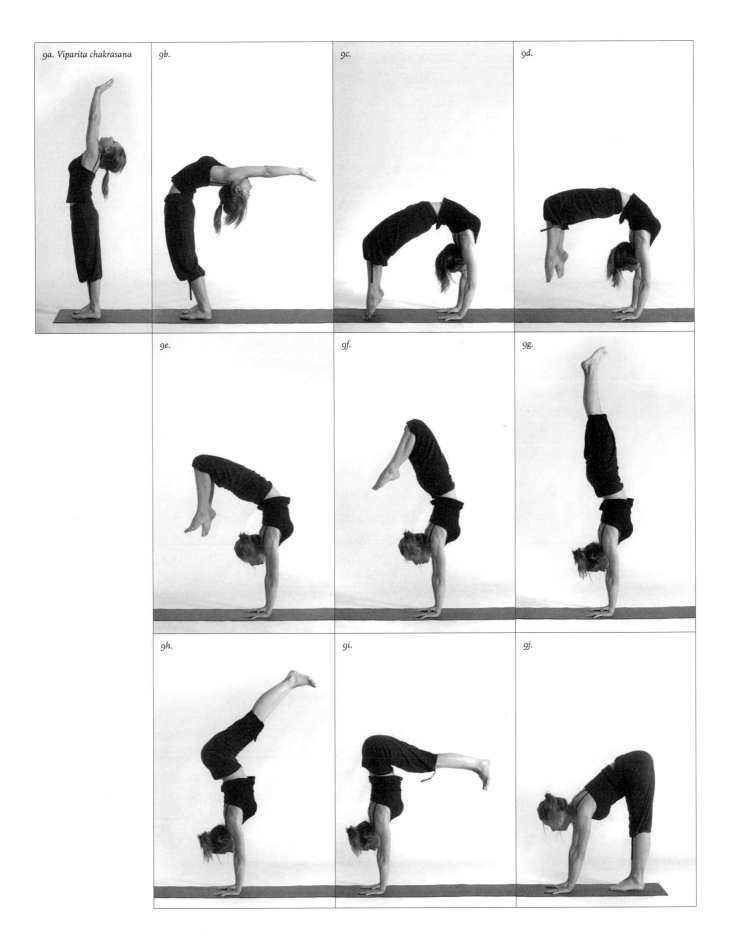

9a. Viparita chakrasana

9b.

9c.

9d.

9e.

9f.

9g.

9h.

9i.

9j.

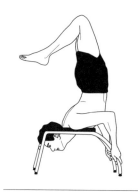

On the headstand bench, it is important to keep your lower ribs connected to your abdomen and to use your lower abdominal muscles to pull your tailbone away from your lower back. Otherwise, your legs will hang from your lower back, and there will be absolutely no question of space.

· Keep your knees together and lower them while rolling over your collarbones toward the top of your chest so that you are standing as shown in figure 11.4-25.

Note: Your sternum is free from pressure on the headstand bench, making it possible to relax the area between your shoulder blades. However, this can only happen when you keep your balance precisely in this area of your back, without relying on your hands to bear the weight.

· Allow your body to roll through from this position, moving with your breath. Pull lightly on the legs of the headstand bench to soften your drop (figures 11.4-26a through 11.4-26c). If you are afraid of dropping back, place a couple of shoulderstand blocks where your feet land to add height.
· Remain in this position for a couple of breaths, then jump back. Keep your legs and knees together, and transfer the movement of your legs to your chest. Pull on the legs of the headstand bench while lifting your head and connecting it to your upper back so that your body can roll back.

Note: It can be difficult to realize that jumping back up is a movement that encompasses your entire spinal column. This means that your body rolls through in a circular form. Nearly everybody thinks from the *legs* when jumping back, causing the body to be positioned as shown in figure 11.4-27a. This position totally blocks any possibility of free movement. Instead of lifting your knees, keep them low and lift your *head* to initiate the roll (figures 11.4-27b and 11.4-27c).   *(continued)*

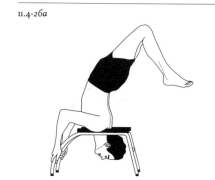

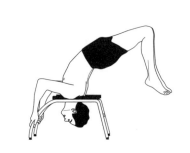

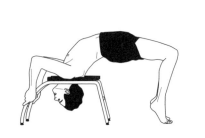

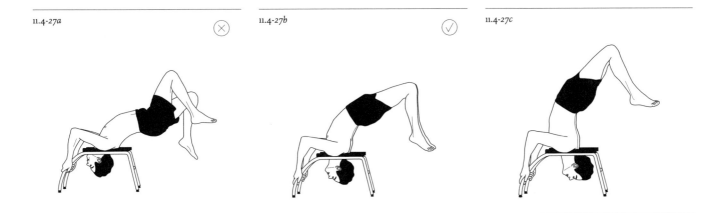

The second problem involving the legs is the position of the thighs and feet. The legs often move apart and too much weight on the outside of the feet causes the ankles to collapse outward (see also figures 11.4-6 and 11.4-7). Then the lower back cannot transfer the movement into the thoracic spine. The movement hangs in the pelvis and blocks the free movement of the SI joints. Because of this, the energy of the jump will not be transferred into the back, and the jump will not be converted into a total movement of the spinal column. If this happens, you can use the support of the belt around your thighs as described earlier for Urdhva Dhanurasana.

Instructions

- From Tadasana, move into Urdhva Dhanurasana as described previously. Make sure your heart gravity point remains open during the drop-back. Keep your hands no farther than 6 inches away from each other so that the movement of your arms can be transferred to your back. If your hands are too far apart, your shoulders will receive a lot of pressure and the connection to your back will be lost.

Note: If you find it difficult to keep your hands together, hook your thumbs when starting the movement from Tadasana, as shown in figure 11.4-28.

- Jump the moment that your hands touch the floor and your chest moves forward, maintaining the control on the insides of your legs and feet. Use the balls of your feet to initiate the jump, while simultaneously initiating the roll from your head. Connect your head to your upper back, then your body will roll through effortlessly. When your heart area gravity point is relaxed in the drop-back, there will be a momentum in the movement that allows your feet to lift spontaneously. Then the jump is effortless.
- As soon as you feel your balance on your hands, extend your body up into Adho Mukha Vrksasana (see chapter 8.4, number 18) and remain in balanced stillness for a moment.

11.4-28

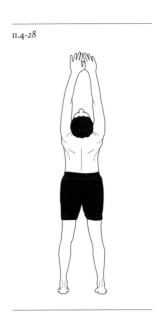

- Rotate your thighs inward. Keep your chest and shoulders open, and on an exhalation, slowly lower your stretched legs to the floor.
- Repeat this asana as often as you can. Rest afterward by sitting on your heels with your knees apart and your head resting on your arms (figure 11.4-29) — or you can stretch your arms forward and rest your head on the floor.

11.4-29

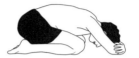

12

TWISTS

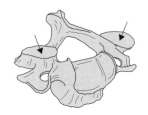

12.1-1   Cervical vertebra

12.1 Introduction

The lower back should be kept stable and not rotate during twists. This allows the upper back to extend easily and the sternum to move forward. Then the sternum, with the assistance of the pressure of the hands or arms against a leg, can be rotated to the left or right.

When practicing twists, the upper body is rotated to the left and right around the spine, which functions as the axis. Only the upper back twists. The shape of the lumbar spine, when extended, prevents rotation. The facet joints of the cervical and thoracic vertebrae are shaped favorably for rotations (see the arrows in figures 12.1-1 and 12.1-2). But the facet joints of the lumbar vertebrae block rotations (see the arrows in figure 12.1-3). The different angles of the facet joints were illustrated in chapter 8.2 (see figures 8.2-23 through 8.2-25). The lower back is stable when compared to the upper back and neck, because the lumbar spine cannot rotate in an extended position. Therefore, it can support free movement in other areas of the body (see chapter 10.2, coordination exercise 1).

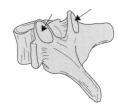

12.1-2   Thoracic vertebra

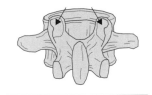

12.1-3   Lumbar vertebra

Because of the different movement possibilities of the spine, twists have two very different effects:

1. They strengthen and stabilize the lower back.
2. They increase the mobility of the thoracic spine, neck, and shoulders.

Twisting enhances relaxation. During a twist, one side of the spine is stretched, which helps those muscles to relax. This relaxation makes it easier for the back to extend. Rotations can be divided into four subgroups. Each has a particular effect on and promotes optimal movement in the spine, shoulders, and pelvis.

1. Straight twists

In these asanas, the back is stacked and aligned in such a way that the body weight can be transported by the small postural muscles that are situated close to the vertebrae. Many of these muscles run from one vertebra to another. Therefore, they are able to transport the rotation at the vertebral level, and it is also possible to develop the movement from this level. To do so, it is necessary to relax the movement muscles. With this relaxation, the spine can lengthen, releasing tension and increasing mobility in the back.

Parivrtta Siddhasana and Parsva Sirsasana (with or without the headstand bench; see chapter 8) belong to this group.

2. Backbend twists

The weight of the upper body moving backward creates pressure in the vertebrae of the mid- and upper back and, consequently, more extension. This enhances the rotational capability of the vertebrae, allowing the flexibility of the back (especially if it is bent and stiff) to increase.

Bharadvajasana (Bharadvaja's Twist) I and II and a coordination exercise belong to this group.

3. Twisting forward bends

When the habitual posture of the back is a forced upright position, or military posture, then twisting forward bends will not only remove the back from its straightjacket and recover the flexibility of the spine, but they will also increase mobility to the shoulders, neck, and chest. This mobility will support the greater strength in the back, which will eventually be directed to the midline of the body—that is, the spine itself.

In Parivrtta Ardha Padmasana (Revolved Half Lotus Pose), the emphasis is placed on correct support from the lower back. Ardha Matsyendrasana and Parivrtta Parsvakonasana also belong to this group, as does the standing pose Parivrtta Trikonasana.

4. Balancing twists

These poses comprise twists that also belong to the previous group. I have placed them in their own subgroup because they are done in combination with Viparita Chakrasana and therefore belong to the dynamic asanas.

Their effect is substantial: mobility of the spine is increased through powerful twists combined with backbends, and the strength of the arms and shoulders is significantly developed by balancing on the hands. When these asanas can be done easily, feelings of freedom, lightness, and energy increase.

Malasana (Garland Pose) is a preparatory pose for this group. Bakasana (Crane Pose),

Parsva Bakasana (Side Crane Pose), Dvi Pada Kaundinyasana (Two-Legged Sage Kaundinya's Pose), and Eka Pada Kaundinyasana (Single Leg Sage Kaundinya's Pose) also belong to this group.

In our daily lives, we twist many times from our habitual postures. We develop preferences for turning to one side and often only use a small part of the spine to do so. This can distort our alignment and seriously disturb the movement chains. Manual therapy aims to increase the mobility of the spine through passive twists that free the facet joints. During Critical Alignment, however, we *actively* free these facet joints ourselves and start to build strength immediately in the new, free position.

A number of twists have already been discussed in this book—Parivrtta Trikonasana (see chapter 9.3, number 9); Parivrtta Parsvakonasana (see chapter 9.3, number 11); and Parsva Sirsasana (see chapter 8.2, number 2). Reread the instructions there for additional information.

12.2 Coordination exercise

Supine twist with the roll placed under the shoulder blades
This is a passive exercise that immediately tells you about mobility in the area of your back that is on the roll. It clearly shows the difference in tension in the left or right side of your spine. If you find that lying on the roll is painful for your back, take time to develop the movement. Do not use force; move slowly and carefully with the rhythm of your breathing. This is a good preparation for the twists that follow, as the area of your spine that is on the roll can be regarded as the base of your neck. This gives you a clear feeling about the connection between your neck and upper back.

Instructions

- Make a thin roll from your felt mat and place it against your back just under your shoulder blades. Lie down and bend your knees. The thickness of the roll can vary, and experience will show what is best for you. If twisting becomes difficult because of the thickness of the roll, make it thinner. If you don't have a roll you can also use the rubber strip—about 1 inch should be thick enough.
- Hold a doubled-up rubber strip between your hands and the back of your head. Lift your head and keep your chin close to your chest; relax your neck and allow it to lengthen. Feel the contraction in your abdominals as your lower ribs are pulled toward your abdomen. Gently press the back of your head against the rubber strip to lengthen your neck.
- Feel the pressure of the roll against your back, and use exhalations to make yourself heavier so that your back can relax. In small increments during exhalations, slowly press your hands toward the floor with your head. Maintain the length and relaxation in your neck. Support your head with your hands as though you were weighing it. When your neck is relaxed, your head will be heavy. When your hands and head touch the floor, wait for a while before you remove your hands and place the strip on the floor. Your hands should lengthen your neck and spine externally. Extend your neck and press the back of your head softly against the strip to produce an internal extension before placing the strip on the floor. Make sure your abdominals are still active.

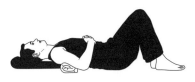

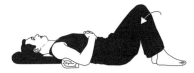

· Place your hands on your lower ribs (figure 12.2-1). Guide your exhalations to that area and spread your elbows wide. Relax your back at the height of the roll, and try to make your back heavier with every exhalation. Do not lose the active extension of your neck.

· Slowly rotate your knees a little to the right, enough to feel the pressure on the muscles at the right side of your spine (figure 12.2-2). These are the movement muscles that cause stiffness in your spine. Feel the pressure and breath in that area, as if your breath is circulating in the muscles, loosening the tension. Stay here for 1 minute, then repeat the same movement on the other side.

Note: Notice whether you feel a difference between your right and left sides. When there is more musculature on one side, it means your spine is more rigid on that side. Spend more time on the stiffer side.

· Rotate to the right again, and become conscious of the use of your breath before continuing the movement. Very slowly, using the rhythm of your breath to accompany the movement, rotate farther to the right. If you experience a sharp pain where your back touches the roll, do not move farther. Wait until the muscles adjacent to your spine relax. By lying still, you give them a chance to release. Once they do, your back will extend, allowing the twist to develop in a natural way. Do not use willpower and force; this will only make matters worse and increase your pain.

Note: The following is the protocol for developing mobility in this group of asanas: extension always precedes twisting. When you feel resistance while twisting, do not continue with brute force but focus on developing length. Direct the extension toward the area of resistance.

· Because the lower back itself cannot rotate, it transfers the movement of your legs and pelvis completely to your midback. The way the rotation of your pelvis is used to coordinate the rotation toward your upper back in this pose is similar to the movement in Parsva Sirsasana (see chapter 8.2, number 8).

· Twisting makes it difficult to breathe completely from your abdomen into your chest. Inhale as lightly and fully as possible, and guide your exhalations toward your back.

· Let your head remain heavy on the strip, and try to extend your neck constantly. Both shoulders should remain on the floor.

· Remain in this position for 30 to 60 seconds, then slowly roll back and repeat the movement on the other side. When your spine feels more relaxed, you can move a little faster.

12.3 Standing twists

Parivrtta Siddhasana and Parsva Sirsasana (with or without the headstand bench; see chapter 8.2, number 8) belong to this group. During these asanas, the relaxation of the movement muscles creates length in the spine and increases mobility.

1. Parivrtta Siddhasana

Parivrtta means "rotated"; *siddha* means "accomplished."

The large muscles of the back usually initiate rotations in daily life. Critical Alignment, on the other hand, limits the use of these large muscles where possible so that movement can develop through relaxation. Relaxation is achieved by aligning the spine correctly; read about Parsva Sirsasana on the headstand bench (see chapter 8.2, number 2) for an extensive discussion of this. The twist must nevertheless be guided and developed, and this occurs through the strength of the arms. How this strength is applied varies in each asana; sometimes it is through the elbow, sometimes through the upper arm. In this asana, the rotation is initiated from the hand. When the arm is activated, the back's movement muscles can relax, and it can extend through the coordinated use of the postural muscles. The importance of this was highlighted in the discussion of the preceding coordination exercise: relaxation and extension free blocked vertebrae and allow the twist to develop fully.

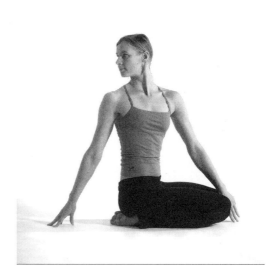

Instructions

- Bend your knees and sit down on your feet and ankles. If your knees feel stiff, put a roll between your ankles and sit bones. If you feel a great deal of pain in your ankles, put the roll between your ankles and the floor to reduce the stretch on your feet. It is also possible to start with your legs crossed (figure 12.3-1). Lean forward so that the weight of your body falls into your groin. This will make it easier to relax your hips and knees. Do this movement without lifting the back of your pelvis. If your lower back has difficulty stretching in a cross-legged position, elevate your seat with a shoulderstand block.

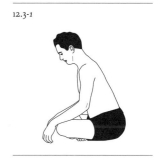

12.3-1

- Place the back of your left hand against your lower back and your right hand against your front lower ribs. Shift your ribs back as if you were pushing a drawer shut. When your pelvis stays in the same position and your hips and knees remain relaxed, you will feel the lower vertebrae in your back move into their natural lordotic curve (see chapter 6.3, connection 9). Your back should feel strong and your abdomen relaxed. Place your hands on your thighs and increase the feeling of spaciousness in your abdomen by breathing into it. If you like, you can shut your eyes.

> **Note:** If you find it difficult to position your lower back in its stable curve when sitting on the floor, try sitting on a chair.

- Breathe into your chest from your abdomen and feel how the upward movement of your sternum pulls your thoracic spine straighter, without requiring engagement of the movement muscles in your back. In fact, the more relaxation in your back, the easier this extension becomes. When your upper back extends, your neck automatically moves into alignment, allowing it to transport the weight of your head to the part of your spine that was on the roll in the coordination exercise. Actively stretch your neck toward the crown of your head at the end of every inhalation, and maintain this stretch during each exhalation.

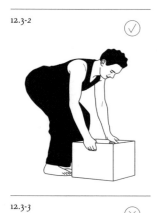

12.3-2

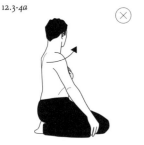

12.3-3

- Relax your shoulders with an exhalation. Extend your neck to push the crown of your head upward, and feel how this movement increases relaxation down your spine toward your pelvis.
- Place your left hand against the base of your sternum and observe the breath moving under your hand toward the top of your chest. When you exhale, the extension of your neck ensures that the base of your sternum does not collapse. If you keep your neck and head aligned on top of your spine, your chest will never collapse. Remain here for a couple of breaths.
- Place your right hand against the inside of your right knee while keeping the upper arm connected to your shoulder blade. Imagine that your shoulder blade is a second hand that pushes the right side of your chest forward into a twist.

Note: This connection was discussed extensively in chapter 6.3, connection 4. It is an important support for keeping your back erect and relaxed when jumping up on the headstand bench. In this pose, your arm is connected to your shoulder blade in a more usual manner, such as when you are lifting something (figure 12.3-2 shows a correct connection) or sitting behind a computer (figure 12.3-3 shows a lost connection).

For the correct development of movement, it is important to realize that your *arm*, not your tensed shoulder and upper back, provides the strength to twist. Often, when the shoulder remains relaxed, hardly any strength develops in the arm. If the hand starts to push, the shoulder has a tendency to move up and forward (compare figures 12.3-4a and 12.3-4b).

For this reason, do not push lightly against your knee while keeping your shoulder relaxed, but push yourself firmly into your end position. When you can recognize coordination problems between your arm and shoulder in this exercise, you can recognize them in your daily movements. Then you can start to make a change in your habitual patterns (figures 12.3-5a and 12.3-5b).

12.3-4a

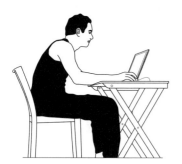

- Keep your breathing slow and deep. Feel the spaciousness in your chest, and align your head and neck. Inhale toward your left hand, and push your right hand against your knee so that the base of your sternum (under your left hand) remains raised and begins turning to the left at the end of your inhalation. Relax your shoulders on an exhalation and pretend to press the back of your head against a strip to actively extend your neck.

12.3-4b

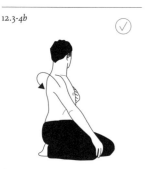

Note: Keep your head straight and looking forward at the beginning of the exercise. Then you can imitate the pressure toward the imaginary strip behind your head from the back of your head. At the end of the movement, your head rotates as well. Then you have to extend your neck to the side of your head. To understand this movement clearly and feel the exact spot on the side of your head, lie down on a doubled-up rubber strip (see chapter 6.3, connection 4). After a while (about 30 to 60 seconds) of allowing your spine to relax, rotate your head to the right side. Relax your neck completely. Inhale into your sternum to produce an inward movement of your spine. Press the side of your head away from your spine during your exhalations. Feel how your neck extends to the side of your head, and reproduce this feeling in all rotations described in this chapter and in standing poses as well.

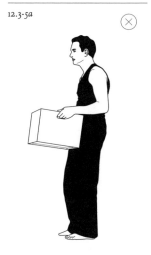

- Twist in small increments together with your breath until you can go no farther. Coordinate your breathing so you rotate at the end of every inhalation. This will keep your back erect, and you will be able to breathe right up to the top of your lungs. Breathing in this way will develop more extension of your spine, even during the static end position of the pose.
- The feeling of the rotation coming to an end often takes place somewhere in the midback, just under the shoulder blades. This end position can feel either natural and elastic or blocked. If the latter is the case, use your inhalations to extend your spine more. This will lengthen your neck toward the crown of your head and help you release the area of tension. Keep pushing your hand firmly against your knee so that, when your back relaxes, the twist can continue by itself.
- When you have developed the twist for 1 to 2 minutes, you can increase the strength to the postural muscles by slowly lessening the pressure of your hand so that these muscles can take over. Hold this position for 20 seconds.

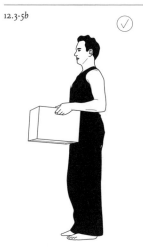

Note: It is a physiological rule that a muscle is able to release more tension after a firm contraction. Therefore, the aforementioned contraction of your back muscles allows more movement in your spine afterward. This pose clearly illustrates this muscular principle. After completing the rotation at the beginning of the exercise, in which your hand coordinates the rotation, you feel that you are unable to move any farther. Then, after holding the contraction in your back muscles for 20 to 30 seconds, the back muscles relax when your hand starts to push again. Your whole spine rotates farther then before. Try it, and experience a substantial improvement of mobility.

- Take your time returning to a neutral spine and feel the difference in your breathing, especially with regard to your posterior ribs. They will be able to broaden and narrow more easily with each inhalation and exhalation.
- Repeat the movement on the other side.

The difference between moving from your breath and moving from strength is significant. When I started to integrate movement with breath in my lessons, I was amazed that almost everyone could maintain an erect seated pose during Parivrtta Siddhasana. Before I began working with the breath, this asana was one of the most difficult to explain, because it is easy to end up misaligned. This misalignment restricts the free movement of the breath immediately. When the focus is not on the breath, it is difficult to realize that you are misaligned. You may think that obstructed breathing is normal in this asana. When breath is integrated into movement from the beginning and you resolve to keep your breathing free, then your body will move naturally into the most advantageous position. Then awareness, breathing, and body intelligence all work together. But be careful—just a single thought, especially if it is related to ambition, can disturb this subtle balance!

12.4 Backbend twists

Bharadvajasana I and II and the earlier coordination exercise belong to this subgroup. The combination of twists and backbends increases the mobility of the back, especially if it is bent and stiff.

2. Bharadvajasana I

The *Mahabharata* tells, among other things, the story of Bharadvaja. He was the father of Drona, who was the weapons preceptor of the Pandavas and the Kauravas, two armies that were fighting against each other. When Bharadvaja was young, he had an insatiable appetite for learning. As a young child, he spent all of his time learning the Vedas and was advised to meditate on the god Indra. After many years of living soberly and meditating, his body became so weak that he had difficulty sitting erect. One day, Indra appeared and asked him what he would do if his life were extended. Bharadvaja answered that he would continue meditating and studying the Vedas. Indra told him that this was already the third life in which he had exhausted his body in understanding the Vedas. Then Indra explained Bharadvaja had gained more knowledge about the Vedas than the gods had themselves. He told Bharadvaja that Vedic knowledge is infinite; it is important to realize that, even though you continue learning, you should not retreat from life. You bring your knowledge into practice by sharing it with others.

This asana is a twist combined with a backbend.

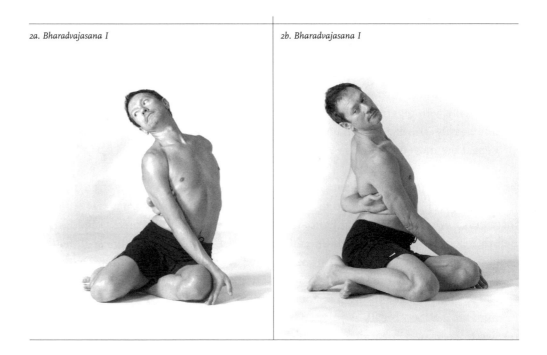

2a. Bharadvajasana I   *2b. Bharadvajasana I*

Instructions

It is helpful to sit on a shoulderstand block so that you can maintain the extension of your lower back and the balance of your pelvis. (If you can maintain these qualities without the block, sit on the floor. I have included the block in the instructions for this asana.)

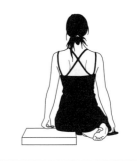

- Sit with your left buttock on the right corner of the block, and place your left foot next to your right foot on the right side of your pelvis. Place your right foot in Virasana (see chapter 13.2, number 2) on top of your left foot, as shown in figure 12.4-1. Feel the balance in your pelvis and keep your right hip heavy so that your lower back remains erect.

- Relax your left shoulder, bring your left hand behind your back, and take hold of your right upper arm. Feel the pressure of your left underarm under your shoulder blades, the place where the roll presses in the coordination exercise and where your neck connects to your back.

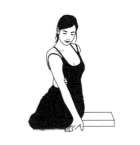

- Lean your upper body forward so that your left knee touches the floor, and take hold of your left knee with your right hand, or slide your hand under your knee (figure 12.4-2). Push your left knee down firmly. This will help you actively extend your lower back through the midline. It also helps you to release tension around your right hip so that your pelvis can remain balanced.

> **Note:** Watch out for your left shoulder elevating when your right hand moves toward your left knee, causing the right side of your chest to be pulled inward. This brings your right hip up and makes your lower back contract. Correct this by doing the exact opposite. Depress your left shoulder so that the right side of your chest can move outward (toward your left hand), allowing tension to be released from your right hip and balance to be maintained in your pelvis. Then you will be able to breathe fully because your body is balanced. This allows movement to a much larger area of your spine.

- Breathe slowly and deeply, and use your inhalations to elevate your chest; this extends your upper back. Push your right hand against your knee so that your chest starts to twist to the left at the end of your inhalations.
- At the end of an inhalation, turn your head to the right and move the side of your face over your shoulder toward your underarm (see the extra exercise that follows). Move your upper back as deep as you can during exhalations. Then your neck can transport the weight of your head into your spine.
- Keep breathing deeply and elevating your chest as your back extends back over your arm like a high jumper jumping over a horizontal bar.

> **Note:** Make sure your left knee and your right hand stay low so that the backward movement can be initiated from the support of your lower back and transferred to your upper back. Your neck and head then acquire space, so they can approach your upper back from the direction of the neck. If your hand lifts, the movement in your back has become blocked and your body has bent backward from your hips.

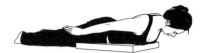
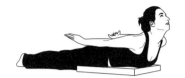
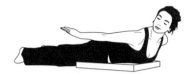

· Remain in this position for 30 to 60 seconds, return, and repeat on the other side.

It is difficult to move your head toward your upper back. The following exercise establishes this movement.

Instructions

· While lying prone on a shoulderstand block, elevate your neck and head so they are aligned with your upper back. Stretch your arms back alongside your body, as shown in figure 12.4-3. Allow your upper back to relax with every exhalation so that it sinks deeper between your shoulder blades.
· Lift your head and move the back of your head toward your upper back. If tension develops in your neck, remember that this will lessen when you extend your upper back through your inhalations. Keep using your exhalations to relax your upper back.
· On an inhalation, elevate your chest to bring the balance of your body toward your lower ribs, and lift your hands as high as you can, with your palms up (figure 12.4-4). Remember that your inhalations extend your upper back every time they lift your sternum. This helps lessen the pressure in your neck.
· Without losing the connection to your upper back, turn your head to the right and look over your right shoulder toward your right palm (figure 12.4-5). Keep breathing deeply, inhale to the top of your lungs, and use your exhalations to release your upper back between your shoulder blades to reduce the pressure to your neck.
· Through the rotation of your head, the transportation of movement becomes more specific. Your neck transports the weight of your head, not to the center of your spine, but to the area between your spine and your right shoulder blade. Visualize the extension of your ribs at the side of your right shoulder blade during inhalations, and use your rotated neck to move toward that area during exhalations.
· Remain in this end position for 20 seconds, return, and repeat on the other side.

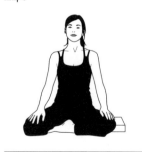

3. Bharadvajasana II

Instructions

· Place your right foot in the Virasana position (see chapter 13.2, number 2) next to the right side of your pelvis, and place your left foot in Padmasana (see chapter 13.2, number 1) on your right thigh. Relax your right hip, knee, and ankle so that your hips remain balanced. If this is difficult, sit on a shoulderstand block as described for

Bharadvajasana I. If it is difficult to place your left foot in Padmasana, place your left heel against your right thigh (figure 12.4-6).

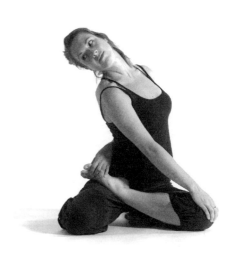

- Relax your left shoulder, and bring your left hand behind your back to take hold of your left foot. Your underarm pushes against your lower back, and you will feel your lower back extending when you shift your body weight toward your knees while actively pressing your left knee into the floor. Slide your right hand under your left knee, or if your back does not allow this, push your hand against your knee. Use the extension of your lower back to support the elevation of your chest with every inhalation. Push your hand against your knee to turn your chest to the left. Move the side of your face over your right shoulder and look at your feet.
- Do this without moving your right hand. If it does move, you are no longer moving back from your lower back and chest (as described in the preceding extra exercise); your body is rotating backward from your pelvis. Use your head to push your upper back, vertebra by vertebra, deeper into extension until the movement reaches the place where your right underarm meets your lower back.
- Use your inhalations to provide space to your two gravity points and your exhalations to extend your lower back, relax your shoulders, and twist farther.
- Remain in the end position for 30 to 60 seconds. Return slowly and repeat on the other side.

This pose not only increases the flexibility of your spine, but it stretches the muscles around your left shoulder intensely.

12.5. Twists combined with forward bends

Parivrtta Ardha Padmasana, Ardha Matsyendrasana, and Parivrtta Parsvakonasana belong to this subgroup, as do the standing pose Parivrtta Trikonasana and the seated pose Upavista Konasana (see chapter 10.5, number 8).

These asanas help you recover the free movement of your spine and increase mobility to your shoulders, neck, and chest. You develop strength in your back, particularly around your spine.

4. Parivrtta Ardha Padmasana

Parivrtta means "rotated"; *ardha* means "half"; *padma* means "lotus." This seated twist is initiated from Ardha Padmasana (Half Lotus Pose)—hence, the name. Relaxation in the hips and shoulders plays an important role in the development of twists. (This was discussed in the section on standing twists in chapter 9.3.) Freedom of movement in the hips makes it easier to extend the lower back, which increases the ease of the twist. The advantage of this pose is that it can be held for a greater length of time than standing asanas.

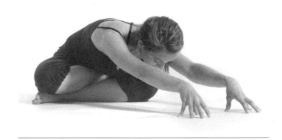

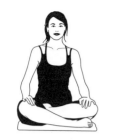

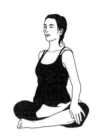

As discussed in chapter 10 (reread the introduction there), mainaining cohesion in the lower back during a forward bend is the main requirement for a healthy forward bend. The same applies here. If the lower back loses its cohesion and bends too far, it can also twist—but into a totally unstable position. In daily life, bending forward and twisting without cohesion in the lower back is the cause of many back problems. The control of the lower back in this group of exercises is the same that is needed in everyday forward bending.

Instructions

- Sit on the front edge of a shoulderstand block, and place your right foot in Padmasana (chapter 13.2, nr. 1) on top of your left leg. Place your left foot under your right knee, as shown in figure 12.5-1.
- Extend your lower back as described earlier, and on an inhalation, position your neck and head directly on top of your spine. Place your left hand against the inside of your left knee and your right hand behind you on the floor. On an inhalation, push your hand against your knee to rotate your chest to the right. Keep looking forward over your right knee (figure 12.5-2.) Breathe from your abdomen to your chest, and keep your abdominal muscles relaxed.
- Keep pushing against your knee, and move your upper body forward without lifting your shoulders or collapsing your chest. Your lower back is no longer erect, but it still carries the weight of your upper body. Your abdomen remains relaxed.
- If you are able to move your hands forward without collapsing the front of your body or contracting your abdominals, place your hands on both sides of your right knee and move them forward slowly. Alternatively, keep your hands in the previous position so that they can support your lower back and move your abdomen and chest toward your thigh while keeping your abdominal muscles relaxed. Again, just as in forward bending, extension to the front of your body precedes the bending of your back. The reason for the placement of your left foot now becomes clear. The foot under the knee keeps your pelvis stable when you start to move forward with your hands. In addition, because your pelvis stays low, the muscles around the hip and in your lower back and thigh receive the stretch and can relax.

> **Note:** If your knees are stiff and painful, take your time moving forward. When you do, try to feel if the muscles around your knees contract when they become burdened with the weight of your body. If so, do not move any farther, but wait for relaxation to occur.

- Breathe freely from your abdomen to your heart gravity point, and use the breath to release areas of tension. Use inhalations to create space in these areas and exhalations to release tension. Stretching the muscles around your hip can be painful. Do not get lost in the discomfort, but use your breath to develop feelings of lightness and let that circulate throughout your body.
- After 1 minute, move your hands back and return with your upper body. Cross your legs the other way and repeat on the other side.

5. Ardha Matsyendrasana

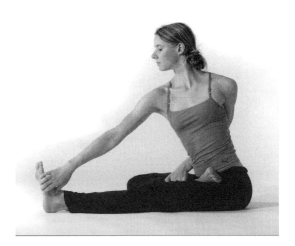

Ardha means "half"; Matsyendra is the Lord of the Fishes.
Matsyendra was also a yogi who is claimed by both Buddhists and Hindus. There are many temples to him in Nepal. Matsyendra's kundalini went up in this asana—hence, the name.

This pose strongly resembles the first coordination exercise in chapter 10.2 and is directed to the extension of the lower back. This extension is the driving force that creates space in the chest, shoulders, and neck.

The positive effects from practicing this exercise are important for everyone who leads a sedentary life. Sitting in daily life can require the same coordination as this asana: the increased stability in the lower back gives an increased freedom for seated work. Everyday activities, such as bending and lifting, will become much more efficient as the extension of the back improves through this pose.

Instructions

·   Sit in Dandasana (see chapter 10.3, number 3), and place your right leg on your left leg in Padmasana (see chapter 13.2, number 1). Place your foot as high as possible on your leg and bring your knees close together. If Padmasana is not possible, place your right foot against the inside of your left thigh as in Janu Sirsasana (see chapter 10.5, number 7).

·   Take hold of the outside of your left foot with your right hand, as shown in figure 12.5-3. Do not take hold of your foot at any cost. If you are able to grasp the outside of your foot but cannot extend your lower back, hold your ankle or lower leg instead so that you can activate your lower back.

·   Place your left hand behind your back and take hold of your right thigh or lower leg. Where your left arm touches your back is exactly where your back should extend.

12.5-3

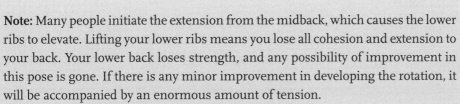

Note: Many people initiate the extension from the midback, which causes the lower ribs to elevate. Lifting your lower ribs means you lose all cohesion and extension to your back. Your lower back loses strength, and any possibility of improvement in this pose is gone. If there is any minor improvement in developing the rotation, it will be accompanied by an enormous amount of tension.

Because of these problems, I will describe this exercise at length. It is a complex movement that should be guided in a tranquil, introspective manner with open attention. Do not develop the movement automatically, as that only strengthens habitual movements.

When your lower ribs are elevated, the extension to your upper back will not develop. The arch of your back moves to your diaphragm, as discussed in the sections on Sirsasana and Salamba Sirsasana I (see chapter 8.2, numbers 1 and 7). Then your neck gets longer, but your upper back does not extend. This obstructs your sternum and nullifies the effect of deep breathing, which no longer affects the extension of your upper back.

- If your back does not change shape, your right arm will not be able to connect with your shoulder blade. Then the initiation of the twist will come from tension in your shoulder instead of strength in your upper arm, or it will come from your left shoulder causing tension to develop in your back (under the left shoulder blade).
- Because your diaphragm has shifted forward and you have lost the extension in your lower back, the integrity of your inner tube is also lost. This has serious consequences for your breath. Often, your breath will become stuck around your diaphragm, compromising relaxation in your abdomen and lightness in your chest. Instead of shifting your diaphragm forward and losing the extension in your lower back, keep your diaphragm relaxed and your lower ribs broad. Only then will strength develop in your lower back.
- Therefore, when positioning your right hand, make sure you keep your ribs low. Then your lower back can be positioned so that you feel pressure in your groin. Reread the instructions for Dandasana (see chapter 10.3, number 3). Then shift your diaphragm back so that the lumbar vertebrae under your left arm move into a deeper curve and you feel that your lower back is actively pushing your pelvis toward the floor.
- This activity in your lower back not only affects your pelvis but your upper back and chest as well. Your lower back creates the foundation from which you can position your chest and upper back with your breathing. It carries the relaxation in your chest so that your shoulders can relax and your neck can extend and connect with the area under your shoulder blades.
- The extension of your lower back increases in this pose. For this reason, place your right hand in a position where your lower back is slightly bent, so the extension can develop. By working on the extension to your lower back, your neck will move back and connect to your spine. This increases the distance between your face and left leg. Imagine that a thread is attached to the middle of your neck and that it is being pulled backward, causing your lower back to extend more. The extension of your lower back depends not only on its strength but also on the relaxation in your hip and the length of your hamstrings. These are the same areas that are worked intensely during forward bends.

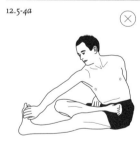

12.5-4a

- The extension of your lower back ensures that your right arm remains straight. Imagine that your arm is a rope that is constantly being pulled taut by your lower back. If your arm looks like those shown in figures 12.5-4a and 12.5-4b, then your lower back is no longer actively extending but has started to bend, causing your arm to bend as well. Any possibility of free, total movement has been lost.
- When your neck can make a better connection to the vertebrae of your upper back, your breathing will be affected immediately. This can cause you to breathe more deeply (and initially also faster). The "extra" breath targets the top of your lungs and results from the activity of the nerves in your upper back. This exercise was also described using the headstand bench (see chapter 8.2, number 1). This is a positive development, so make the most of it! Ensure that your shoulders remain low when you inhale and your chest stays high when you exhale.

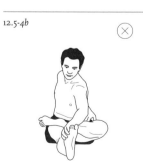

12.5-4b

- Remain here for 30 to 60 seconds. Sometimes, when your concentration is extremely lucid, it is worthwhile to remain in the pose a little longer. You are aware of time, but it no longer dominates. Stay in this asana as long as you want, but remember to do the other side for the same length of time.

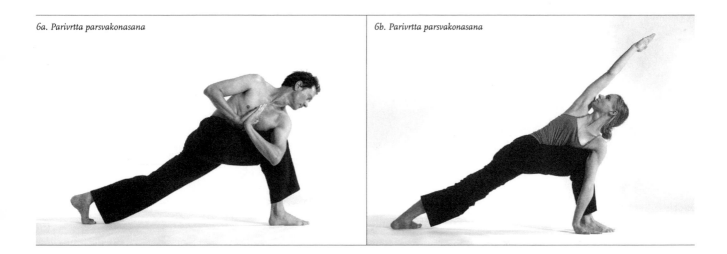

· Return slowly. Your ribs and vertebrae can feel somewhat twisted, as sometimes occurs after lying on the roll (described in the coordination exercise at the beginning of this chapter). When returning, you will feel the effect of this asana on your skeleton. Take time to allow your breathing to normalize before moving into the next asana.

6. Parivrtta Parsvakonasana

This pose was described with the standing poses (see chapter 9.3, number 11). Within the context of twists, it is important to note that the upward movement of the diaphragm is blocked during this movement. The development of cohesion in the extension of the spine as described in the previous asana, Ardha Matsyendrasana, is subtle. Balance is achieved here through a continuous subtle awareness of connections. Strength plays a much larger role in Parivrtta Parsvakonasana, and this can be helpful for breaking through and releasing very stiff structures. The strength is transferred from the arm to the lower back without the danger of the diaphragm losing its connection to the abdomen.

12.6 Balancing twists

Astavakrasana (see chapter 10.6, number 14) belongs to this subgroup, as do Bakasana, Parsva Bakasana, Dvi Pada Kaundinyasana, and Eka Pada Kaundinyasana. Malasana is a preparatory exercise.

These poses are very active and have a considerable effect on the flexibility of the spine. Feelings of freedom, lightness, and energy increase enormously when these asanas can be done easily.

7. Malasana

Mala means "garland."
In this pose, the arms are placed around the body as a garland (figure 12.6-2). The pose is done in three phases and ends with Bakasana. It forms the basis for a number of twists that are also balance poses; the body is balanced on the hands.

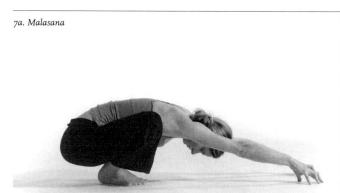

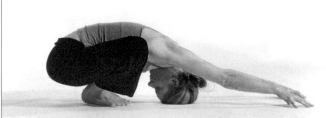

Malasana frequently occurs in combination with forward bends. Viewed from the perspective of forward bending, this stretch is targeted toward the pelvic rim, sacrum, and SI joints; these are areas that are difficult for people with stiff hamstrings to stretch, as that stiffness prevents the pelvis from tilting freely.

Instructions

Phase 1

- Squat with your feet touching. Find your balance by relaxing your ankles and your insteps. When you relax the latter, the crease between the top of your foot and the front of your ankle moves deeper, allowing your calves to stretch. Remain in this position for a short time so that your calves can relax, improving your balance. When your ankles sink toward the floor, they become the anchor for the pose—the stable point from which the stretch develops.

- Lift your arms so that they connect with your lower back (figure 12.6-1a) and your lower back can extend. Try to arch your lower back as much as possible, and connect your lower ribs with the arch by pulling them in. Make sure you do not extend your spine from the lift of your lower ribs, as that will weaken your lower back. From a proper extension of the midline of your lower back, your pelvis and hips should stretch backward, away from your lower back, so that your ankles and heels can come closer to the floor. The extension in your lower back creates space in your abdomen. Pull the area just below your navel up toward your navel and hold that position for a few breaths. Breathe into your inner tube. Maintain the connection between your arms and lower back, and stretch your abdomen forward between your legs during exhalations. Remain in a horizontal position for a few breaths (figure 12.6-1b), keeping your heels anchored in the same position. Breathe from your abdomen to your chest.

- Without bending your back, place your fingertips on the floor and start to walk forward with your fingers (photo 7a). Apply the rule of forward bending: lengthen your abdomen and chest before bending your back. When you have reached the end position with your fingers, do not lift your heels to go farther forward. Many people make this mistake, and it causes the stretch to be lost immediately. The act of stretching is then lost in both directions; instead of stretching to the front and the back, you only shift your weight forward.

- You can now keep your neck in line with your upper and lower back or allow it to bend

12.6-1a

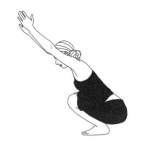

12.6-1b

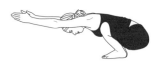

(photo 7b) so that your chin moves toward your sternum. Two areas of your back that are sensitive to overload can now relax—your neck and the lowest part of your back. It is particularly pleasant to relax your legs and knees during and after standing poses. You can stop here or increase the extension.

- To go farther, move as if you were going to lift your fingertips from the floor, and allow the initiative for this movement to originate from your lower back. This causes the bend in your lower back to flatten somewhat, and then extension and stretching can develop in an active manner. This intensifies the pose because of the active participation of your lower back. If your ankles became unbalanced during the development of the movement, they will now be able to recover stability.
- Remain in this position for 1 minute, and breathe slowly and freely. Return by elevating your arms or move into the following phase.

Phase 2

- Move your arms back, one at a time, under your knees and join your hands behind your lower back. Use the connection of your arms, through your hands, to apply pressure to your shins with your upper arms. This pressure stimulates the stretch of your lower back under your hands.
- Keep your head low so that you feel like the stretch of your lower back is pushing the middle of your neck forward, as indicated by the arrow in figure 12.6-2.
- Breathe as freely as possible, and remain in this classic end pose for 30 to 60 seconds. Return from this pose or move into the following phase.

12.6-2

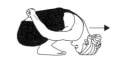

Phase 3

- Place your upper arms as low as possible against your shins. Move your legs as close as you can to your upper body. Connect your arms with your shoulder blades. The pressure of your upper arms guides the stretch of your lower back and gives the feeling that your pelvis is being pushed farther away, while your chest moves in the other direction, creating more space there.
- Place your hands on the floor in front of you, breathe freely, lift your head, and look straight ahead (figure 12.6-3). This pose is called Malasana II in the lesson plans.
- Remain in this end position for 30 seconds, or move into the next pose.

12.6-3

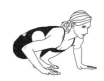

8. Bakasana

Baka **means "crane."**
This is the first asana from the series of balance poses. They are beautiful movements that can be practiced together with Viparita Chakrasana at an advanced level. Here, I will give beginner's instructions, and later in this chapter, I will describe the entire series.

Instructions

- From the end position of phase 3 (see Malasana II), move a little farther forward so that you can lift your feet off the floor. Use the pressure of your arms against your legs to extend your lower back. This immediately gives your abdomen and chest more space and allows you to lower your shoulders.

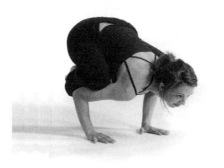
8a. Bakasana

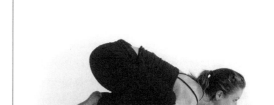
8b. Bakasana

> **Note:** You must make quick use of the pressure of your arms against your legs; otherwise, your shoulders will do what they always do in times of tension—contract and rise. Then your gravity point will shift toward your shoulders and disturb your balance. Place a shoulderstand block in front of you for protection in case you fall. If you lose your balance, pull your chin toward your chest so that you end up on the crown of your head and not on your face.

- Increased relaxation in your hips allows your lower back to extend farther backward and provides space to your upper body. Relaxation in your hips and lower back results in less space between your legs and trunk, which allows greater extension in your back. Lift both your feet and chest so that they support the stretch in your lower back.
- Remain in this end position for 20 to 30 seconds. Keep your breathing free and regular. Lower your feet back to the floor.

9. Parsva bakasana

Parsva means "side"; *baka* means "crane."
You can develop the flexibility necessary for this pose by practicing it against a wall (figure 12.6-4). This will be discussed before Parsva Bakasana. When you can do that exercise easily, you can practice balancing on your hands. You develop the strength necessary for this pose during Bakasana and Nakrasana (Crocodile Pose; see chapter 13.3, number 6).

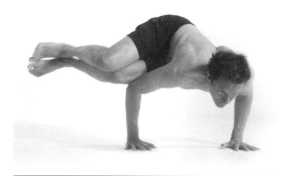
9. Parsva bakasana

Preparation exercise against the wall

- Squat with your left side approximately 8 inches from the wall. If you cannot place your heels on the floor easily, place a shoulderstand block under them to facilitate your balance. Then you can be sure that your heels stay at the same height.
- Lift your pelvis slightly. Place your right arm behind your left thigh and twist as far as you can to the left. Lifting your pelvis lengthens the front of your trunk so that the twist can work through your abdomen.

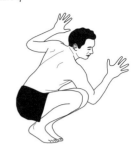

- Place the palm of your right hand against the wall and lower your pelvis so that your back can extend all the way up to your crown. The pressure of your upper arm helps this movement.
- Place the palm of your left hand against the wall, and make sure that your heels remain level. If your knees and ankles are uneven, then you have twisted in your pelvis instead of your back. Therefore, make sure your pelvis is balanced first and then increase the extension and twist from the pressure of your arm.
- Use the wall as your point of reference. See that your left hip is aligned above your feet, and measure the distance of your face from the wall. The pressure of your upper arm transfers to your lower back. This allows your entire spine to extend and your neck to connect with your upper back, which moves your face farther away from the wall.
- Fill your abdomen and chest with an inhalation, and use the exhalation to extend your lower back and neck, as if you are pushing the side of your head against an imaginary strip, as described in the exercise with the doubled-up strip under Parivrtta Siddhasana (see page 308). Rotate farther at the end of the inhalation. When you inhale, push your left hand against the wall to maintain the twist you have developed.
- Initially you can look at the floor, but when your neck feels stable in extension, start to look upward.
- Remain in this position for 1 to 3 minutes, return slowly, and repeat on the other side.

Instructions

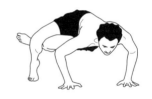

- If you are unsure about your balance, place a felt mat in front of your yoga mat. From a squat, place your right arm over your left leg and bend your body forward to slide your hands under the felt mat. Lift your left foot from the floor and stabilize the strength and position of your left shoulder by remaining here for a few breaths (figure 12.6-5).
- Lifting your left foot and stabilizing your shoulders places the gravity point of the pose in your lower back. Then you can extend your lower back. This provides space to your abdomen and chest. Use this space, and move your chest forward so that you can also lift your other foot. During this movement, the position of your left shoulder is the most uncertain factor. I often see people collapsing in this area. If that happens, try changing the position of your hands; sometimes a broader base can help.
- If you can balance with both feet lifted, place your right foot on top of your left, and push the lower foot against the top one. Lift your chest higher.
- The strength of this movement allows your lower back to extend even farther when your hip joints relax more. Then your entire spine develops the optimal twist and extension.
- Look straight ahead and breathe freely. Remain here for 20 seconds. Return your feet to the floor and repeat on the other side.

10. Dvi pada kaundinyasana

Dvi means "two"; *pada* means "foot."
Kaundinya is the name of the holy person to whom this pose is dedicated. He was regarded as the foremost of the Buddha's five initial disciples. He travelled around India spreading the dharma.

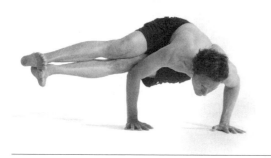

10. Dvi pada kaundinyasana

In this asana, which is an extension of Parsva Bakasana, both legs are extended sideways.

Instructions

- Place your legs as high as you can on your upper arm when doing Parsva Bakasana.
- Extend both legs, while keeping your chest at the same height from the floor.
- Remain in this end position for 20 seconds, breathing deeply and regularly. Bend your legs and return your feet to the floor. Repeat on the other side.

11. Eka Pada Kaundinyasana

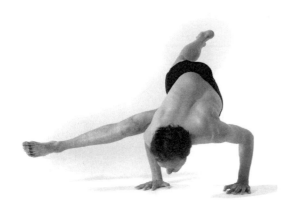

11. Eka pada kaundinyasana

Eka means "one"; **pada** means "foot."

During this asana, which is a variation of Dvi Pada Kaundinyasana, the legs are extended and crossed. The basis for this pose is Parsva Bakasana, and it is described from that asana.

Instructions

- From Malasana (see chapter 12.6, number 7), place your right arm over your left thigh and place both hands diagonally in front of you on the floor. Shift your body weight forward. Lift your left foot and shift your balance into your hands. Lift your right foot and balance in Parsva Bakasana.
- Lift your right leg off the left and extend it backward, in line with your trunk, while simultaneously straightening your left knee.

> **Note:** When you can align your right leg with your trunk, you will be able to extend your lower back. This extension will also increase the extension to the front of your trunk. The rule applies here too: extension precedes rotation. The extension intensifies the rotation of your spine so that more vertebrae are involved in the movement. This increases the flexibility of your spine.
>
> As in the preceding variations, this pose increases the strength in your wrists, arms, and shoulders, alleviating the load to your shoulders and neck.

- Remain in this pose for 20 seconds. Return your feet to the floor via Parsva Bakasana, and relax before repeating on the other side.

12. Moving asanas for advanced students

You should now be able to do a number of asanas in one fluid movement—hence, the name "moving asanas."

Lift your legs into Salamba Sirsasana II (see chapter 8.2, number 12), then move into one of the four balance poses (see asanas 8 through 11 in this chapter), and return back to

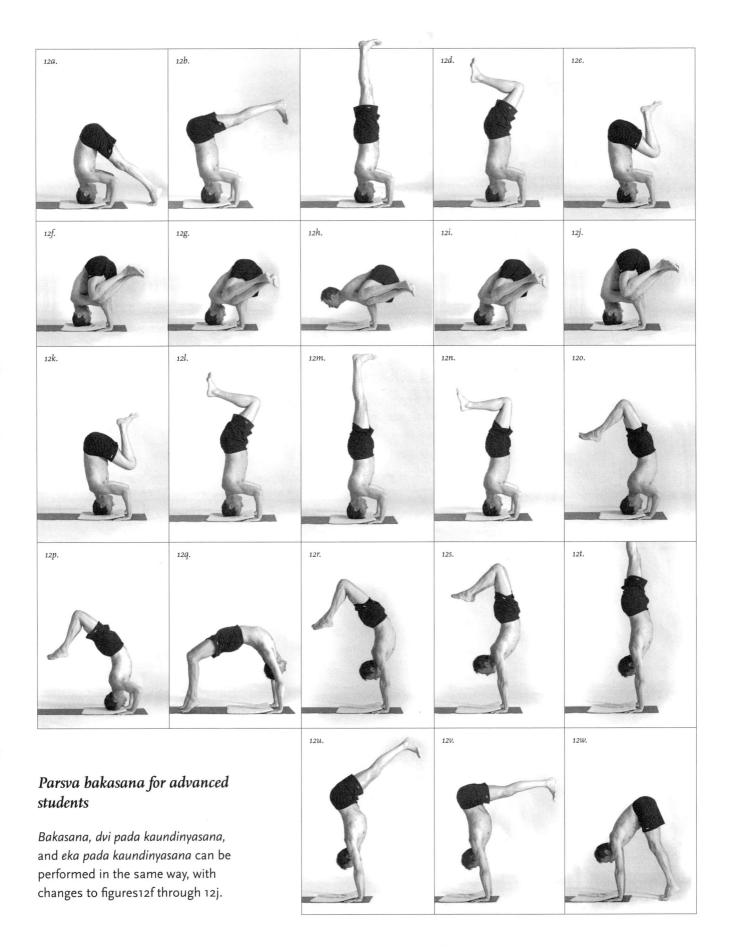

12a.	12b.		12d.	12e.
12f.	12g.	12h.	12i.	12j.
12k.	12l.	12m.	12n.	12o.
12p.	12q.	12r.	12s.	12t.

Parsva bakasana for advanced students

Bakasana, dvi pada kaundinyasana, and *eka pada kaundinyasana* can be performed in the same way, with changes to figures12f through 12j.

12u.	12v.	12w.

Salamba Sirsasana II. Drop back into Urdhva Dhanurasana and move through Viparita Chakrasana into Adho Mukha Vrksasana. From there move into Uttanasana (photos 12a through 12w).

This series of asanas forms the climax. Not many people are able to complete these movements. Because it is such a difficult series, it should only be learned from an experienced teacher. I will now describe some alternative exercises that can be practiced without the help of a teacher. Keep in mind that this series includes some strong backbends. You must prepare and warm up your back (see chapter 11).

Bakasana

Instructions

- Place a felt mat on the front of your yoga mat, and kneel on the floor in front of the felt mat. Slide your hands under the felt, as shown in figure 12.6-6. Place the crown of your head on the felt mat so that a triangle is formed by your head and the palms of your hands. Extend your neck and walk in (figure 12.6-7).
- Extend your lower back and lift both legs simultaneously. Balance on your head (figure 12.6-8); after a few seconds, bend your knees and place your shins on your upper arms (figure 12.6-9). Try not to have any space between your thighs and trunk.
- Lower your pelvis slowly and feel the increase in pressure from your legs to your arms. Use this pressure to extend your lower back. Lift your feet and point your toes.
- Keep your arms strong, and lift your head. While you do, move your abdomen and chest forward without changing the position of your forearms. Otherwise, you will lose your balance and fall (see the arrows in figure 12.6-10). Push your fingertips into the floor and follow the instructions for Bakasana or Parsva Bakasana in one fluid movement, while keeping your shoulders low.

> **Note:** If you keep falling when you try to lift your head in Bakasana, then try to practice the pose from Malasana. When you can do that, try the asana again as described here by placing your head on the floor and lifting your legs back up into Salamba Sirsasana II. When your arms and back get stronger, you will be able to carry your body weight easily when lifting your head from the ground.

- Remain in this end position for 15 seconds, then return the crown of your head to the floor. Contract the muscles of your lower back, and lift your legs back up into Salamba Sirsasana II.

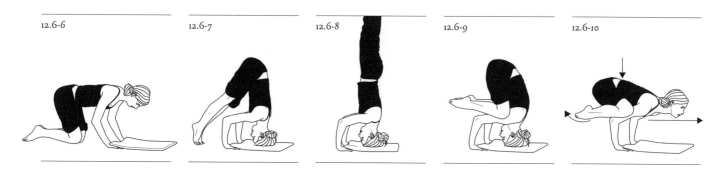

12.6-6   12.6-7   12.6-8   12.6-9   12.6-10

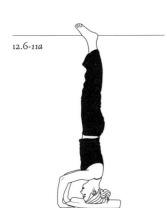

12.6-11a

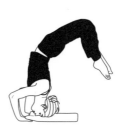

12.6-11b

12.6-11c

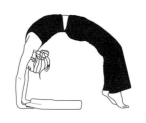

12.6-11d

12.6-12a

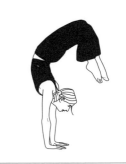

12.6-12b

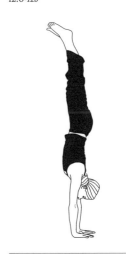

- Remain in this pose for a few seconds, then bend your legs and lower your feet as far as you can by relaxing your back from your tailbone, vertebra by vertebra, as described in the headstand bench variation for Viparita Chakrasana (see chapter 11.4, number 9). During the last phase of the movement, roll your head forward so that your weight is balanced on your forehead, neck, and hands. Shift your weight entirely to your hands after you drop back so that you can push youself up into Urdhva Dhanurasana. Directly after the drop, the gravity point will move into your heart region. Study figures 12.6-11a through 12.6-11d carefully, and make sure you do not let too much weight fall into your neck.

> **Note:** Many people keep their neck stiff; bend only in their lower back; and when they drop back, they bend their knees. Try to engage your entire spine continually in this movement, and keep extending your upper back between your shoulder blades. The preparatory exercise for the aforementioned headstand bench variation is appropriate for learning this movement.

- From Urdhva Dhanurasana, move your chest forward and your head toward your upper back three times. During the third time, jump up into Adho Mukha Vrksasana (figures 12.6-12a and 12.6-12b).
- Stand on your hands for a moment of tranquillity, then return with straight legs to Uttanasana.

> **Note:** If you cannot do Viparita Chakrasana, do the following variations. The cycle will not be as fluid.
>
> 1. Move from Salamba Sirsasana II to Bakasana and back to Salamba Sirsasana II.
> 2. Stand in the headstand bench, drop back, and jump back up (see figures 11.4-26a and 11.4-27b–c) and return with straight legs. Or return from Salamba Sirsasana II and only do Urdhva Dhanurasana.

- If you are able to complete these asanas in succession, repeat the sequence two or three times to increase your strength. Do not work hastily. Take time to rest between poses.

Parsva bakasana

Instructions

- From Salamba Sirsasana II (see chapter 8.2, number 12), bend your knees and lower them toward your abdomen. Keep your neck stable, and place your left thigh on your right upper arm. Sometimes this movement will be fluid; other times, you may have to push your legs in with force or use the momentum of the movement to bring your thighs close enough to your shoulder. Make sure that your right elbow does not move to the right. Keep moving it inward; otherwise, your leg will miss your arm.
- Push your left foot against the right to stimulate the extension in your lower back when you lift your head.

> **Note:** When lifting your head, you can start to use your spine again and extend from your lower back into your pelvis and toward your neck.

- Remain in this end pose for 20 seconds and keep breathing freely. Place the crown of your head back on the floor. Use your lower back muscles to lift your legs back up. Remain balanced for a moment in Salamba Sirsasana II. Bend your knees, and repeat the movement on the other side. Return back to Salamba Sirsasana II, and finish the movement with Viparita Chakrasana, as described for Bakasana (photos 12a through 12w).

Dvi Pada Kaundinyasana

Instructions

- Follow the instructions for Parsva Bakasana, and after you have placed your thighs on your upper arm, lift your head and extend your legs.
- Remain in this end position for 20 seconds. Bend your legs and return to Salamba Sirsasana II, or move from Salamba Sirsasana II with extended legs to the halfway position and place your left thigh, with the leg extended, on your right upper arm.
- Lift your head and extend your spine from your lower back to the top of your chest. Remain in this end position for 20 seconds, then lift your extended legs back into Salamba Sirsasana II. Bend your legs and move through Viparita Chakrasana. Jump into Adho Mukha Vrksasana, and return back to Uttanasana (see photos 12a through 12w).

Eka Pada Kaundinyasana

Instructions

- Place your hands under the felt mat and move from Salamba Sirsasana II to Parsva Bakasana. Extend your right leg back and your left leg sideways, as described earlier in this chapter.

- After 20 seconds, return your legs to Parsva Bakasana and move back into Salamba Sirsasana II. Repeat the movement on the other side, and complete the cycle by moving from Salamba Sirsasana II to Urdhva Dhanurasana (see chapter 11.4, number 8) and through to Viparita Chakrasana (see chapter 11.4, number 9, and photos 12a through 12w).

13

SEATED POSES, SHOULDER AND ABDOMINAL EXERCISES, AND RELAXATION PRACTICES

13.1. Introduction

If your hips, knees, ankles, or shoulders are stiff or if your abdominal muscles are weak, then the exercises in this chapter can be beneficial. They can be done separately from the asana series. For example, the shoulder exercises can easily be done at work and the abdominal exercises before going to bed or on awakening; the seated poses can be done while watching television. These three types of exercises will be discussed extensively in this chapter, concluding with Savasana, the relaxation exercise that is done at the end of every lesson.

1. Seated poses
In this group of asanas the lower back transfers the movement into the pelvic floor, hips, and legs. This way it is easier for the hips and legs to relax, especially during forward bends and backbends in a seated position.

The exercises in this group are used during seated pranayama and meditation practice. If you have stiff legs, hips, and ankles, it may be a long time before you can do the exercises correctly. Therefore, it is better to practice them independently, outside of the classroom situation, so as not to disrupt the flow of the lesson.

The Critical Alignment principle of relaxation preceding movement is very important when practicing seated poses. It is necessary to recognize the difference between tension and relaxation in the leg joints, especially when assuming positions that involve stress to the knees. Here, movement must be slow. Tension and resistance in the knee joints from hasty movement often stems from the back of the knee and can lead to injury. The principle of using body weight to create relaxation applies when relaxing the joints. When these poses are done from relaxation, the knees, hips, and ankles can relax more than in any other position. Then the muscles around the hips and legs are stretched.

Malasana (see chapter 12.6, number 7), Siddhasana, Padmasana, Virasana, and Baddha Konasana belong to this subgroup.

2. Shoulder exercises

The arms transfer movement into the shoulders, which pass it on to the lower back. This rule is nonnegotiable; it applies whether the pose is aimed at relaxing or strengthening the shoulders.

Three shoulder exercises will be described in this chapter. The shoulder stabilizing exercise of lying on a doubled-up rubber strip (see chapter 6.3, connection 4) is done in a seated position instead of a supine one, and two other exercises are introduced. These exercises stretch the arm muscles and the muscles around the shoulder joints. Gomukhasana (Cow Face Pose) and Garudasana (Eagle Pose) belong to this group.

3. Abdominal exercises

A special point of attention here is that the contraction of the abdominal muscles must not disturb the stability of the natural lumbar curve. The supine abdominal exercises described are important, because they support this natural curve. Building up strength in the abdominal muscles is conducive to a balanced diaphragm and proper alignment of the pelvis. The deeper postural muscles of the lower body (the transverse abdominals and those of the lower back, pelvic floor, and diaphragm) form the inner tube.

Mayurasana, as well as a group of supine abdominal exercises, belong to the category of abdominal exercises.

4. Relaxation exercise

Savasana is done at the end of every lesson. It neutralizes tension and, after the activity of the lesson, allows a return to consciousness created from total relaxation.

13.2 Seated poses

1. Padmasana

Padma means "lotus."
Even though Padmasana is a classic yoga pose, it is not easy. Individual differences influence a person's ability to accomplish this pose. Some people are able to do it right away; for others, it can take years, and they will always have to warm up first. When sitting in

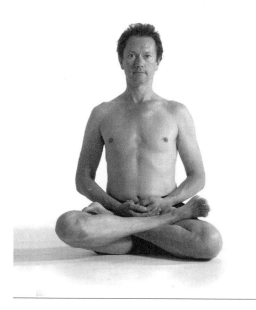

1. Padmasana

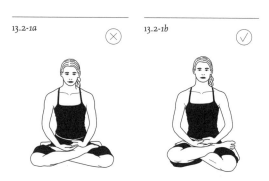

13.2-1a ⊗   13.2-1b ✓

Padmasana for longer periods during pranayama or meditation, pain can dominate. If this happens, you can slowly and consciously move into Siddhasana (number 2 of the alternative poses that follow).

Instructions

· Sit with your legs stretched out in front of you. Place your right foot as high as possible on your left thigh and your left foot as high as possible on your right thigh.

Note: Try to place your ankle rather than your foot on your thigh. This prevents your ankle from twisting and keeps your foot aligned with your lower leg. Then your knees can move closer together, and one knee will lift off the floor (compare figures 13.2-1a and 13.2-1b). Lean slightly forward so that the weight of your upper body shifts to the front of your pelvis, allowing you to relax your groin and the sides of your hips. If you sit with a collapsed lower back and lean back with your upper body, both knees will lift, creating tension in your knees. By shifting your weight from your lower back to the front of your sit bones, your knees will lower and be able to relax.

It is important to lean slightly forward when crossing your legs. Leaning back and pulling on the legs, combined with tension in the knees, can cause injury and unnecessary pain. This applies particularly if you have stiff knees that need to be warmed up first.

· Follow the instructions for sitting upright in Dandasana (see chapter 10.3, number 3).

Note: If you cannot extend your lower back in this pose, sit on a shoulderstand block with a strip underneath as described in the sitting meditation exercise (see chapter 7.2, number 2). Then you will be able to extend your lower back and transfer the weight of your upper body to your groin.

Even though your knee makes a specific movement during Padmasana, the external rotation of your leg actually occurs in your hip. This rotation of your femur protects your knee. The following exercise, described in two phases, prepares and frees up your hip.

Warming up the hips and knees

Phase 1

· Sit with the soles of your feet together and your knees wide and bent at 90-degree angles.

- Take hold of your feet and extend your lower back as much as you can. Place your hands on the floor without bending your back and start to move your fingertips forward until your head is above your feet (figure 13.2-2). Remember that the extension to your abdomen and chest that is initiated from your hands moving forward, precedes the bending of your back. You can also take hold of your feet to strengthen the extension to the front of your body. For this movement, follow the instructions for Paschimottanasana (see chapter 10.5, number 6).
- Remain in this pose for 1 to 2 minutes, and use your breathing to relax any tension you encounter.

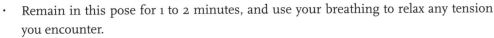

Phase 2

- Sit with the soles of your feet together as in phase 1. Pull your left foot in so that the heel touches your pelvis.
- Extend your upper body forward in a diagonal line without losing the connection between your neck and lower back. If you lose that, you will also lose the strength in your lower back. Move your hands forward to increase your forward bend. (You may choose to take hold of your right foot instead of walking forward with your hands.) Relax your hips and knees during exhalations.
- Remain in this pose for 1 to 2 minutes, then repeat with the left leg stretched out and the right leg pulled in.

If Padmasana is still not possible, try the following poses. They are good alternative end positions.

1. Cross-legged

Instructions

- Pull your left foot toward your right hip and your right foot toward your left hip (figure 13.2-3) under your knees.
- Extend your lower back as described for Padmasana. When your core is properly aligned, your knees and hips will be able to relax.
- Remain in this pose for as long as you can, then repeat with your legs crossed the other way.

13.2-3

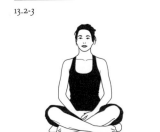

2. Siddhasana

Siddha means "accomplished."

Instructions

- Place your left heel against your perineum (the bottom of your pelvic floor), and place your right foot between your left calf and thigh.
- Extend your lower back as described for Padmasana so that the weight of your body moves into the front of your sit bones and you can relax your hips and knees (figure 13.2-4).
- Remain in this pose for as long as you can, then repeat with your legs crossed the other way.

13.2-4

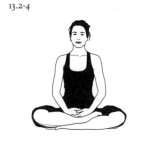

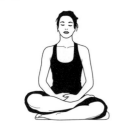

3. Ardha Padmasana

Ardha means "half."

Instructions

- Place your right foot on your left thigh and slide your left foot under your right thigh (figure 13.2-5).
- Extend your lower back as described for Padmasana.
- Remain in this pose for as long as you can, then repeat with your legs crossed the other way.

2. Virasana

Vira means "strong."

Instructions

- Sit with your legs extended. Bend your knees and place your right foot next to your right hip and your left foot next to your left hip. Align your feet with your lower leg.

> **Note:** If you cannot place your buttocks *between* your feet on the floor, you can start by sitting *on* your feet. Slowly start to shift your feet to the sides until you end up with your buttocks on the floor, as shown in figures 13.2-6a through 13.2-6c.

There are now two possibilities to improve the position of your legs and knees:

1. In the end position, the inside of your calf should touch the outside of your thigh. To relax your knees, lift your pelvis slightly and take hold of your calf, just under the knee. Use your hand to pull your calf away from your thigh. You can also place a belt around your calf and use this to pull it away from your thigh (figure 13.2-7). Keep using the belt to create space if this helps your knees to relax.
2. Place your hands over your knees and pull the skin under your knees upward. This can ease tension in your knees.

- If your *ankles* are stiff and painful, place a rolled-up felt mat under your ankles to lessen the stretch in your feet (figure 13.2-8). The thicker the roll, the easier it is for your ankles. As your ankles become more flexible, lessen the size of the roll.

2. Virasana

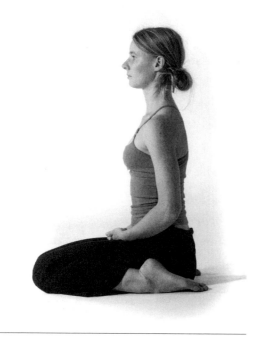

13.2-6a

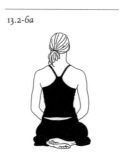

13.2-6b

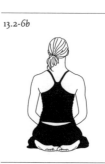

13.2-6c

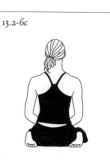

- If you feel pain in your *knees,* place a rolled-up felt mat between your sit bones and ankles (figure 13.2-9). This lessens the bend of your knees and eases tension. Here too, the thicker the roll, the easier it is for your knees. As your knees become more flexible, reduce the size of the roll.
- Remain in this position for as long as you can. Relax your legs slowly, or do the exercise for a shorter period of time and then do Supta Virasana (Reclining Hero Pose).

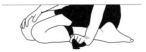
13.2-7

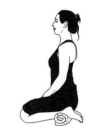
13.2-8

Supta Virasana

Supta means "asleep."
This exercise is completed in two phases. In the first, you try to flatten your lower back as much as possible toward the floor with the use of your inner tube; the back of your head rests on the floor. In the second phase, you arch your back and place the crown of your head on the floor.

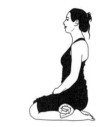
13.2-9

In the first phase, the emphasis is on stretching your thighs. During the second phase, your back learns how to bend backward correctly—that is, with your legs rotated inward. The combination of these two variations is an excellent preparation for the backbends in chapter 11.

Instructions

Phase 1

- Sit in Virasana and place your hands behind you on the floor. Look at the distance between your lower ribs and pelvis, and keep observing this distance while you develop the movement. Your abdomen should not lengthen when your trunk moves farther down. Lean back and keep your lower abdominal muscles working so that your tailbone stretches away from your lower back and your pelvis tilts backward. Keep your diaphragm relaxed and connected to your abdomen. In that position, your lower ribs coordinate the transport of movement through the arch of your lower back toward your pelvis.
- If your thigh muscles become more flexible you can intensify the stretch by leaning on your elbows, keeping your hands close to your feet, by putting your hands on your lower ribs and allowing them to move down, or by stretching them over your head (figures 13.2-10a through 13.2-10d).
- Remain in this pose for as long as you can, or do it for a shorter period and then move into phase 2.

13.2-10a

13.2-10b

13.2-10c

13.2-10d

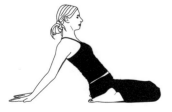

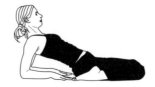

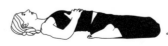

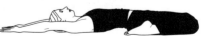

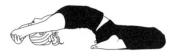

Phase 2

- From the preceding position, place your fingertips on the floor next to your head. Push your back and shoulders off the floor and place the crown of your head on the floor.
- Hold your elbows and place your arms over your head on the floor, as shown in figure 13.2-11.
- Remain in this end position for 30 to 60 seconds and return. Relax your legs slowly.

> **Note:** Push your head and pelvis into the floor so that your back forms a bow. Breathe into the front of your body and use every exhalation to extend your back. The movement of your back is initiated from the midline. Your tailbone pushes into the floor to strengthen the arch of your lower back, while the crown of your head pushes into the floor to strengthen the extension of your upper back. This activates the deep postural muscles.
>
> In this pose, you learn how to bend backward with inwardly rotated legs. Try to keep your knees together. This leg position activates the midline of your body and frees your lower back. For these reasons, it is an excellent preparation for the backbend exercises described in chapter 11.

3. Baddha Konasana

Baddha means "bound"; *kona* means "angle."
In this pose, the soles of the feet are placed together and brought as close as possible to the pelvis using the hands. Then the knees are lowered as far as possible. This is how shoemakers sit in India.

Instructions

- Sit with bent knees and take hold of your feet. Pull them, one at a time, toward your pelvis so the soles touch. Extend your back as described for Padmasana.
    - Lower your knees out to the sides as far as possible.
    - If your lower back cannot extend, it will be impossible to relax your groin. Then you must elevate your seat so that your lower back can extend and your groin can move toward the floor. From your groin, stretch your inner thighs toward your knees and push your knees actively toward the floor.
    - Remain in this pose for as long as you can; return, and relax your legs.

3. Baddha konasana

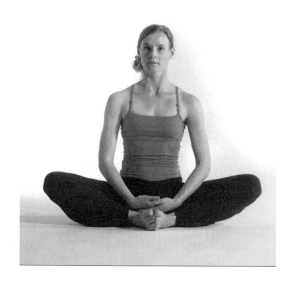

> **Note:** It can help to sit on a roll (on top of the shoulderstand block) against the wall, as shown in figure 13.2-12. Lean forward, relax your knees, and position your pelvis correctly; stretch and lower your knees as much as you can. Then, without allowing your knees to lift, extend your back so that your shoulder blades touch the wall but your lower back

doesn't. Sit here for a while (about 30 to 60 seconds), then place your hands on your knees and push them slowly toward the floor.

There is a depression on the inside of each knee, where the thigh and lower leg meet. Place your hands on these depressions to push your knees out and down. This will stimulate the outward rotation of your thighs and the stretch to your inner thighs.

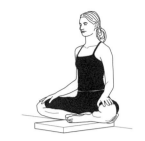

13.2-12

13.3 Shoulder exercises

In chapter 6.3, connection 4, a shoulder exercise (lying on a rubber strip) was introduced to connect the arms and shoulders. This exercise increases the strength to the upper arms. Reread the comments and instructions written there. In this chapter, we will develop this exercise further. It will be done seated without the support of the rubber strip on the upper back, which stays straight.

During normal everyday circumstances, the body often resists the act of lifting the arms: the shoulders tighten, and the back muscles contract. This breaks the connection between the arms and the shoulder blades. The reflexive tension in the shoulder girdle totally blocks the transfer of movement from the arms to the back. The underlying cause of this is an inability to keep the upper back straight. It is important, therefore, to extend the upper back before raising the arms. You can use a belt to help your shoulder girdle relax; tighten it to the width of your shoulders so that it keeps your wrists and arms at this breadth when you extend your arms (figure 13.3-1).

Preparation exercise

Instructions

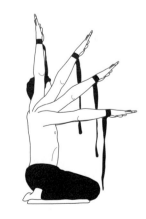

13.3-1

·   Sit so that you can keep your lower back extended for some time, and place your hands on your thighs. Position your lower back and pelvis by following the instructions given in chapter 6.3, connection 9.
·   On a deep inhalation, align your neck and head on top of your upper back; relax your shoulders on an exhalation. If it is difficult for you to extend your upper back, start with the supine version of this exercise.

13.3-2

·   Place the belt around your wrists, and extend your arms straight out in front of you. Push lightly against the belt so that your shoulders can relax. Straighten your elbows completely, and keep your shoulders relaxed. Pull your upper arms toward your body to connect to your shoulder blades.
·   Breathe freely from your abdomen into your chest, and lift your arms slowly until they form a straight line with your back (figure 13.3-2). The end position will be defined by the shape of your upper back. If you were able to keep your spine straight and your shoulders relaxed, then if you move your arms forward and backward slightly, you will feel a resilient movement around your shoulder blades.
·   Breathe deeply three times and then stretch your arms as far as you can toward the ceiling. Visualize your arms stretching your shoulders and upper back, providing length. Do not lose the structure of your inner tube when lifting your arms or hold your breath in your chest.

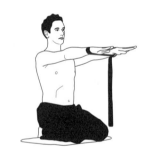

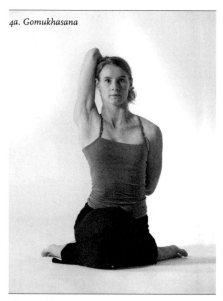

4a. Gomukhasana

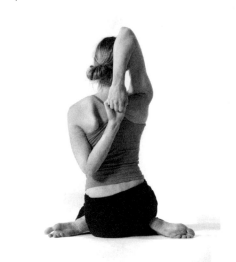

4b. Gomukhasana

- Keep your elbows extended and your breathing open and free. Be aware of the space around you, and fill this space when you make the movement.
- Slowly lower your arms back into the horizontal position and repeat the exercise until your upper arms tire.

4. Gomukhasana

Go means "cow"; *mukha* means "face."

Instructions

- Sit on the floor with your legs extended in front of you. Bend your left leg and place your left foot next to your right hip. Bring your right leg over your left, placing your right foot next to your left hip.
- Bend your left arm and slide your hand as far as you can up your spine between your shoulder blades. Lift your right arm, placing your upper arm next to your head, and slide your hand down between your shoulder blades to take hold of your left hand.
- If your hands will not meet, use a belt to connect them.
- Breathe slowly and deeply, use your breathing in the following manner: breathe in and feel your breath moving under your left hand, along your upper back. Keep your upper back as erect as possible and position your neck directly above it. You may feel your back sinking deeper between your shoulder blades, because your inhalations pull your spine straighter. When your back straightens in this way, your shoulder and arm muscles can relax more fully. By keeping your back erect, your inhalations stretch the front of your chest toward your left collarbone. The relaxation of your shoulder and arm muscles will not feel good to start with, but that is common when stiff muscles are stretched and stiff joints become mobile.
- In the beginning, there will be a lot of resistance in the muscles of your left (lower) arm and shoulder. This will lessen if you keep your forearm and elbow heavy and your neck in alignment with your back.
- Your right (upper) arm moves toward your head. This softens the muscles of the shoulder in the same area that you rest on the headstand bench.
- Remain in this end pose for 1 to 2 minutes, then switch arms and legs to repeat on the other side.

There are not many exercises that show the difference in tension between the left and right sides of your body caused by left- or right-handedness so clearly. If you are right-handed, your right arm and shoulder will generally be stronger and stiffer than the left, and vice versa. If you look at the position of your shoulders in a mirror, you will probably see that one is lower and slightly more forward than the other (for right-handed people, this will generally be the right shoulder). This is caused by a combination of rotation and bending in the upper back. For this reason, it is recommended that you prepare for this exercise by lying on a doubled-up rubber strip for 5 minutes. This will relax and stretch your upper back.

Gomukhasana can be done supine as well.

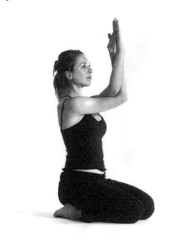

- Sit on your yoga mat with your legs extended in front of you. Place your arms in the Gomukhasana position with your left arm down. Keep your left elbow close to your side and slowly lower yourself, with a hollow back, to the floor. Lean your head on your right forearm.
- Relax your left shoulder and arm. Use your breath to broaden this area from your collarbone.
- Your upper arm (in this case, the right) extends away from your chest: the upper arm stretches toward the elbow, while your lower ribs move toward your abdomen. This stretches the area around your right armpit. Lying on your arms applies pressure to your wrists and can be likened to lying supine with the rubber strip between your shoulder blades. This pressure stretches your arm muscles and relaxes your wrists, and it is a reference point for your breathing. When your breathing moves past this place, you can feel clearly whether or not your back is relaxing and extending.
- Remain in this pose for 1 to 2 minutes, and come out by rolling slowly to your right side; relax and repeat on the other side.

5b. Garudasana

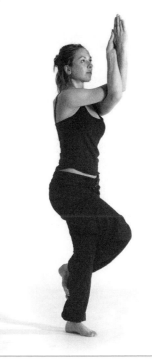

5. Garudasana

Garuda means "eagle."

Garuda is a mythical bird, the vehicle of Vishnu. This pose comprises two phases, the first of which is aimed at relaxing your shoulders. This phase can best be done while seated in Virasana. In the second phase, your legs are crossed while you balance on one foot.

Instructions

Phase 1: seated

- Sit in any position in which you can keep your lower back extended for some time. Bend your right arm and bring it in front of you, with your elbow at shoulder-height. Place your left elbow on your right arm. Twist your forearms around each other so that the fingers of your right hand rest on the palm of your left. Your left hand is at a right angle to your face.
- Breathe slowly and relax your shoulders. Breathe deeply into the area between your shoulder blades without lifting your shoulders. "Massage" the area between your shoulder blades, shown in figure 13.3-3, with deep inhalations. This stretches the muscles under your shoulder blades.

13.3-3

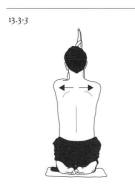

Note: This area often causes problems for people who work at computers, which can result in a prolonged, nagging pain in this section of the back. It is caused by small "knots" in the muscles (trigger points) that cause chronic pain. Some doctors say that 75 percent of all chronic pain is caused by these trigger points, which can be found all over the body.[1] Stretching muscles and applying *(continued)*

- Use your left elbow to push your right arm higher, keep your shoulders low, and do not allow your hands to move toward your head. Do not lose the twist in your arms; keep your right hand at a right angle to your face.
- Relax your arms after 1 minute, and repeat the exercise on the other side.

Phase 2: standing

- From Tadasana, bend your left leg and cross the right leg around the top of it. Hook your right big toe behind your left calf.
- Maintain your balance by focusing your gaze on one point on the floor and concentrate on relaxing your left foot.
- When your balance is stable, position your arms as described for phase 1 and straighten your left leg a little more, without losing the grip of your right big toe. Push your left arm up as described for phase 1.
- Remain in this pose for 30 to 60 seconds. Return, relax, and repeat on the other side.

This pose stabilizes the postural muscles of your ankles and feet and stretches your legs.

6. Nakrasana

Nakra means "crocodile."

Whereas the preceding poses relax the shoulders and arms, Nakrasana strengthens the arm, chest, and shoulder muscles. For this reason, it is an excellent preparation for the balance poses in chapters 10.6 and 12.6.

Some people dislike poses that require strength, while others have difficulty relaxing. The confrontation with strength (or the lack of it) in this asana often causes a lot of laughter and a lack of concentration, both of which are detrimental for any pose. This occurs because (for many) the end pose is not immediately attainable. It is important to find a position in the buildup of this exercise where you can remain for some time and increase your strength. Make sure that you do not stay in the pose for too long,

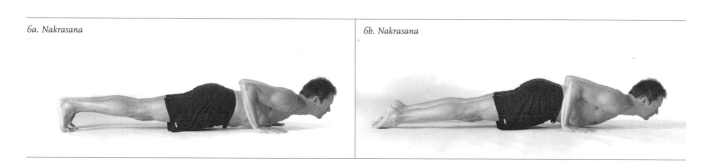

6a. Nakrasana   6b. Nakrasana

as you will eventually collapse on the floor. Retain enough energy so that you can return properly.

The exercise is written in three phases: for absolute beginners, for those who are stronger, and for advanced students. The first two phases are initiated from standing on hands and knees; the third is built from Adho Mukha Svanasana.

Instructions

Phase 1

- Standing on your hands and knees, allow your upper back to relax so that your upper arms can connect with your shoulder blades. Breathe toward your sternum, lift your head, and look forward. Your hands should be at shoulder-width.
- Slowly bend your arms into an end position that you can maintain for a short time. Push yourself back up to your hands and knees. Repeat this, moving slightly farther forward and a little lower each time until your sternum ends an inch above the floor between the line of your hands. It is not necessary for your lower arms to end at right angles to the floor initially.
- Keep your shoulders low, look straight ahead, and bring your elbows close to your body (figure 13.3-4). Keep breathing regularly and feel the tranquillity in the areas of your body that you can keep relaxed. Your knees should still be touching the floor.
- Push yourself back up to the starting position and pause. Repeat this movement until you are tired.

13.3-4

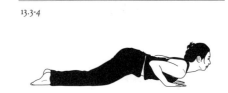

Phase 2

- From the end position in phase 1, stretch your legs out so that you are balancing on your hands and toes.
- Keep your pelvis slightly higher than your shoulders. Maintain this position for as long as you can. Reserve enough energy so that when you place your knees back on the floor you can push back up to your hands and knees.
- From this end position, you can increase the strength and flexibility of your wrists by stretching your feet so that your entire body moves farther forward between your lower arms. Then move back with your heels, place your knees on the floor, and push yourself back up to your hands and knees.
- Repeat this movement until you become tired.

Phase 3

- Standing on your hands and knees, move into Adho Mukha Svanasana (see chapter 9.2, number 4). Lift your head and bend your arms so that your body moves forward and lowers between your arms. Do not allow your chest to touch the floor. Remain in this position with your toes on the floor or move farther into the variation with stretched feet. Keep your pelvis slightly higher than your shoulders. Breathe in and out deeply a few times.
- Move back into Adho Mukha Svanasana, imagining that someone is pulling your pelvis back and up. Your chin and chest should remain close to the floor when you move back. Stretch your arms. Keep your elbows as close as you can to your trunk

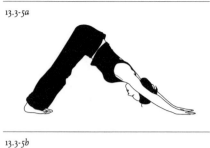
13.3-5a

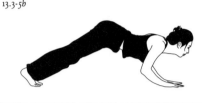
13.3-5b

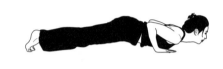
13.3-5c

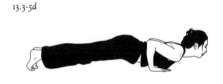
13.3-5d

during the entire movement. This is a difficult way to return (figures 13.3-5a through 13.3-5d). The easier version is to move back into Adho Mukha Svanasana via a straight diagonal position (figures 13.3-6a through 13.3-6c).

· Repeat the movement until you tire.

13.4 Abdominal exercises

The exercises described here strengthen the large abdominal muscles that are necessary to keep the pubic bone and lower ribs connected during complex movements. They act as the constraint that keeps the inner tube intact. This is necessary for many groups of asanas, such as moving into inversions, extending the back for standing poses, and creating the air bag effect in backbends. These supporting muscles are also called the outer core, because the muscles are located on the surface of the body.

Once movement has been completed and a tranquil end position has been accomplished with the skeleton aligned, the superficial abdominal muscles can gradually relax. Then the postural muscles of the abdomen, the transverse abdominals (see page 118), take over. These muscles are referred to as the inner core.

This process of changing from movement muscles to postural muscles was described in the discussion for going up in the headstand bench (see chapter 8.2, number 1). The transverse abdominals will be exercised separately so they can be felt clearly. This will be done after Urdhva Prasarita Padasana.

7. Urdhva Prasarita Padasana

Urdhva means "facing upward"; *prasarita* means "extended apart"; *pada* means "foot."

Abdominal exercises are often done at the expense of space to the two gravity points of the body—the hara and heart region. The space in either of these two points can then be compromised, causing the physical experience of lightness and relaxation to evaporate. When you overwork your core muscles, your gravity points are compressed.

In addition, many abdominal exercises interfere with the free, extended position of the lower back. During supine exercises, when the stomach muscles contract, the lower back is often pushed into the floor. I have had numerous clients with injuries caused by these types of exercises. To understand exactly what is meant here, it is important to reread the discussion about problems that can occur in the lower back (see chapter 6.3, connections 7, 8 [inner tube], and 9).

The key is to avoid losing the natural lordotic curve of the lower back. This arch keeps the lower back strong when lifting and the vertebrae mobile while walking.

Many people go overboard when training their abdominal muscles. Well-formed abs (the six pack!) are often the goal. No attention is given to the position of the lower back, which can suffer from such training. From the

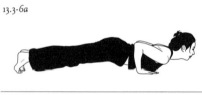
13.3-6a

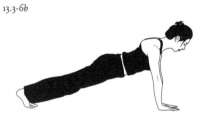
13.3-6b

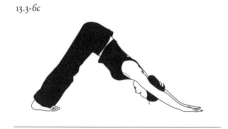
13.3-6c

340   LEARNING THE EXERCISES

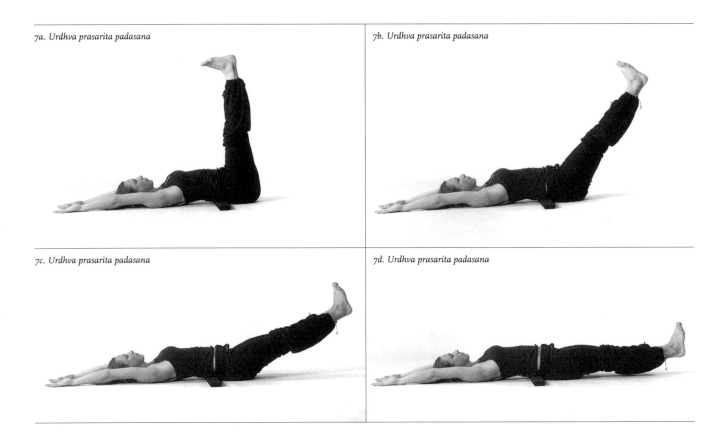

7a. *Urdhva prasarita padasana*

7b. *Urdhva prasarita padasana*

7c. *Urdhva prasarita padasana*

7d. *Urdhva prasarita padasana*

perspective of Critical Alignment, exercising the abdominals is very important, as they strengthen the inner tube. But the strength of the abdominals must never be accomplished at the expense of the natural curve and free movement of the lower back. A rubber strip is used during the following exercise to allow you to observe and constantly maintain your natural lordotic curve.

Do the exercises carefully in the following two phases, which move from easy to difficult, making it possible for you to build up strength safely.

Instructions

Phase 1

- Lie on your yoga mat with your knees bent and your arms stretched out on the floor above your head. Position the rubber strip horizontally under your lower back; your back should touch the strip lightly, just above your pelvis, even when you move your lower ribs toward your abdomen. This contact is constant during this exercise; pressure should not increase or decrease when you lift your legs. Place your hands on your abdomen and feel that the muscles are relaxed.
- Extend your right leg upward, keeping your knee bent. Straighten it only if you can do so without increasing the pressure of your back on the strip. When you lower your right leg, straighten your knee and end with your right heel 1 inch above the floor. Allow your left foot to become lighter on the floor as if you were going to lift it. Press your tailbone firmly into the floor so that your abdominal muscles contract strongly. Note that your abdominal muscles move upward to form a column between your pubic bone and diaphragm. If you push your fingers against your stomach, it will feel

firm, like an inner tube that has been correctly inflated, but not so hard that it cannot move. Keep the contact pressure of the strip on your lower back constant.

· Breathe into your abdomen and observe if tension arises in your shoulders and neck. This can be a consequence of this exercise; the strength of your abdominals shifts the bend of your upper back into your shoulders and neck (figure 13.4-1). The tension in your neck and shoulders will lessen when your upper back straightens.

· This is the easiest part of this exercise and can be done by everyone. Remain in the end position for a few breaths. Bend your right leg and return. Repeat on the other side. Keep repeating until you tire, or move into the next phase.

Phase 2

· From the end position in phase 1, you can increase the intensity of this exercise depending on your ability.

13.4-1

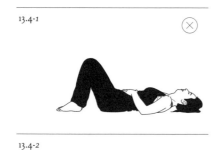

13.4-2

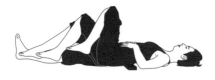

   1. When you have straightened your right leg with your heel 1 inch above the floor, lift your left foot ½ inch off the floor, and push the inside of your foot against the inside of your right thigh. Remain here for two or three breaths, keeping the pressure from the rubber strip constant on your lower back. Feel how breathing into your stomach does not weaken your abdominals.

   2. From this position, you can slowly start to extend your left leg, sliding your foot along the inside of your right leg (figure 13.4-2). Choose a position in which your lower back still touches the strip and where you can remain for a few breaths.

   3. Ultimately, you will be able to stretch your left leg completely, keeping both heels 1 inch above the floor. Repeat the movement on the other side.

   4. When you can complete this phase with ease, you can move both legs together (bent or straight, depending on the length of your hamstrings).

This exercise gives you insight into the strength of your abdominal muscles in relation to the position of your lower back. It helps you to recognize the neutral position of your inner tube.

You strengthen not only your abdominals but also your leg muscles and (if you feel an intense extension in your lower back) your lower back muscles.

The slow buildup with one leg is especially good if tension develops in your groin when you lift both legs together.

13.4-3

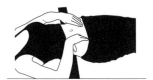

13.4-4

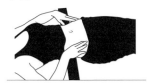

The transverse abdominals

- Lie on your back with the rubber strip lightly touching your lower back, as in the previous exercise.
- Feel your hip bones with your fingertips (figure 13.4-3). Push your thumbs firmly against the outsides of your hip bones, and push your fingertips as deep as possible into your abdomen (figure 13.4-4). Keep your abdomen totally passive during this movement.
- To activate your transverse abdominals, pull the area of your lower abdomen, 1 inch under your navel, up toward your navel. When you do this, your transverse abdominals push your fingers out of your abdomen.

> **Note:** Make sure that you do not push your lower back into the rubber strip, because this means you have activated your abdominals.

- Stay in this end position for 5 to 15 minutes, and keep breathing into your abdomen without your fingers sinking in (this shows the muscles are relaxed).
- Take a couple of weeks to train these muscles while supine so that you begin to recognize them in action. Then you can practice this exercise in a seated pose. Finally, you will maintain this control when standing, walking, and practicing all asanas.

The effect of this exercise was described in chapter 6.3, connection 8.

8. Mayurasana

Mayura means "peacock."
This is the ultimate abdominal exercise. Not only do the abdominals get stronger, but so do the wrists, arms, shoulders, lower back, and legs.

8. Mayurasana

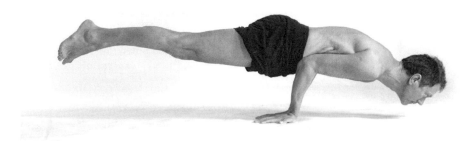

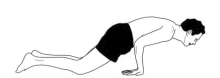

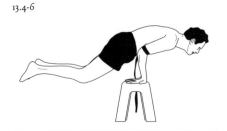

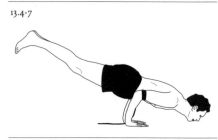

Instructions

- Standing on your hands and knees, twist your arms so that your fingers face your knees. Bend your arms slowly while keeping your elbows together. Push your elbows firmly into your upper abdomen and look straight ahead (figure 13.4-5).
- Move your upper body farther forward until you can lift your feet off the floor. Straighten your knees, and remain in this end position for as long as you can, breathing regularly.

> **Note:** If your elbows slide apart, place a belt around your upper arms to keep them in position. If the load on your wrists is too much, try balancing on a stool (figure 13.4-6).

There is a similar pose called Hamsasana (Goose Pose). The instructions for this asana are the same as for Mayurasana, only your fingers now point forward and your elbows push lower into your abdomen (figure 13.4-7). Because the pressure on your wrists is much greater in this variation, it can greatly increase their flexibility.

13.5 Relaxation practice

9. Savasana

Sava means "corpse."

During Savasana, you lie "dead" still—hence, the name. Savasana is the final pose of every yoga session. Relaxation must not be confused with falling asleep. If you fall asleep during Savasana, your alert consciousness will disappear, and you will move unconsciously. There is no question of a relaxation exercise in such a state, because the relaxation is no longer consciously developed. The open, nonthinking consciousness will be taken over by the stream of thoughts that occurs during sleep.

In the first phase of the exercise, you give attention to placing your body in a

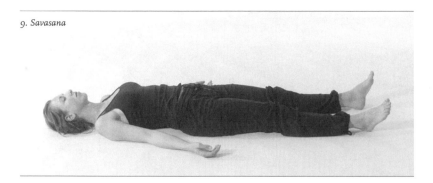

9. Savasana

balanced position. During the second phase, you can realize a higher consciousness. Reread chapter 5 for a detailed description about realizing higher consciousness. Also re-read the last remark made in chapter 7.2 in which the interaction between the yoga class, a relaxation exercise, and their connection with daily activities was discussed.

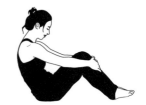

Instructions

Phase 1

- Sit in the middle of your yoga mat with your knees bent, and take hold of your knees. Push your lower vertebrae toward the floor (figure 13.5-1); lower yourself, vertebra by vertebra, until you are lying on your back.

> **Note:** If your lower back is stiff, then lowering yourself gradually may not be possible, and you will drop to the floor quickly. Try to prevent this for as long as you can. If it does happen, make sure you exhale as you drop.

- Lying on your mat, your lower back is now extended properly, even though it is too close to the floor because your legs are still bent. Keep your shoulders low and hold the back of your head with your hands. Lift your head from the floor and relax your neck. Place your head back on the floor without contracting your neck muscles. Keep your throat soft.
- Extend your legs, one at a time, by lifting them up and stretching your heel away from you. When you have placed the first heel on the ground, keep the foot flexed; repeat this movement with the second leg. Allow your legs to become heavy and feel how the arch of your lower back elevates. Your tailbone stretches away from your lower back, but the extension of your legs allows your lower back to return to its natural lordotic curve. Do not move your pelvis when you relax your legs, and allow your feet to fall outward slowly.
- Stretch your arms alongside your body, and turn the palms of your hands up so that your shoulders can broaden and relax. Shut your eyes.

Phase 2

- Observe and relax the different areas of your body together during exhalations.
- Begin with your legs, and feel how your exhalation relaxes each leg from the top side to the floor. This makes your body feel increasingly heavy. Resolve not to move anymore. Relax your pelvis, back, shoulders, arms, and finally your neck and head in the same way.

> **Note:** The pressure that builds in certain areas of your body when you lie still can become uncomfortable, causing small movements like the twitching of a hand or shoulder. If you notice the discomfort and do not react to it, the deeper postural muscles will finally be able to relax, and the urge to move will disappear. This means your relaxation has increased.

- Relaxing your neck makes your head feel heavier. Observe your facial muscles, especially those around your eyes and in your forehead, and allow tension to flow away through the back of your head where it rests on the floor. Your eyes will fall deeper into their sockets and the contact between your eyeballs and eyelids will start to feel light.
- When facial tension dissipates, you will be able to observe your body from the back of your head, a nonthinking part of your brain (manonmani; see page 62). Keep observing your body from this area of your head.
- Without focusing on what you see, open your eyes and observe the space above and around you in a completely relaxed way. Instead of interpreting the meaning of what you see, which will activate your thoughts, use the awareness to connect your body to your surroundings. Keep observing from the back of your head. Start to become aware that the space is limited. There is a ceiling, walls, and so on. Close your eyes slowly and enter the darkness in front of you. Darkness is infinite. The universe is darkness. Connect your body with the awareness of that endless space.

> **Note:** As soon this awareness is broken, conscious thoughts take over your attention, and your eyes develop tension, causing them to move back and forth. This often happens because the nature of the mind is to be active. Take time to observe this, and try to return to your relaxed connection with infinite space in a gentle way. Do not *feel* disturbed when you notice that the activity of thinking interferes with your concentration.

- When you have achieved mental tranquillity, bring your attention back to your body and observe your right arm. By keeping your attention there, you will find that warmth (energy) develops. This subtle energy, which expands slowly into the rest of your body, becomes the carrier of your attention.
- Without lessening your attention on your right arm, include your left arm in your observation until you feel the stream of energy manifest. Then you can connect your arms and shoulders through your chest so that they form an open entity where the energy flows freely.
- Expand the awareness of your body into your abdomen, pelvis, legs, and finally your head.
- When you become aware of your entire body by passively observing from the back of your head, mental awareness and body awareness melt into higher consciousness. To achieve this, you must become aware of the openness and transparency of the space around you. Through this awareness, you may feel that the space around you is filling your body and that your body is filling the space. Then you will be totally present in the here and now, and thoughts such as "I am in this space," become "I am this space."
- Maintain this awareness for as long as you can, remaining in Savasana for 5 to 15 minutes. To come out, start to make small movements with your hands and feet. Take a few deep breaths, and open your eyes. Roll to your side before getting up.

Note: When you bring awareness back to the concept of space, do not think in terms of infinite space immediately. First explore the space a few inches around your body. This will make it easier to connect your body with your surroundings. Once your body produces a feeling that there is actually no difference between the space around you and your body, expand your breathing.

PART FIVE

TEACHING YOGA AND BUILDING LESSON PLANS

The preceding parts of this book have extensively discussed various concepts of Critical Alignment, such as the protocol, the connections, the groups and subgroups of asanas, the props, various aspects of awareness, a higher consciousness, and so on. However, I have saved the combination of these concepts for this last part devoted to lesson plans and teaching.

All of the concepts and instruments of the Critical Alignment method come together in the lesson plans to create a positive and dynamic experience that leads toward a higher consciousness. To give more depth to this process, I will explain certain aspects that are necessary when planning a lesson. Special attention will be given to the following points:

1. *Creation of a starting point.* The lesson should unite and deepen attention, relaxation, awareness, and so on. A clear starting point is necessary to initiate this dynamic construction and attempt to break through constant, repetitive, negative thoughts and feelings. Students come to class with these thoughts and feelings from their daily lives. It is important for the teacher to draw students' attention to these processes at the start of the lesson. Only then can they distance themselves from their negative attitudes. If the teacher succeeds in this, the danger of the lesson getting bogged down in negativity will diminish, allowing a positive experience to develop.

2. *Organization of positive development through stages.* Every lesson comprises seven stages that are arranged in a particular sequence. These stages are necessary to provide structure, focus, and momentum. They make it possible for every lesson to develop innovatively. Each stage is unique and is characterized by the practice of certain asanas with a focus on the connections involved. The goal of each stage is to optimize and continue the development of higher consciousness.

3. *The gradual increase of speed while doing asanas and the addition of more asanas and connections.* This is an important rule for:
   a. Penetrating into deeper layers of muscles and joints
   b. Increasing the strength and coordination of the postural muscles
   c. Coordinating the development of a higher consciousness

4. *Application of the cause-and-effect relationship.* This important rule prescribes that asanas and other exercises be done in a strictly sequential order. This is necessary to deepen relaxation of the movement muscles, increase coordination, strengthen the postural muscles, and increase the mobility of the joints. It dictates that simple exercises must come first so that the superficial muscles can relax. These are followed by more complex movements that increase relaxation, strength, and coordination.

5. *Use of creativity when planning lessons.* The enormous variety of connections and subgroups of asanas makes it possible to create lessons suited to individuals or certain groups of students. Creative lessons are planned in the same way as "normal" lessons, by adhering to the preceding concepts and rules.

14

PLANNING THE LESSONS

14.1 Introduction

The lessons are the quintessence of the Critical Alignment method. All of the concepts are combined in the lesson, making a positive, dynamic development of consciousness possible. This can never be achieved by practicing yoga asanas in a random sequence, as you will be unable to develop either focus or momentum. Attention and relaxation cannot deepen, and this will prevent you from realizing a higher consciousness. You can achieve this consciousness only by combining the aspects of Critical Alignment—focus, relaxation, and attention—in such a way that they interact dynamically with each other.

An important point should be considered in developing a class and must be dealt with in a sensitive way. It is my experience that nearly every student begins the lesson with a negative attitude. If this is not immediately recognized and discontinued, then the lesson will languish in negativity with absolutely no chance of anything positive developing. The easiest way to break through this negativity is to confront students with their own negative feelings and thoughts. Recognition of your attitude initiates the dynamic process from which a higher consciousness can develop.

Negativity
Despite the fact that I have been teaching yoga for many years, I am still astounded at the negative reactions of both beginning and advanced students. I do not mean that students do not arrive cheerfully for their lesson; they do, for the most part. I am talking about a basic attitude that is revealed as soon as they encounter tension and pain. These negative feelings are coupled with negative thoughts and often take the form of self-pity ("I told you so. These sorts of exercises are not meant for me." "I'm far too stiff to do this." "I can't do this. I couldn't even do this as a child."); resistance ("This hurts; it can never be good for me."); or ambition ("I must do my best and push myself as far as I can." "Look how good I am. I am the best in the class, and I want everyone to see me.").

These negative thoughts and feelings are not recognized as negative thoughts; they are totally unconscious and result in inadequate concentration. They are repetitive and habitual.

The body has ingrained negative movement patterns that are also largely unconscious. They manifest as soon as the body is confronted with tension, stiffness, and pain. Fast or heavy breathing, sighing, restless movements, movement into habitual postures, and an increase in muscle tension are all clear examples of this. These negative physical reactions and negative feelings and thoughts all continue to arise at inopportune moments, whenever tension and resistance become excessive. Negative feelings and movement patterns are usually experienced together and expressed simultaneously.

It is very important that students be made conscious of their negativity. This confrontation must take place at the beginning of the lesson; otherwise, their negativity will block any sort of positive development. Both the student and the teacher have a responsibility in accomplishing this, and it will be discussed further in chapter 14.2. Breaking through the negative barrier marks the beginning of a successful and positive lesson.

Further developments of the lesson

The lesson must be structured. Generally, this means that every lesson starts with a meditative attitude and an awareness exercise that is conducive to the first stage in realizing higher consciousness. Subsequently, there are simple exercises that lead to increasingly complex movements. This allows a deeper stabilization of the postural muscles and, at the same time, an increase in higher consciousness. The mental and the physical come together.

After this, insight, warmup, repetition, rhythm, and pleasure all play important roles in developing and maintaining consciousness while doing increasingly difficult asanas. Because related asanas are practiced in every class, the spine is used in a one-sided manner. Therefore, the lesson ends with one or two inversions to return the spine to a neutral, erect position.

The connections, props, protocol (relaxation, movement, and strength and coordination), grouping of related asanas and their division into subgroups, and different forms of attention are important instruments for planning the structure of a lesson. Their application during the lesson allows them to interact so that they strengthen the gradual development of openness, positivity, and consciousness. This will be discussed in chapters 14.3 and 14.4.

Creativity

The division of the asanas into subgroups allows for variety when creating lesson plans. Variety prevents boredom and increases the alertness of both student and teacher, making it easier for attention and consciousness to develop.

But there is another aspect to this, and that is creativity. The concepts of Critical Alignment are used for both personal practice and teaching. This means it is possible to develop your own program and apply these concepts to your own teaching program. The examples in chapter 14.6 can be used as an example to inspire your creativity in this area.

Of course, variety and creativity are bound by certain rules, which will be discussed in chapter 14.5.

14.2 Teacher and students are responsible for recognizing a negative situation.

The teacher must realize that students will (almost) never express angry or hurtful feelings and thoughts during class. On the contrary, after many years of observation, I am sure that most negative attitudes are caused by situations in daily life. I am also sure that these are brought into the lesson in a passive, covert way. Beginners and advanced students express this negativity in various ways. During beginner lessons, I often hear comments about discomfort, pain, and so on. Beginners are often restless in their movements, while advanced yoga students have a tendency to work with ambition and willpower.

Purely mechanical causes of physical tension—like sitting incorrectly for long periods of time—as well as stressful and emotional situations at work and at home disturb our normal, healthy resilience, causing negative feelings and attitudes to develop and become habitual. Sadness, fear, anger, and so on start to dominate and are taken into the lesson.

This negativity must not be tackled with willpower, as that causes a vicious circle of action–reaction. The negativity and reactions must be seen; the student must become aware of them. Both student and teacher have a responsibility in this.

At the start of the class, students are literally prisoners of their own negativity. This makes it impossible for them to recognize their moods. It is the explicit task of the teacher to make them aware of their negativity—not verbally, but by using an appropriate exercise. The student must learn to recognize negative situations and the methods available to neutralize them. It is the teacher's task to show students the way using the instruments of Critical Alignment.

The yoga exercises give students an opportunity to get a handle on their negative attitudes. Habitual negative thoughts and feelings do not have to be discussed; students merely have to observe their physical reactions. These reactions can be the development of tension, the use of compensatory movements, heavy and irregular breathing—all are connected with negative thoughts and feelings. In addition, lessons always contain confrontations with discomfort, pain, and lack of ability. Through these confrontations, students are repeatedly invited to look in the mirror, to see their reactions and which negative feelings they are indulging in. The exercises are opportunities for students to become aware of their negativity.

It is also important for the teacher to set the learning process in motion by considering the following questions: Is the confrontation with tension related to our natural limitations, or is it caused by a buildup of chronic tension? Are the asanas breaking through our limitations and creating new possibilities?

It would be misguided to expect students to provide answers that are fully cognizant of the source of their limitation or its possible solution. They would look at the problem as a fact, which would close any avenue to further investigation. By keeping the question open, students can investigate various means to release the tension. Thus, they are able to observe themselves in a much more authentic and objective way. Students must take responsibility in this process by remaining open to the instructions of the teacher so that positive developments can be realized. Students should develop an attitude of "I *want* to follow the instructions given by the teacher," instead of "I *have* to follow the instructions given by the teacher." If students *want* to follow the instructions, they are able to interact with every new situation or state of development in their own personal way. Only then are they able to research their (negative) behavior patterns. If students attend a class with an attitude that they *have* to do what the teacher tells them, they are just waiting for the next instruction.

This is about an interaction between teacher and student: both work toward the same goal.

14.3 The concepts of Critical Alignment support lesson structure.

The main characteristics of the Critical Alignment method are the connections (see chapter 6); the props (see chapter 2.5); the protocol (see chapter 2.4.1); the asanas (see chapters 7 through 13); and the various forms of attention and fulfillment of consciousness (see chapter 5). Here I will limit myself to discussing only a few of these characteristics—those aspects that clearly contribute to the structured development of the lesson.

Practicing connections and subgroups of asanas
Connections and subgroups of asanas play a major role when developing the full movement of an asana. The full movement is generally developed as follows: at the beginning of the lesson, the asanas from the subgroups are practiced using only a few connections; as the lesson progresses, asanas with more connections are introduced in which the end poses become full movements.

For example, a forward bend lesson starts with a few asanas from the subgroup of standing forward bends to practice the cohesion of the connections between the lower back, hips, and legs. Then the neck should be positioned in relation to the upper back to engage the next set of connections. Finally, students practice the end poses, in which all the connections are used to develop the full movement of the forward bend.

The lesson plans are designed to support the gradual development of each exercise. Only one or two specific points should be taken up and applied consistently in subsequent exercises in the session. Excessive scattered information is not incorporated into the body.

Relevant muscle groups and joints are warmed up through the gradual increase of pressure or stretching, and this creates relaxation and more mobility. The lower back roll is a good preparation for a forward bend lesson (see chapter 6.3, connection 7). Lying on the roll and slowly pulling the legs toward the abdomen warms up the hips. This prepares them for the increase in pressure that will be applied later in the lesson when the same movement is done from a standing position. If the pressure on the joints or the stretch to the muscles is too intense to start with, the body will resist, preventing relaxation. On the other hand, if the movement is repeated throughout the lesson and gradually fleshed out within one or two connections, it will develop with ease. Then it can be absorbed into students' consciousness, allowing the next connection to be introduced. In this way, asanas and attention can interact and develop optimally.

The gradual stabilization of asanas through the postural muscles
As the lesson progresses, strength and coordination of the postural muscles must be developed gradually to stabilize the asanas. Only then can openness, relaxation, and consciousness develop.

The deeper postural muscles can only be activated by relaxing the superficial movement muscles, which is done by focusing on one or two specific connections as already discussed. The application of the protocol (see chapter 2.4.1) is crucial here. If it is applied carefully during the lesson, it will lead to greater stabilization in the asanas. It must be understood that specific movement and postural muscles work together in the practice of certain asanas. Not *all* of the movement muscles can be relaxed. For example, during Trikonasana, the postural muscles of the lower back and hip are activated simultaneously with certain movement muscles that are necessary to transfer the weight of the body to the lower back and hip (see chapter 2.4.1).

Higher consciousness

The passive stretches at the beginning of the lesson have two purposes. They show which connection(s) are central for the lesson, and they lay the groundwork for consciousness to develop. I will now discuss this latter objective.

The passive stretches function as the starting point for the development of a higher consciousness. They can be characterized as consciousness exercises, as they enable students to incorporate areas of the body that have become insensitive due to stiffness. Lying on a roll or a rubber strip for an extended period of time ensures that the consciousness of stiff areas remains in the body for a long time. Since this feeling then becomes part of students' movement intelligence, it functions as a memory support and can then become a foundation on which to lay groundwork for the next phase of consciousness. In this next phase, (simple) asanas are practiced. It is important that attention be directed toward the entire body in a relaxed manner; that attention is brought to specific areas of the body and then back to the entire body. A second, more general attention is necessary to accomplish this zooming in and out of attention and to coordinate it with movement. This attention can oversee the complex and dynamic totality from a distance.

The onset of this general attention marks the next phase of the development of consciousness. It makes it possible to recall the memory of feelings brought to consciousness from the previous exercises that have been absorbed into the new body awareness. The images created from that can be used to accomplish more complex movements. An example of this is the feeling of mobility gained in the whole lower back from the passive stretching exercise on the roll and from the use of the abdominal muscles to support it. The memory of this can then be applied during the standing poses that follow.

As the lesson develops with increasingly complex and active asanas, consciousness develops via a number of phases. First, a functional relationship grows between thoughts, the body, and feelings pertaining to the practice of the exercises. Then, total attention that is carried by a subtle, circulating energy develops. Finally, a higher consciousness can be realized. Consciousness must be constantly renewed in the end poses (see chapter 5 for a detailed description of the various stages of consciousness).

14.4 Dividing lessons into stages builds energy within the practice.

Every lesson consists of different exercises that must be completed in a specific order. The sequence is dictated by cause-and-effect relationships and interactions between the exercises. For example, a common interaction is where one exercise relaxes the superficial muscles in a certain area of the body, allowing a deeper layer of tension to manifest. The next exercise penetrates into this deeper layer of tension to allow it to relax, and so on.

The preceding example illustrates how cause-and-effect relationships define the type and sequence of the exercises that can be selected. Generally, simple exercises are used at the beginning of the lesson and difficult exercises toward the end. As we progress in the exercise, we need to incorporate new connections and deepen the connections already in use to gain more flexibility and deeper penetration of the postural muscles.

By placing the exercises in a cause-and-effect relationship, the lesson can be divided into stages. Then, the focus on increased relaxation and awareness can constantly be renewed, deepened, and passed on from stage to stage. This ensures that the development and intensity of consciousness can be maintained.

During my lessons, I use seven stages, but for the sake of clarity, I will discuss the three main ones here: beginning, middle, and positive transformation at the end of the class.

The *start* has a direct relationship to the middle and transformation stages and to the theme of the lesson (the sort of connections and exercises practiced). This first stage defines the background and tone; that is, it introduces the most important connections and exercises that are central to the lesson. It clarifies which direction the lesson will be taking. This is not indicated verbally but through the exercises. At this point, the question about whether negativity can be confronted and dissolved or not should be considered. The answer to this question can only be found in the middle part of the lesson. If negativity is not eliminated, then a satisfactory transformation can never be achieved at the end of the lesson. In addition to breaking the negative pattern complex, this ensures that the initial steps toward higher consciousness are taken.

These objectives make it clear why the simple exercises at the start of the lesson must be chosen carefully. They define which exercises should follow in the middle and transformation stages. The focus, impact, and momentum all contribute to the effectiveness of the lesson.

The *middle* is the most difficult stage and the longest part of the lesson. Because of this, it can be difficult to maintain a constant focus throughout. Both teacher and students must realize that the battle is won or lost at this stage. If hardly any activity is developed or if an important exercise is overlooked in which a key connection is missed, the lesson will lose its impact.

It is important to continue the theme introduced during the first stage. The exercises chosen for the middle stage must flow from those done in the first. Otherwise, there is a chance that the cause-and-effect relationship between the exercises and the various stages will be broken. The purpose and supporting intelligence of the lesson will be lost. If necessary, this middle stage can be divided into smaller units that allow a continuity in the lesson. I will discuss this shortly.

The *transformation* is the goal, the ambition, and the reason why students are participating in the lesson. It is the state of flow, which can be defined by the following characteristics.

Students have a constant goal in mind.
Students know what has to be done and are sure of their end goals.

Every action is followed by a response.
Movement is continuously adjusted in order to create optimum balance and alignment.

There is a balance between challenge and ability.
Students feel that their capacity is suited to the action undertaken. This increases their satisfaction when more complex actions are practiced.

The awareness of time and space changes.
When students are totally absorbed in the action, time flies by. An hour can be experienced as only 20 minutes.

Action and consciousness are united.
During the transformation, it becomes clear to students why they have been practicing in this specific manner. Good lessons provide more than just the feeling of a workout. They promote optimism, positive feelings, and so on. These can only be experienced if the stages that lead to higher consciousness have been developed. Thus, ultimately, it is about consciousness.

During my lessons, within the three main stages, I make use of seven stages that follow each other in this order: negativity → awareness → presence → deepening → connection → turning point → higher consciousness (diagram 2). Negativity and awareness belong to the first stage; presence, deepening, and connection belong to the middle stage; and turning point and higher consciousness belong to the transformation.

The benefit of more stages is that smaller intervals of tension can be created to keep students alert. Then they can concentrate on the specific exercises and connections that belong to each stage. This supports the dynamic development and intensity of relaxation and consciousness.

I will discuss each stage briefly and explain which combination of exercises, connections, and awareness are necessary to continue from one stage to the next.

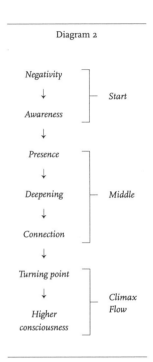

Diagram 2

Negativity
↓
Awareness ⎤ Start

↓

Presence
↓
Deepening ⎤ Middle
↓
Connection

↓

Turning point
↓
Higher consciousness ⎤ Climax Flow

Negativity
Negative situations occur instantly at the beginning of the lesson, and students must be made aware of this as soon as possible. This negativity is produced because of the confrontation with discomfort and pain. To stimulate the process of awareness, the teacher must move quickly into the following stage. Otherwise, students will remain hanging in judgment, fear, ambition, and so on.

Awareness
The teacher verbalizes the reactions of the student's body and thoughts, pointing out that the body prefers to compensate in another place to avoid pain: muscles start to contract to avoid movement and, therefore, pain; breathing becomes restricted; the student is sunk in negative thoughts like, "This is not a healthy movement for my spine"; and so on. In this manner, the student becomes conscious of the negative situation of the body, thoughts, and feelings. This realization makes it possible to observe these reactions with open attention.

During this stage of the lesson, students are lying down for the passive stretch and are asked to relax the body. This exercise can be the lower back roll, upper back roll, the rubber strip, and so on, depending on the particular theme of the lesson. The teacher explains the pain and makes it clear that the point of these exercises is to relax the muscles so that the position and shape of the vertebrae and their discs can return to natural alignment. The teacher also clarifies how this improved spinal alignment will make certain simple asanas easier. These asanas are carried out after the passive stretches. They are aimed toward the transfer of movement in a small part of the body so that only a few small connections are activated.

Presence

During this stage, students should focus on their breath. Breathing can allow or block relaxation. Willpower must not be used to achieve relaxation. Students' attention must remain open so they can observe movement. This makes the experience of being in the here and now possible. You are present in the moment in a positive way. Your answer to the (painful) situation is no longer automatic and negative, but it is based on feelings of relaxation and space produced by developing your breath. If this is not the case, your body will take control, and you will again become the victim of habitual movements.

The connections from the previous stage are now practiced during simple movements. Deeper levels of tension are addressed. A number of asanas are introduced and repeated so that this tension can be dealt with. This allows movement to become increasingly supple without losing the previously developed skeletal structure.

Deepening

New exercises that provide a more intense confrontation with tension are introduced here, leading to deeper relaxation. These exercises include new segments and connections in addition to those from the previous exercises. The emphasis moves to other areas of the body and to working on their associated connections so that new movements can be completed with ease. Open body awareness spreads out to these new areas.

Connection

Breathing is directed toward activating the hara and heart gravity points. These points can counter feelings of discomfort and pain with feelings of relaxation and lightness. Because of the increasing relaxation of the movement muscles and the stabilization of the joints and spine through the postural muscles, students will realize that the body has developed preferential movement patterns. With this realization, students immediately receive the tools needed to break through these patterns. Then the gravity points can be balanced, allowing feelings of space and relaxation. When relaxation in the hara gravity point can be maintained during movement and in the end position, these feelings of lightness will intensify and spread from the hara into the rest of the body. These feelings will start to dominate students' attention. Thus, the development of awareness moves toward consciousness. Awareness expands to its full potential.

During this stage, end movements are introduced. These include new exercises in addition to movements from the previous stages. The number of connections used in these exercises combines all the connections practiced during the previous stages.

The balance between the two gravity points is vital. A precise awareness of the connections must be maintained to support the balance between these points. The end movements must be renewed continually until a general relaxation occurs.

Turning point

When relaxation increases, it leads from negativity to positivity. Concentration is now united with the rhythm of movement. This leads to deeper relaxation. Connections, breathing, and movement sequences enter the here and now. Then the body starts to produce positive signals: we start to feel lighter and more open, and there is a clear experience of space, unity, and relaxation. These experiences lead to a nonthinking consciousness (manonmani). We become spectators of our own movements where unconscious corrections begin to occur. The body spontaneously takes the initiative to improve posture and balance. The gates open to positive thinking: positive body feeling, creativity, clear thinking, humor, and decisiveness. Feelings of confidence and independence support our practice.

This brings us to a turning point where we can include the space around us in our observation. The rhythm of the activity itself keeps us in the here and now. The body and mind start to work together in a unique way. The body has let go of its negative attitude and has begun to seek openness and relaxation in a positive way. Because of this, relaxation is intensified, providing us with an experience that is beyond our cognitive knowledge—it is a new, intuitive type of learning. We act from a state of flow. It is important not to become distracted here; even the smallest disturbance can break this process.

Higher consciousness

The stages before the turning point are developed through the interaction between our thoughts, our situation, and the feelings that arise and steer our actions. Asanas are meant to break our tension patterns. Whenever we feel disturbed during the physical transformations during practice, we have an opportunity to analyze our automatic (negative) thinking patterns and body reactions in a cognitive way.

In this final stage (manonmani), we act beyond thinking. Thinking cannot be controlled when all forms of awareness come together: the awareness of performing the asana with the right technique, the awareness of our behavior when confronted with stress and pain, the awareness of the adjustments we make to develop a pose, the awareness of the space around us, the awareness of the balance between our two centers of gravity, the awareness of our breathing, and so on. Then our activities are not dominated by tense behavior but by totally open concentration based on an intense appreciation for change. Maybe that appreciation derives from the intuitive fact that we actually know that state of being from our early years, when we were playful and full of energy.

Then we enter a new state of consciousness that cannot be forced in any way. It comes to us or it doesn't. When it comes, we just "are" and observe our own actions. We can conclude that through this intense, involved positive attitude, our mind and body can start to take over and make the right decisions on their own, that new steps in our development come from our relaxed, easy, and sharp awareness. People may offer comments such as, "I felt that a very old tension started to loosen up. I just witnessed it without interfering. I did not even know it was there, but afterward I actually knew how much tension I had been holding all these years. I have no idea why it happened, but I felt very grateful afterward."

This presence, where consciousness has developed through action, forms the basis for the final exercises of the class, but it can come in earlier stages too. It is continued and experienced as absolute tranquillity during Sirsasana and Sarvangasana. From this development, asanas attain a spiritual dimension in our experience of the here and now.

If we are successful in maintaining this contact, our body will keep seeking correct alignment, and all the connections we practice will melt into a totality where we can constantly experience the consciousness of being here and now. Inversions are delicate balance poses in which the slightest disturbance can cause pain and discomfort. They force us to maintain our consciousness.

14.5 Creativity in lessons depends on variations in asanas and connections.

The lesson plans discussed in this chapter start at a beginner's level, move to an advanced level, and are completed with one or two inversions. It is interesting to try out the exercises in the order given in these lesson plans. This will give you good insight into your strong and weak areas—whether you are a beginner or a more advanced practitioner, whether forward bends or backbends are your forte, and so on.

You can use your creativity to change the structure of your own practice and develop your own themes based on your new understanding. You can concentrate on one specific subgroup of asanas or one specific connection, giving more attention and time to your personal needs. Use your creativity to bring variety into your practice.

Creativity is necessary, because everyone has their own specific starting point, with corresponding limitations and movement and postural preferences. This is the case with teaching as well.

I will now discuss some ways of creating variety. The ground rule is that the body must be warmed up gradually so that the connections can be fully used to establish freedom of movement through the postural muscles. Thus, only one or two connections should be worked on at a time (see chapter 14.3). Obviously you must consider other aspects, such as structure (in terms of designing a class or practice), stages of development, and so on (discussed earlier), when developing your own lesson plan whether for teaching or practice.

1. One key asana
The asana selected must be a total movement, an end pose (see chapter 14.3) from a specific group of asanas. Examples are Urdhva Dhanurasana from the backbends and Paschimottanasana from the forward bends. Certain standing poses or Sirsasana can also function as an end pose.

The lesson works toward this end pose, and the end pose defines which connections and points for attention are primary. Since every end pose has multiple connections, the teacher must choose which connections are fundamental for that lesson. For example, if the end pose is Urdhva Dhanurasana, the lesson can start with a single connection for the upper or lower body.

2. One central connection
Any connection can be chosen as the primary one for the lesson. For example, the connection between the arms and shoulder blades may be selected and applied in various poses like the shoulder exercises on the strip, Adho Mukha Svanasana, twists, Sirsasana, and so on. There are many possibilities for various exercises.

3. One central group of asanas
When practicing forward bends or backbends, this point seems to be the same as point 1. However, it works out differently during standing poses, inversions, and twists, because

the subgroups have such different characteristics. For example, the hips are mobilized in various ways during standing poses. Similar differences are present within twists (from a backbend, a forward bend, or a straight position) and inversions (in the large variety of neck positions). Because of these variations, these groups of asanas are not necessarily developed from one constant and gradual buildup.

4. A focus on linking groups of asanas
During one lesson, for example, simple standing forward bends can be followed by backbends. However, not all combinations are possible, so it is important to make logical transitions. This means that one aspect of the exercise or action within a certain movement must be taken into the following movement. The potential for variety exists here too, because multiple points for attention and/or connections can be used as the basis for the lesson.

14.6 Lesson plans

The lessons in this chapter, which come from my teaching experience, have been written concisely, so you can use them as a framework for your own lesson plans. A few points have been noted for each exercise and how these develop during the lesson. For detailed descriptions of the asanas and the connections, see the related chapters. The seven stages for developing lessons are indicated in the lesson description. A beginner's lesson takes about an hour and an advanced lesson approximately two hours.

Key points for inversions
In the following lesson plans, I have given suggestions for practicing inversions, Sirsasana on the headstand bench, Halasana, Sarvangasana, and Sirsasana.

This is a general idea. You must make your own plan, which depends on the speed of your development. You can create variation by switching from the headstand bench to Sirsasana on the floor. If you are a beginner, you can start with the headstand bench to relax your shoulders and prepare for Salamba Sirsasana, but you can also begin with Salamba Sirsasana to see how long you can stand on your head without tension and then finish on the headstand bench.

It is important that when you are practicing Sirsasana, you do not see the headstand bench version as a lesser or weaker form of the pose. The effect of both versions is equally intense. If you have the feeling that Salamba Sirsasana is too difficult for you, wait a few months before including it in your lesson plan.

There is one important rule that you must bear in mind: when you begin with Sarvangasana or Halasana, you must never do Salamba Sirsasana afterward, as your neck has been stretched out. You may stand in the headstand bench.

Comment regarding advanced poses
In the descriptions of the advanced poses, I have given no specific points for attention. The list of names in the lesson plan reflect end poses. The description of these asanas can be found in the relevant chapters.

LESSON 1: FORWARD BENDS

To start the forward bend lesson, your upper lower back is mobilized by lying on the thin lower back roll. When practicing forward bends, it is essential for the development of the asanas that your lower back bends while simultaneously being kept flat. This is the only way to create movement in your hips and sacrum.

The position of your lower back is maintained with strength while moving in and out of the asanas. For example, during Utkatasana, you keep your lower back straight through the strength of your lower back muscles, while its shape and coordination of movement in the transition from Utkatasana to Uttanasana is guided through the pull of your hands on your ankles.

Once that part of the movement chain is activated, your legs can be included. This coordination between your lower back and leg muscles makes it possible to develop the movement further. This is the central connection of forward bending that you must work on continuously.

Beginner's level

Stages 1 and 2: negativity and attention

1. Lower back roll (thin; approximately 5 minutes)

This opening exercise can be used to awaken consciousness when the lower back needs to relax. Try to limit the development of this awareness to 3 to 5 minutes. The exercise also develops your understanding of how to transfer movement through your lower back and legs into your hips, sacrum, and SI joints. You can achieve this cooperation between your legs, lower back, and hips when your lower back is fully extended (phase 1), as well as when it is bent in the end poses of forward bends (phase 2).

Phase 1

After a few minutes on the roll, once your lower back has relaxed, lift your right foot from the floor and pull your right knee toward your abdomen (you can place the rubber strip or a belt over your knee if you cannot reach it with your hands). Make sure the muscles in your groin remain relaxed, so there is a shift from the movement muscles that initially resist the movement to the deeper postural muscles of your hip. Thanks to this relaxation, more space and movement are available in your lower back, SI joints, and hips. Repeat this movement on the other side.

Phase 2

Lift both feet and pull your thighs as close as possible to your abdomen. Your lower back bends without losing the pressure directed to your hips, as shown in the illustration. Your lower back retains its cohesion even though it is bent. Remember that this cohesion is achieved by the pull of your hands during many forward bends.

Insight into the connection between your lower back, hips, and the back of your pelvis is important when stretching your hamstrings. If you lose this cohesion because your lower back bends too far, then you will lose the stretch as well. Apply the insights from the introduction to the exercises.

The following instructions are in addition to those given in the introduction of the lesson. They are presented here to clarify the whole process of movement. It is not possible to focus on all the points. I have limited myself to those that describe the essence of the movement.

Stage 3: presence

2. Utkatasana (30 to 60 seconds)

- When you bend your knees, make sure your hamstrings relax so that your sit bones move away from your feet.
- Relax your hips by carrying your weight on the front of your heels.
- Extend your lower back and stay aware of the inner tube shape of your abdominal muscles. Place your hands on your knees.
- Slowly bend your lower back so that the pressure in your hips is maintained, and gently push your abdomen against your thighs.
- Without losing the cohesion of your lower back, take hold of your ankles and pull with your hands so that your back flattens. This increases the contact of your abdomen with your thighs.
- Maintain these connections while slowly stretching your legs into the next pose.

3. Uttanasana (1 to 3 minutes)

- When moving into this asana, observe the position and shape of your lower back as if looking at yourself from the side to create an image of what you are doing. As soon as your lower back threatens to lose its cohesion, you will start to lose the pressure in your hips. When that happens, stop moving and wait until your hamstrings and/or hips relax before continuing.
- When returning out of this pose, bend your knees into Utkatasana.

Stage 4: deepening

4. Utkatasana (10 to 20 seconds)

- Place your hands on your upper thighs, close to your hips (see the illustration).
- Feel how the extension of your lower back activates your hips and thigh muscles. (Your hips comprise your pelvis and thighs).
- Slowly stretch your legs into the next pose.

5. Dandasana (standing; 1 minute)

- Contract your thigh muscles under your hands so that you feel your legs are transferring movement from your ankles through your knees and into your hips.
- The weight of your body is transferred through the strength of your lower back into your hips. This strength recedes in the next exercise, but the feeling of pressure in your hips continues when you place your hands on the front of your mat and step into the next pose.

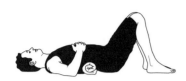

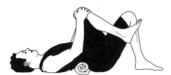

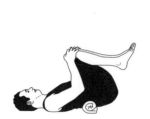

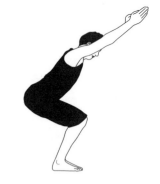

1. Lower back roll

3 minutes

p. 112

Phase 1

1 minute

Right and left

Phase 2

1 minute

2. *Utkatasana*

30–60 seconds

p. 195

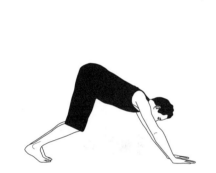

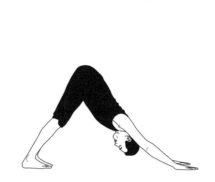

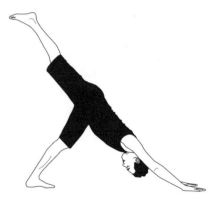

Move from your hips to:

6. *Adho mukha svanasana I*

1 minute

p. 201

7. *Adho mukha svanasana II*

20–30 seconds

Right and left   p. 203

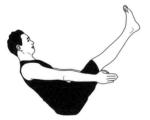

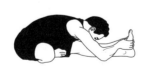

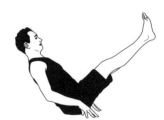

11. *Navasana*

1 minute

p. 251

12. *Janu sirsasana*

30–60 seconds

Left leg extended   p. 264

13. *Navasana*

1 minute

p. 251

Or place your hands next to your hips
on the floor and move through to:

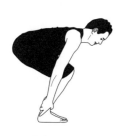

Pull your abdomen against your
legs and move through to:

10–20 seconds   p. 258

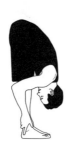

3. Uttanasana

1–3 minutes   p. 257

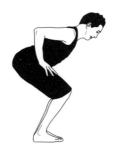

4. Utkatasana

10–20 seconds   p. 195

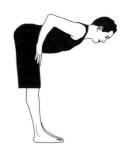

5. Dandasana (standing)

1 minute   p. 199

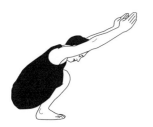

Connect your arms with your lower
back and move through to:

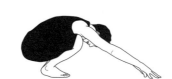

8. Malasana I

1–2 minutes   p. 318

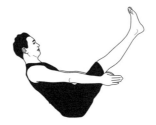

9. Navasana

1 minute   p. 251

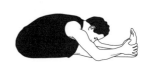

10. Janu sirsasana

30–60 seconds
Right leg extended   p. 264

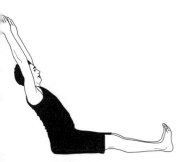

Lift your arms and move through
to the following pose:

20–30 seconds   p. 263

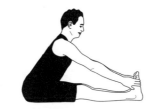

20–30 seconds   p. 262

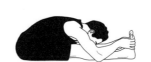

14. Paschimottanasana

1–5 minutes   p. 261

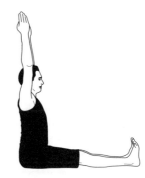

15. Dandasana

30–60 seconds   p. 254

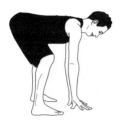

and move through to:

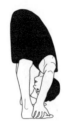

16. Prasarita padottanasana I

1 minute

p. 252

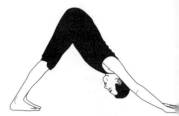

17. Prasarita padottanasana II

1–2 minutes

p. 260

18. Adhomukha svanasana I

10–20 seconds

p. 203

Advanced level » » »

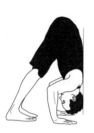

21. Paschimottanasana (standing)

1–3 minutes

p. 264

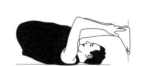

Paschimottanasana (supine)

1–3 minutes

p. 263

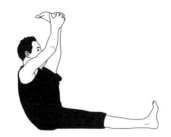

22. Kraunchasana

30 seconds

Right and left   p. 268

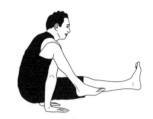

23. Eka hasta bhujasana

30 seconds

Right   p. 271

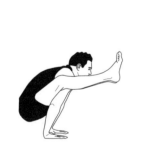

29. Titibhasana I

15 seconds

p. 270

Titibhasana II

15 seconds

p. 270

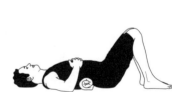

30. Kurmasana (supine)

1 minute

p. 209

31. Lower back roll

2 minutes

p. 112

32. Adho mukha vrksasana

1 minute

p. 184

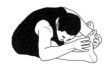

19. *Upavista konasana*

30–60 seconds

Right leg   *p. 266*

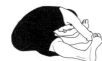

30–60 seconds

Left leg

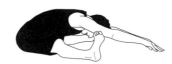

1–3 minutes

Forward and center

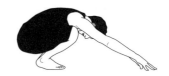

20. *Malasana I*

1 minute

        p. 318

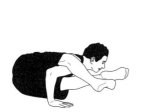

24. *Astavakrasana*

15 seconds

Right   *p. 272*

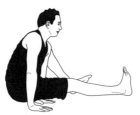

25. *Eka hasta bhujasana*

30 seconds

Left   *p. 271*

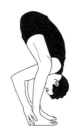

26. *Astavakrasana*

15 seconds

Left   *p. 272*

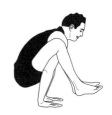

27. *Kurmasana* (standing)

30–60 seconds

Right and left   *p. 269*

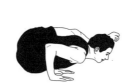

28. *Dvi hasta bhujasana*

20–30 seconds

        p. 269

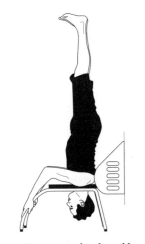

33. *Sirsasana* on headstand bench

1–15 minutes

        p. 144

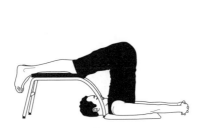

34. *Halasana*

5 minutes

        p. 174

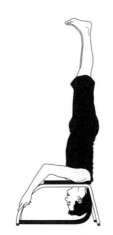

35. *Sirsasana* on headstand bench

1–3 minutes

        p. 144

36. *Savasana*

5–15 minutes

        p. 344

6. Adho Mukha Svanasana I (1 minute)

- Start the pose with bent knees and your shoulders over your hands.
- Give priority to stretching your lower back, and through this, feel the pressure in your hips. Activate your inner tube by connecting your lower ribs to your abdomen and extended lower back. Move your hips back until your upper arms connect with your shoulder blades.
- Straighten your legs by moving your thighs backward and relaxing your calves and ankles while lowering your heels.
- The lower back often bends in this pose. Extension can be improved by practicing Adho Mukha Svanasana II.

7. Adho Mukha Svanasana II (right and left: 20 to 30 seconds each)

- Lift your right leg as high as necessary to feel the extension in your lower back. This feeling will not be in the lower back itself but in the stretching of your left hip. You will feel more pressure there.
- Make sure you complete the movement with stability in your lower ribs; otherwise, the movement will transfer into your midback.
- Lower your leg and repeat on the other side, ending in Adho Mukha Svanasana I.
- Move your shoulders over your hands, bend your knees a little, and jump forward into the next pose.

Stage 5: connection

8. Malasana I (1 to 2 minutes)

- Lift your arms high so they connect to your lower back. Relax your ankles so that your heels can move toward the floor. You will feel the same sort of stretch in the back of your pelvis as you do when lying on the lower back roll with your pelvis lifted (exercise 1, phase 2).
- Do not lower your heels too far, or you will lose the connection of your arms with your lower back. This connection supports spaciousness in your abdomen.
- Move your abdomen forward at a diagonal between your legs. Stop as soon as you feel your lower back breaking the movement, and place your hands on the floor. Keep your neck aligned with your lower back.
- Remember that the lengthening of the front of your upper body precedes the bending of your back. Walk forward with your fingers and follow the movement with your abdomen. Do not allow your heels to lift or your entire body to move forward. When you cannot go any farther, relax your back without allowing it to break into its habitual posture.
- Pull your arms in and sit down for the next pose.

9. Navasana (1 minute)

- Take hold of your thighs and lean your upper body back as far as possible so that your lower back extends. This causes your neck to move back and your lower back to extend actively.

- Remember that this movement occurs in every forward bend.
- The pull of your hands supports the extension of your lower back. Extend your legs. When your legs, lower back, and abdomen are strong enough, stretch your arms alongside your knees, parallel to the floor, without losing the neck–lower back connection.
- Pull your left leg in and place your right leg on the floor for Janu Sirsasana.

10. *Janu Sirsasana (right leg straight; 30 to 60 seconds)*

- Raise your arms, extend your lower back, and move forward. When moving into this pose, your trunk moves faster then your arms.
- Stretch your arms forward to return. Here, your arms move faster then your trunk.
- Place your fingertips on the floor and lift your legs up into Navasana.

11. *Navasana (1 minute)*

- Pull your right leg in and place your extended left leg on the floor for Janu Sirsasana.

12. *Janu Sirsasana (left leg stretched; 30 to 60 seconds)*

- Stretch your arms forward to return.

13. *Navasana (1 minute)*

- Keep your upper body at a diagonal, and place your fingertips on the floor beside you. Slowly lower your legs to the floor.
- Extend your lower back farther, and connect your lower ribs to the arch of your lower back while lifting your arms above your head. Bend forward in a diagonal line without losing the strength in your lower back. Your arms remain connected to your lower back, just like when you squat.
- Take hold of your feet or lower legs without bending your back any more. Relax your shoulders, and breathe into your abdomen.
- Pull your abdomen forward (lengthening preceding bending) and start to relax your back, vertebra by vertebra, to end in the next pose.

Stage 6: turning point

14. *Paschimottansana (1 to 5 minutes)*

- You can keep Paschimottanasana static, or if you prefer, you can alternate it with Halasana and Dandasana (30 to 60 seconds), leaning backward in order to roll back into Halasana (1 minute). In Halasana, your entire back and neck are stretched. Roll back slowly into Paschimottansana (1 to 2 minutes) without losing the open position of your neck. Repeat this movement three times.
- Stretch your arms forward and lift them so that your lower back activates to return to Dandasana. Arch your lower back by leaning backward, and connect your lower ribs to the arch of your lower back.
- From the space in your hara area, move forward until your spine reaches the perpendicular position in Dandasana.

15. Dandasana (30 to 60 seconds)

· Sit very still, keeping your arms, legs, and back as straight as possible in this pose.
· Relax your arms and pull your legs in. Move into a squat, place your hands on the front of your mat, and jump into the next pose.

16. Prasarita Padottansana I (1 minute)

· End with bent legs and your back parallel to the floor.
· Slowly move the weight of your body back into the front of your heels, extend your lower back and connect your core. Feel the pressure in your hips.
· Bend around your hips without losing the strength in your lower back, and move your abdomen toward the plane of your thighs.
· Take hold of the outside of your feet and pull, while slightly lifting your upper body; this will flatten your lower back. Move into the next pose.

17. Prasarita Padottansana II (1 to 2 minutes)

· Lengthen your spine and move the crown of your head toward the floor. Slowly start to straighten your legs.
· Remember that the connection between your hands and lower back has priority over the stretching of your legs.
· Lift your upper body, place your hands on the front of your mat, and jump back into Adho Mukha Svanasana I.

18. Adho Mukha Svanasana I (10 to 20 seconds)

· Take the time to position your lower back and move back with your hips.
· Jump forward into Malasana, and from there, sit with spread legs.
· Stretch into Upavista Konasana.

19. Upavista Konasana (right and left legs: 30 to 60 seconds each; middle front: 1 to 3 minutes)

· After having stretched toward the middle front, walk back with your hands to return.
· Pull your legs in and stretch forward into Malasana I.

20. Malasana I (1 minute)

This is the beginner's level. You can finish the lesson with the inversions described at the end of the lesson. First, neutralize your lower back with a thin lower back roll or by jumping up into Adho Mukha Vrksasana. This stops your body from wanting to maintain the forward bend pose when standing upright.

Or you can carry on with the advanced section.

All important points for forward bends have been discussed. You must carry these points through when completing the advanced series.

Advanced level

21. Two variations of Paschimottanasana: standing with your back against the wall (1 to 3 minutes) and lying on your back with your feet against the wall (1 to 3 minutes)

22. Kraunchasana (right and left: 30 seconds each)

23. Move to Eka Hasta Bhujasana (right: 30 seconds)

24. Astavakrasana (right: 30 seconds)

25. Eka Hasta Bhujasana (left: 30 seconds)

26. Astavakrasana (left: 15 seconds)

27. Kurmasana (standing; 30 to 60 seconds)

28. Dvi Hasta Bhujasana (20 to 30 seconds)

29. Tittibhasana I and II (15 seconds each)

30. Kurmasana (supine; 1 minute)

31. Lie on a thin lower back roll until your back relaxes.

32. Adho Mukha Vrksasana (1 minute)

Inversions

Stage 7: higher consciousness

33. Sirsasana on the headstand bench with the backbender against the wall (1 to 15 minutes)

34. Halasana with the legs on the headstand bench (5 minutes)

35. Sirsasana in the headstand bench without the backbender (1 to 3 minutes)

36. Savasana (5 to 15 minutes)

LESSON 2: TWISTS

Beginner's level

Stages 1 and 2: negativity and awareness

1. The thin roll just under the shoulder blades (5 minutes)

- Use the thin roll as a preparation exercise. Lean against the roll with the area just below your shoulder blades. Hold your head with both hands and place a folded rubber strip between your shoulder blades to support the back of your head. Slowly lower your head to ½ inch above the floor. Bend your legs. Maintain the strength in your abdominals and the extension in your neck during this movement. Breathe into your stomach, and relax your back where it rests on the roll. Remember that this movement is similar to when you stand up or sit down; it aligns your head and neck with your upper back.

- Place your head on the floor and your hands on your lower ribs. Slowly guide your inhalations to your chest. Keep breathing out toward the roll and into your chest to develop awareness.
- Without losing that awareness, allow your left foot to lift off the floor, and slowly start to rotate your legs and pelvis to the right. Take 1 or 1½ minutes to develop the rotation.
- Slowly return to center and repeat to the other side.
- If you feel resistance in your back while twisting, stop moving and wait for your muscles to relax. Through relaxation, your back will lengthen, and this length will allow you to twist farther. This principle of lengthening before twisting applies to all twists.
- Repeat the movement two or three times and return by rolling to your side.

Stage 3: presence

2. Lying prone with your chest and abdomen on the shoulderstand block (1 minute)

- Place your forehead on your arms.
- Even though you are no longer lying on the upper back roll, you can probably still feel its impression in your back. Keep exhaling to this area to relax your back. Use your inhalations to extend your upper back. This will elevate your neck and connect it to your upper back. Your crown moves directly forward.

3. Turn your head to the right without allowing it to lower (30 to 60 seconds)

- If you encounter resistance during this rotation, stop moving and use your inhalations to extend your spine farther. Relax your upper back; exhalations should allow it to sink in more. This will allow your back to lengthen, providing extension to your neck. It will dissolve the resistance and allow the twist to go farther.
- Repeat the movement to the other side, then rest with your forehead on your arms.

The rule of lengthening before twisting also applies here, but now the most important point is that the length in your neck can only develop from extension in your upper back. Take this point with you into the next exercise.

4. Turning the head while lying on the stomach (30 seconds)

- On an inhalation, extend your upper back and elevate your neck; align the two. Using exhalations, relax your upper back so that it sinks deeper between your shoulder blades.
- Breathe in deeply toward your chest and lift your head, moving the back of your head toward your upper back. Use every inhalation to lift your chest higher and every exhalation to relax your back between your shoulder blades. Keep your lower ribs against the floor.
- Lift your arms so that they apply pressure against your shoulder blades, and turn your head to look over your right shoulder toward the palm of your right hand. Stay in this position for 30 seconds.

- Move back toward the center, and repeat the movement on the other side.
- Bring your hands and forehead back to the floor. On an inhalation, lift your neck. Repeat this movement three times. Imagine that you are doing it seated.
- Move into Virasana.

5. *Parivrtta Siddhasana (1 minute)*

- On an inhalation, sit up straight. On an exhalation, relax your shoulders. Place your left hand on the base of your sternum and your right hand on the inside of your knee. Connect your right arm with your shoulder blade.
- Your back should be erect and relaxed, and your right arm initiates the twist. The relaxation of your back allows it to lengthen continuously.
- With one or more inhalations, twist to the left. Keep your neck aligned with the area of the upper back roll during your exhalations. If the movement feels blocked, do not turn farther, but work on developing length to free your back.
- Repeat the movement on the other side.

6. *Bharadvajasana I (30 to 60 seconds)*

- Sit with your left hand holding your right upper arm, your right hand holding your left knee, and turn as far as you can to the left while looking straight ahead.
- Breathe in deeply, right up to your collarbones, three times and feel how your breath lifts your upper ribs. The inhalations extend your spine. This pulls your neck on top of your upper back and directs the weight of your head to your back below your shoulder blades.
- Slowly turn your head to the right and look over your right shoulder toward your feet. Keep breathing deeply into your chest and moving your head farther backward to relax your upper back. Remember that the tension in your neck will be relieved by the extension in your upper back.
- Return slowly and repeat on the other side.

7. *Bharadvajasana II (30 to 60 seconds)*

- When elevating your chest, ensure that your lower ribs keep moving toward the lower arm that is against your lower back.
- When you have done both sides, move into the following coordination exercise.

Stage 4: deepening

8. *Coordination exercise 1 (see chapter 10.2; 1 minute)*

- Pay close attention when doing this exercise, and recall the importance of the correct use of your lower back. Remember that your lower back can bend in a stable, safe way but also in an unstable, collapsed way. The stable way retains coherence, as in the stretched position of this coordination exercise, whereas the unstable position can cause you to contract your abdominals and push your lower back backward. This last movement is especially risky when the bend is combined with a twist.

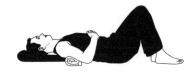

1. Thin roll

5 minutes

p. 306

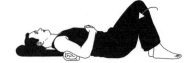

Twist

30–60 seconds

Right and left   *p. 306*

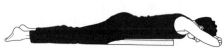

2. Block

1 minute

p. 103

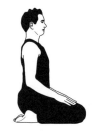

Virasana

20 seconds

p. 332

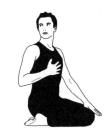

5. *Parivrtta siddhasana*

1 minute

Left and Right   *p. 307*

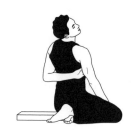

6. *Bharadvajasana I*

30–60 seconds

Left and right   *p. 310*

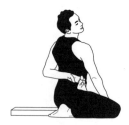

7. *Bharadvajasana II*

30–60 seconds

Left and right   *p. 313*

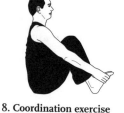

8. Coordination exercise

1 minute

p. 243

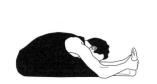

13. *Paschimottanasana*

1–2 minutes

p. 261

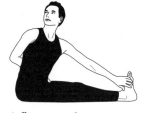

14. *Ardha matsyendrasana*

30–60 seconds

Right   *p. 315*

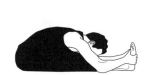

15. *Paschimottanasana*

1–2 minutes

p. 261

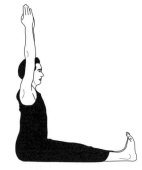

16. *Dandasana*

30 seconds

p. 254

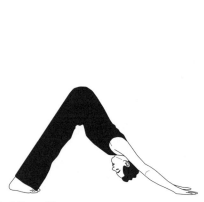

18. *Adho mukha svanasana I*

1 minute

p. 201

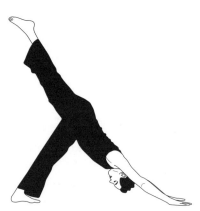

19. *Adho mukha svanasana II*

10 seconds

Right   *p. 203*

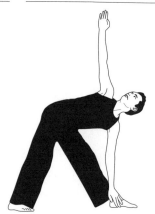

20. *Utthita trikonasana*

30 seconds

Right   *p. 210*

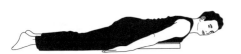

3. Turn your head

30–60 seconds

Right and left

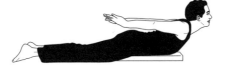

Lift your chin and arms

15 seconds

p. 312

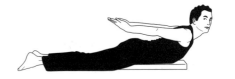

4. Turning the head

30 seconds

3 times to the right and the left   p. 312

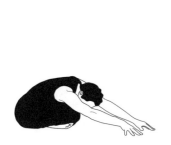

9. *Parivrtta ardha padmasana*

30–60 seconds

Left and right   p. 313

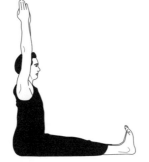

10. *Dandasana (sitting)*

30 seconds

p. 254

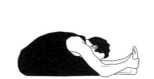

11. *Paschimottanasana*

1–2 minutes

p. 261

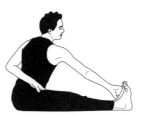

12. *Ardha matsyendrasana*

30–60 seconds

Left   p. 315

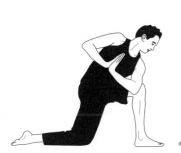

17. *Parivrtta parsvakonasana*

30 seconds

Left and right   p. 317

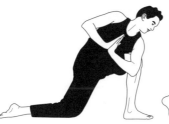

End position 2

30 seconds

Left and right

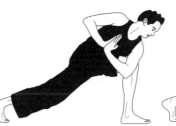

End position 3

30 seconds

Left and right

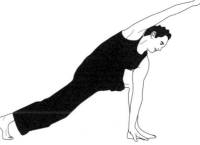

End position 4

30 seconds

Left and right

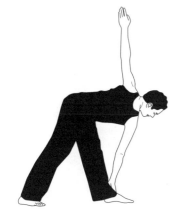

21. *Parivrtta trikonasana*

30 seconds

Repeat steps 20 and 21, 3 to 4 times   p. 215

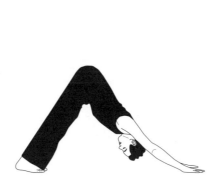

22. *Adho mukha svanasana I*

1 minute

p. 201

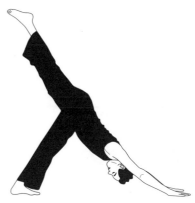

23. *Adho mukha svanasana II*

10 seconds   Link and repeat steps 20 and 21

with your left leg in front   p. 203

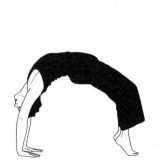

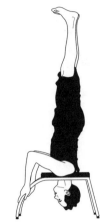

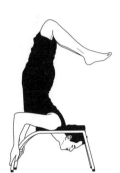

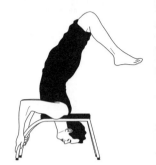

24. *Urdhva dhanurasana*

20–30 seconds

5 times   *p. 291*

25. Jumping up and dropping back from the headstand bench

5 times front and back

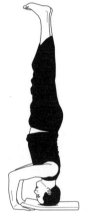

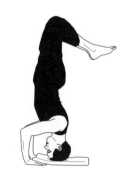

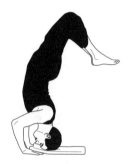

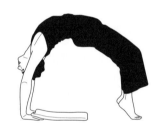

Headstand II

15 seconds

      p. 167

Headstand II and fall through to *Urdhva dhanurasana*

And jump through to *viparita chakrasana*   *p. 299*

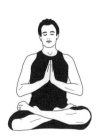

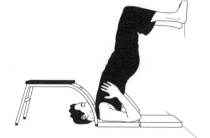

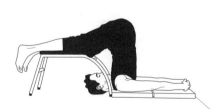

31. *Padmasana*

5 minutes

      p. 330

32. *Sarvangasana* **against the wall**

5 minutes

      p. 172

33. *Halasana*

5 minutes

      p. 174

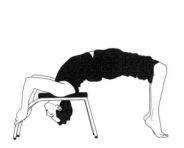

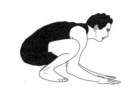

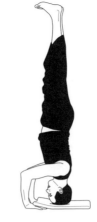

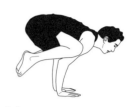

	26. *Malasana II*	From headstand II to:	27. *Bakasana*
	15 seconds	15 seconds	15–30 seconds
p. 300	*p. 342*	*p. 167*	Move back to: *p. 310*

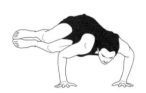

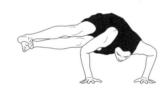

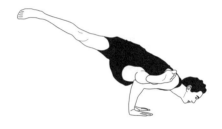

28. *Parsva bakasana*

Plus *viparita chakrasana*

Right and left   *p. 320*

29. *Dvi pada kaundinyasana*

Plus *viparita chakrasana*

Right and left   *p. 322*

30. *Eka pada kaundinyasana*

Plus *viparita chakrasana*

Right and left   *p. 322*

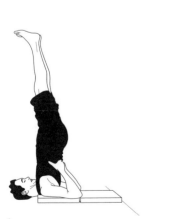

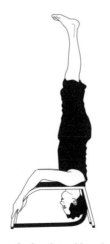

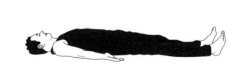

34. *Salamba sarvangasana*

1–15 minutes

p. 168

35. *Sirsasana* on the headstand bench

1–15 minutes

With variations   *p. 144*

36. *Savasana*

5–15 minutes

p. 344

9. Parivrtta Ardha Padmasana *(30 to 60 seconds)*

- Experiment in the end position with maintaining the cohesion of your back. Contract your lower back so that your upper body elevates slightly. This connects your neck to your lower back and pelvis, allowing you to lengthen the front of your body and move your fingers farther forward. Using the strength of your lower back and not your abdominals, lift your hands until only the very tips of your fingers are on the floor. This activity strongly increases the pressure to your hips, allowing relaxation to develop.
- When you have done both sides, extend your legs and move into Dandasana.

10. Dandasana *(30 seconds)*

Stages 5 and 6: connection and turning point

11. Paschimottanasana *(1 to 2 minutes)*

- With your right hand, take hold of the outside of your left foot or lower leg so that you can elevate yourself from your lower back into Ardha Matsyendrasana.

12. Ardha Matsyendrasana *(left: 30 to 60 seconds)*

- The increase of strength in your lower back is central for this pose. Only through this strength can you develop space in other areas of the body. Your extended arm constantly tells you whether or not this strength is present. If your arm bends, your lower back has lost its strength.
- Use the correct technique to connect your two gravity points. Fill the space you developed with your breath.
- Move back to Paschimottanasana.

13. Paschimottanasana *(1 to 2 minutes)*

- Move back to Ardha Matsyendrasana.

14. Ardha Matsyendrasana *(right: 30 to 60 seconds)*

- Return to Paschimottanasana.

15. Paschimottanasana *(1 to 2 minutes)*

- Move back to Dandasana.

16. Dandasana *(30 seconds)*

- Relax your arms.

17. Parivrtta Parsvakonasana *(left and right: 30 seconds in both end positions)*

- Five end positions were described in the book. Complete all five on one side in a fluid manner, then repeat to the other side.
- Place your hands on the front of your mat and step back to Adho Mukha Svanasana I.

18. Adho Mukha Svanasana I (1 minute)

- Give your attention to the position of your lower back before moving into the end pose. Bend your knees to relax your hamstrings, and arch your lower back. Connect your lower ribs to the arch. This exerts pressure in your hips. Slowly move backward, leading with your core and thighs, until your arms have connected to your shoulder blades.
- Lift your right leg up to Adho Mukha Svanasana II.

19. Adho Mukha Svanasana II (10 seconds)

- Step into Utthita Trikonasana.

20. Utthita Trikonasana (right: 30 seconds)

- Use this pose to stabilize the extended position of your lower back. This is necessary to return the back to neutral, after having completed the twists with a bent back.
- Moving asanas follow. Pay attention to the space around you, and allow your movements to fill this space.
- Turn your face toward your right foot, and without losing the stable position of your lower back, move with your left hand to your right foot and into Parivrtta Trikonasana.

21. Parivrtta Trikonasana (right: 30 seconds)

- Turn your upper body to the right and make sure that, when you switch hands, your face remains at the same height over your right foot.
- Move fluidly back into Utthita Trikonasana and return immediately to Parivrtta Trikonasana.
- Repeat this movement three or four times, keeping your head in the same position.
- Step back to Adho Mukha Svanasana I.

22. Adho Mukha Svanasana I (1 minute)

- Lift your left leg up to Adho Mukha Svanasana II.

23. Adho Mukha Svanasana II (10 seconds)

- Repeat the entire movement (asanas 18 through 23) on the left side.

Advanced level

The following can be done immediately after the preceding sequence, or it can be done as a separate lesson. To complete the advanced balance poses, your back must first be prepared for Viparita Chakrasana, which ends this series.

You can prepare and warm up your back with coordination and preparation exercise 1 (see chapter 11.2), then coordination and preparation exercises 2 and 3 (see chapter 11.3), and follow with the rest of the asanas listed here.

24. Urdhva Dhanurasana *(20 to 30 seconds, five times)*

25. Jumping up and dropping back from the headstand bench *(five times)*

- Read the introduction to Viparita Chakrasana (see chapter 11.4, number 9) for this exercise.

26. Malasana II *(15 seconds)*

- The next four asanas are done from Salamba Sirsasana II and are completed with Viparita Chakrasana. To develop strength and flexibility, you can repeat the poses once or twice.

27. Bakasana

28. Parsva Bakasana

29. Dvi Pada Kaundinyasana

30. Eka Pada Kaundinyasana

31. Padmasana *(5 minutes)*

- Remain in this (or a simpler) seated position for a while to recover and allow higher consciousness to develop.
- Then move to the following inversion sequence.

Inversions

Stage 7: higher consciousness

32. Salamba Sarvangasana with your feet against the wall *(5 minutes)*

33. Halasana with your feet on the headstand bench *(5 minutes)*

34. Salamba Sarvangasana plus variations *(1 to 15 minutes total)*

35. Salamba Sirsasana on the headstand bench plus variations
(1 to 15 minutes total)

36. Savasana *(5 to 15 minutes)*

LESSON 3: BACKBENDS

You begin this lesson lying on the thick lower back roll, after which the exercises that are directed toward your lower body are introduced. When you can do these movements easily, it is time to practice exercises that are directed toward your upper body. Finally, you perform the total movement. The beginner's level ends with Urdhva Dhanurasana; after that, the advanced sequence works on Viparita Chakrasana.

Beginner's level

Stage 1 and 2: negativity and awareness

1. Thick lower back roll (approximately 5 minutes)

· Lean against the lower back roll, and rest on your elbows. When lowering yourself to the floor, keep your lower ribs connected to your abdomen and feel how they move toward the floor. This keeps your posterior ribs balanced and free.

· Take time to develop mobility in your lower back. Move slowly and increase your speed toward the end of the exercise, checking that your pelvis is moving directly up and down. The arch in your lower back is necessary for transferring the movements that follow into your pelvis. With the upward pull of your lower abdomen, lift your pelvis toward your navel. Your lower back should be in a neutral extension, allowing you to feel the cohesion of your inner tube (air bag). Breathe into your abdomen without losing the control over your abdominal muscles. Make sure you maintain your core while breathing feelings of openness and space into your chest. Take this consciousness into the next exercise.

Stage 3: presence

2. Virabhadrasana I (left and right: three times and 30 to 60 seconds each)

· The first time you enter Virabhadrasana I, push your fists against your tailbone while keeping your abdominals contracted so that your back is over your tailbone when you bend your front leg. Keep breathing into your abdomen, and repeat the movement on the other side.

· Repeat the movements to both sides, but breathe from your abdomen up into your chest. Develop a feeling of lightness above your diaphragm without losing the contraction in your abdominals.

· Increase the pressure of your back foot on the mat so that you feel your back leg sinking deeper toward the floor. Keep breathing deeply from your abdomen into your chest, and repeat the movement on the other side.

· Repeat the directions under step 2. At the end of an inhalation, lift your head and move the back of your head toward your upper back. Keep breathing into your stomach and contracting your abdominals. Keep your posterior ribs in their balanced and free position as discussed for the thick lower back roll. Lift your arms toward the ceiling to pull length into the arch of your lower back. Push your left foot firmly into the floor so that your tailbone moves down, pulling length into your lower back from this direction.

· Breathe in deeply, from your back into the highest part of your chest, and repeat the movement on the other side.

· Repeat the variation in step 4 but straighten your back leg.

3. Urdhvamukha Svanasana (30 seconds)

· Move from standing on your hands and knees to the end position.

· The difference between this pose and the third phase of Virabhadrasana I is the position of the arms. But even here, your arms (via your shoulder blades) are able to provide space to the top of your chest. Keep the emphasis on the upward movement of your lower abdomen; this strength ensures that your tailbone remains the lowest part of your back.

- Relax your lower back and allow it to "hang," as though someone put weights on your tailbone. Breathe from your lower abdomen up to your collarbones. Extend your upper back with each inhalation, and allow it to relax with every exhalation. Then move into Ustrasana.

4. Ustrasana (30 seconds)

- Feel the pressure of the top of your feet against the floor, and direct the strength of your hamstrings toward stretching your thighs and hips so that your tailbone moves forward.
- Elevate your chest with your breath.

Repeat this exercise three or four times so that ease develops during the movement.

5. Bhujangasana (three times, 30 seconds each)

- Direct your attention mainly toward your lower body.
- Concentrate on the position of your pelvis. Allow it to lift off the floor so that movement can be transferred through your lower back into your tailbone.
- Move slowly and breathe deeply to connect your two gravity points.

Up until this point, your attention has mainly concentrated on developing space in your hara gravity point. In the exercises that follow, it is concentrated on developing space in the heart gravity point so that it can balance the hara. Connect the two areas and use the experience of relaxation and lightness to dissolve feelings of stiffness that you may encounter in your body. What you learned in the previous exercises will keep returning in relation to total movements.

Stage 4: deepening

6. Consciousness exercise with the rubber strip (2 to 3 minutes)

- Remember when completing this exercise that the area where the strip presses is the same area toward which the back of your head must move to develop space in your chest. Breathe deeply into this area, visualizing that your inhalations are able to lift your spine off the strip.

Stage 5: connection

7. Salabhasana (30 to 60 seconds)

- Slowly work on opening your heart gravity point, and get used to keeping your head moving toward your back. To start, keep your lower ribs pressed into the floor, and lift your legs to create space in your hara and strengthen your lower back.
- Keep your head moving toward your upper back, and feel the pressure of the floor against your lower abdomen. Remember that the position of your head remains the

same, and you must actively maintain the upward pull in your lower abdomen when you push yourself up into the next pose.

8. Urdhva Mukha Svanasana (30 seconds)

- Make sure that, when you straighten your arms, you keep moving your head toward your upper back. Breathe into the top of your chest, and relax your back between your shoulder blades during exhalations, then your head will be able to move closer to your upper back.
- Continue the movement of your head and the contraction of your abdominals when you move into the next two poses.

9. Ustrasana (30 seconds)

10. Bhujangasana (30 seconds)

Repeat the exercises 7 through 10, three times each, to develop ease in your lower back and neck during movement. Then do the following three total movements.

11. Bhekasana (30 seconds)

Stage 6: turning point

12. Dhanurasana (30 seconds)

- Focus on the pressure of your body on your hara. Send your exhalations to that spot, while visualizing how this pressure opens your lower back in both directions. Length develops toward your tailbone and in the direction of your upper back; more space is created toward your chest. This movement can lessen discomfort in your lower back. Use your abdominals to provide this same pressure during Urdhva Dhanurasana to dissolve stiffness and pain.

13. Parsva Dhanurasana (left and right: 20 seconds each)

14. Urdhva Dhanurasana (five to ten times)

- Lie on your back and take hold of your ankles. Push your thighs up without losing the cohesion in your core, and move your chest toward your chin. Wait until calm develops in this position before moving farther.
- Use your breathing to connect yourself to the space around you.
- Take this connection and calm with you when moving into the end pose.

Advanced level

The following can be done immediately after the preceding sequence, but it can also stand as a separate lesson. If you do it separately, then you must warm up thoroughly and prepare your back. The exercises that follow flow from exercises 1 through 14.

LESSON 3 *Beginner's level* » » »

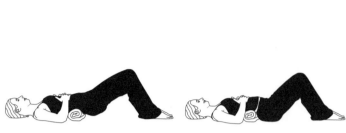

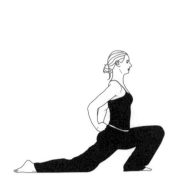

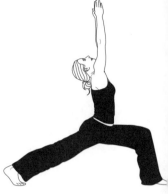

1. Thick lower back roll

5 minutes

Move your pelvis up and down   *p. 113*

2. *Virabhadrasana I*

30–60 seconds

3 times to the right and the left   *p. 232*

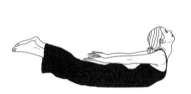

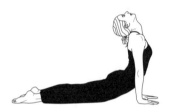

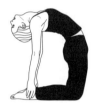

7. *Salabasana*

30–60 seconds   *p. 277*

Repeat exercises 7 through 10, 3 times   *p. 279*

8. *Urdhva mukha savanasana*

30 seconds

9. *Ustrasana*

30 seconds   *p. 286*

10. *Bhujangasana*

30 seconds   *p. 282*

Advanced level » » »

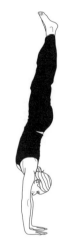

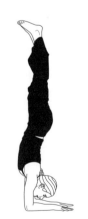

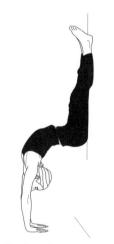

15. *Adho mukha vrksasana*

1 minute

p. 184

16. *Pincha mayurasana*

1 minute

p. 189

17. Handstand (variation)

20–30 seconds

3 times   *p. 294*

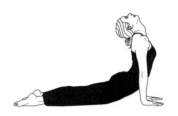

3. Urdhvamukha svanasana

30 seconds p. 279

Repeat exercises 3 and 4, 3 to 4 times

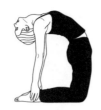

4. Ustrasana

30 seconds

p. 286

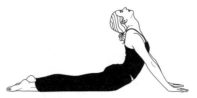

5. Bhujangasana

30 seconds

3 times p. 282

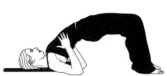

6. With the rubber strip

2–3 minutes

p. 100

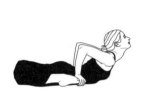

11. Bhekasana

30 seconds

p. 289

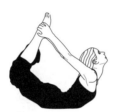

12. Dhanurasana

30 seconds

p. 288

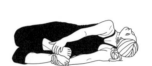

13. Parsva dhanurasana

20 seconds

Right and left p. 289

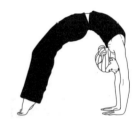

14. Urdhva dhanurasana

As long as you want

5 to 10 times p. 291

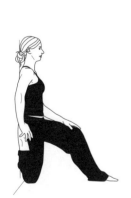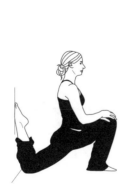

18. Coordination exercise 2

2–3 minutes

Right and left p. 284

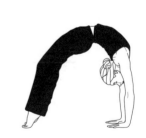

19. Handstand (variation)

20–30 seconds

3 times p. 294

20. Urdhva dhanurasana

Lift up immediately

10 times p. 291

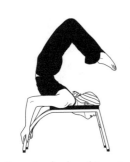

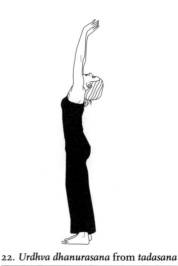

21. Dropping back and jumping

3 times   *p. 300*

22. *Urdhva dhanurasana* from *tadasana*

Repeat the drop-back 5 times and push up in the end position 5 times

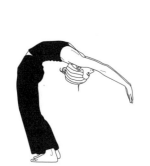

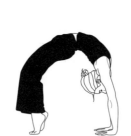

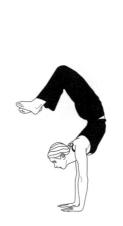

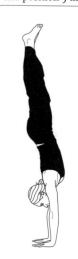

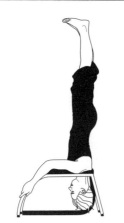

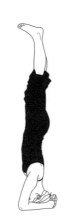

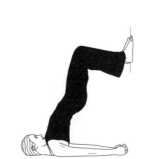

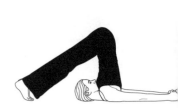

25. *Sirsasana* on headstand bench

5–10 minutes

With variations   *p. 144*

26. *Salamba sirsasana*

1–10 minutes

                                                          p. 157

27. *Sarvangasana* against the wall

3–5 minutes

                                                          p. 171

28. *Halasana*

3 minutes

                                                          p. 174

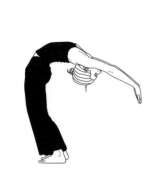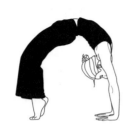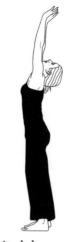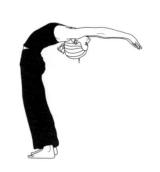

23. Viparita chakrasana

p. 291

1 to 108 times   >>>

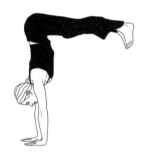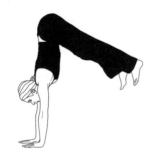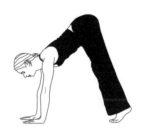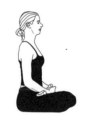

24. Padmasana

5 minutes

p. 299   *p. 134*

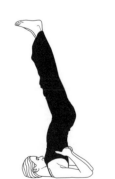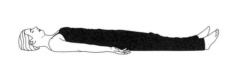

29. Salamba sarvangasana

3–15 minutes

p. 168

30. Savasana

5–15 minutes

p. 344

15. *Adho Mukha Vrksasana (1 minute)*

16. *Pincha Mayurasana (1 minute)*

17. *Adho Mukha Vrksasana with the pelvis against the wall (two times, 20 to 30 seconds each)*

18. *Coordination exercise 2 (see chapter 11.2; left and right: 2 to 3 minutes each)*

19. *Adho Mukha Vrksasana with the pelvis against the wall (three times, 20 to 30 seconds each)*

20. *Urdhva Dhanurasana (ten times, or 2 sets of five in a fluid manner, without holding the end position or resting in between—crown touches the floor and immediately moves back up)*

21. *Dropping back and jumping up from headstand bench (three times)*

22. *Urdhva Dhanurasana from Tadasana (five times); after every drop-back, complete Urdhva Dhanurasana five times in a fluid manner (shoulders to the floor and immediately moving back up)*

23. *Viparita Chakrasana (1 to 108 times)*

24. *Padmasana (5 minutes)*

- Remain in this (or a simpler) seated position for a while to recover and develop consciousness.
- Then move on to the inversions.

Inversions

Stage 7: higher consciousness

25. *Sirsasana on the headstand bench with variations (5 to 10 minutes)*

26. *Salamba Sirsasana (1 to 10 minutes) (I)*

27. *Sarvangasana with feet against the wall (3 to 5 minutes)*

28. *Halasana (3 minutes)*

29. *Salamba Sarvangasana (3 to 15 minutes)*

30. *Savasana (5 to 15 minutes)*

LESSON 4: STANDING POSES

This lesson is used to develop the concept of moving asanas, which has only been used during Viparita Chakrasana until now. In this lesson, there are moving asanas and repetition of the sequence of asanas. The standing poses are well suited for this. They are held for shorter periods than the asanas in the previous lessons, and the movement can be seen as a dance in space. Therefore, they are ideal for including the space around you in your consciousness.

Higher consciousness

The first exercise, Tadasana, is used to develop awareness toward relaxation, lightness, and space. Spend 3 to 5 minutes in this when starting the lesson. After that, a shorter time will be sufficient; otherwise, it will break the flow of movement. When the rhythm of your movements produces a flow, you can skip Tadasana and repeat the series without pausing. Then you can experience higher consciousness through movement.

Speed

The series is repeated three times. Use the first time to develop the technical aspects of movement, the second to integrate your breath, and the third to pay more attention to the fluidity of the movement. As soon as you achieve the end position of one pose, you move immediately to the next. Then it is pure movement; you do not hold end poses. You must know the series by heart when you move this way. Otherwise, there will be no fluidity between the movements; you must be able to prepare yourself for each one.

The speed with which you move depends on your own experience. Ideally, movement should strengthen your experience of the space around you. Free breathing plays an essential role in that. Use your breath to develop and strengthen feelings of lightness and space within your body. If this is your goal, then you will realize that easy, slow breathing contributes to it much more than fast, heavy breathing. Tune the speed of your movement to your breathing so that they are synchronized. Moving too slowly can build awareness but block feelings of space and lightness.

Within this series, a few sections are repeated. Use these repetitions to develop ease in movement so that feels effortless.

Phases

It is not advisable to complete the entire series immediately; start with phase 1. Subsequently, you can add phase 2 and finally phase 3.

Phase 1

Stages 1 and 2: negativity and awareness

1. Tadasana

- If you like, shut your eyes and bend your knees slightly so that you can relax your lower back. Activate your transverse abdominals by pulling your lower abdomen, 2 inches under your navel, upward. Breathe into your abdomen without losing this contraction, and straighten your legs.
- Breathe into your chest, and align your neck and head with your upper back.
- Take time to contact the various areas of your body and connect them to your breathing, as when you are realizing consciousness. Allow your breath to circulate freely through your body and become aware of the space around you. Connect yourself to this space and resolve to maintain this connection during the series.
- Prepare yourself for lifting your arms into the next movement, and try to find a speed at which you can maintain your awareness of the space around you. Try to keep this speed constant when completing the series.

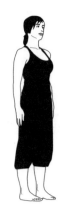

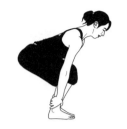

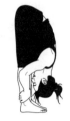

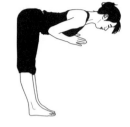

1. *Tadasana*

p. 193

2. *Utkatasana*

p. 195

Hold your ankles and move through to:

3. *Uttanasana*

p.257

4. *Dandasana* (standing)

p. 199

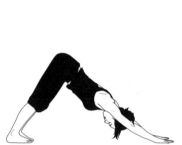

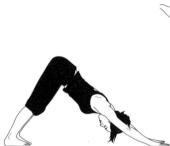

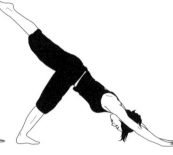

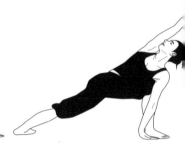

Step back to Adho Mukha Svanasana and repeat steps 6 through 8 on the other side

9. *Adho mukha svanasana I*

p. 201

10. *Adho mukha svanasana II*

Right   p. 203

11. *Parivrtta parsvakonasana*

Right   p. 223

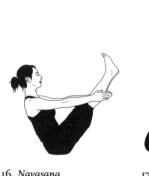

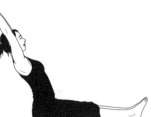

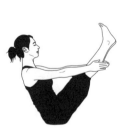

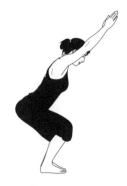

16. *Navasana*

p. 251

17. *Paschimottanasana*

p. 261

18. *Dandasana*

p. 254

19. *Navasana*

p. 251

20. *Utkatasana*

p. 195

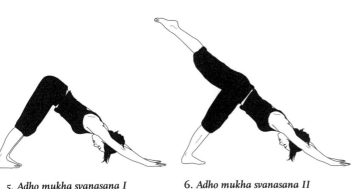

5. Adho mukha svanasana I

p. 201

6. Adho mukha svanasana II

Right   *p. 203*

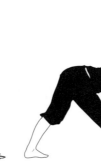

7. Utthita trikonasana

Repeat steps 7 and 8, 3 to 5 times

Right   *p. 210*

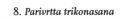

8. Parivṛtta trikonasana

Right   *p. 215*

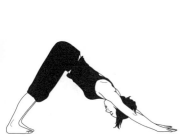

12. Adho mukha svanasana I

Repeat steps 9 through 11
on the other side   *p. 201*

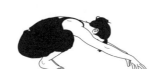

13. Malasana I

p. 318

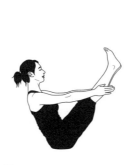

14. Navasana

Repeat steps 14 and 15, 3 times

p. 251

15. Utkatasana

p. 195

Phase 2 » » »

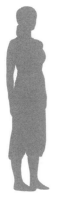

If you want to stop after phase 1,
finish here in Tadasana

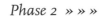

21. Adho mukha svanasana I

p. 201

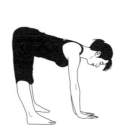

22. Prasarita padottanasana I

p. 252

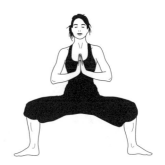

23. Virabhadrasana II (variation)

p. 206

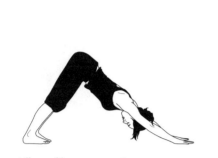

24. Adho mukha svanasana I

_____

_____

_____   _p. 201_

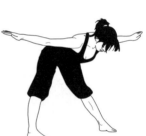

25. Adho mukha svanasana II

_____

Right   _p. 203_

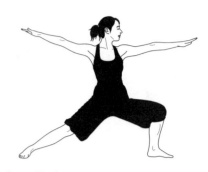

26. Virabhadrasana II

Repeat steps 26 and 27, 3 times

Right   _p. 206_

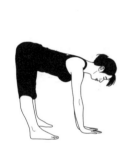

**30. Prasarita padottan-
asana I**

_____

_p. 252_

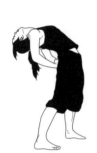

**31a. Backbend with wide-
legged stance**

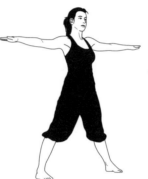

31b. Wide-legged stance

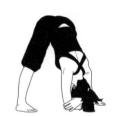

**31c. Prasarita padottan-
asana I**   "the bird"

**31d. Prasarita padottan-
asana II**

_p. 260_

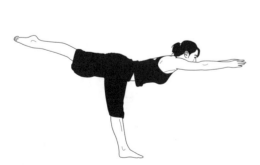

35. Virabhadrasana III

1 minute

Right   _p. 204_

Move from step 35 to 34 and back to
32 and repeat steps 32 through 35 on
the other side. Repeat this 2 times.

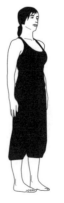

36. Tadasana

_____

_____   _p. 193_

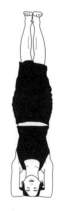

37. Salamba sirsasana

5–15 minutes

With variations   _p. 157_

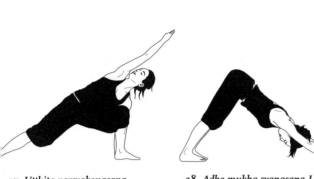

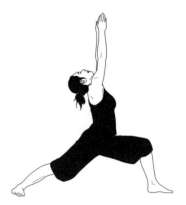

27. *Utthita parsvakonasana*

Right   *p.219*

28. *Adho mukha svanasana I*

                                    p. 201

If you want to stop after phase 2, finish here in Tadasana. Otherwise, carry on to phase 3 and step out to:

29. *Virabhadrasana I*   *p. 232*

Right, repeat steps 29 and 30 on the other side, ending in 28, then jump to:

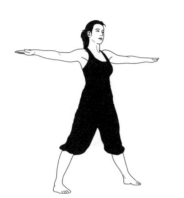

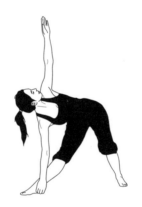

32. Wide-legged stance

Then move to:

33. *Utthita trikonasana*

Right   *p. 210*

34. *Ardha chandrasana*

Right   *p. 229*

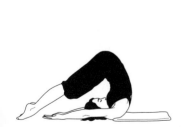

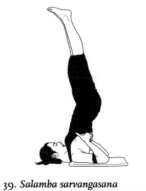

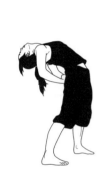

38. *Halasana*

2–5 minutes

                                    p. 174

39. *Salamba sarvangasana*

5–15 minutes

With variations   *p. 168*

40. *Savasana*

5–15 minutes

                                    p. 344

Stage 3: presence

2. Utkatasana

- Bend your knees and take hold of your ankles. Move as if you were going to lift your feet off the floor with your hands, and slowly straighten your legs. The complete extension of your legs does not have priority in this movement; the strength of your hands pulling on your ankles and the flatness of your back does. Move into Uttanasana.

3. Uttanasana

- If moving into this pose with straight legs is difficult for you, bend your knees slightly. Work out the leg stretch at a later stage, when your legs are warmed up.

4. Dandasana (standing)

- Feel how the extension in your lower back provides pressure to your hips. Use that feeling when you move into the next pose.

5. Adho Mukha Svasanasa I

- Keep using this pose to observe your body in its entirety. After completing the more demanding poses in this series, your attention can be pulled into a sort of emptiness where you are no longer conscious of your body because you feel tired. Recover the contact with your body with attention, allowing your breath to circulate freely and being conscious of the space around you.
- Remain conscious of the speed with which you lift your leg into the following pose. Keep the movement open.

6. Adho Mukha Svanasana II (right leg lifted)

- Take a small step forward with your right foot into the next pose.

Stage 4: deepening

7. Utthita Trikonasana (right)

8. Parivrtta Trikonasana (right)

- Repeat poses 7 and 8 three to five times, making sure that your body turns while your head remains in the same position, exactly over your front foot. Ensure that your face also stays at the same height. Remember that if your face lowers, your back has lost its stable extended position.
- As you repeat poses, try to develop a fluid swing.
- Step back into Adho Mukha Svanasana I and repeat poses 5 through 8 on the other side.
- Then, step back into the next pose.

9. Adho Mukha Svanasana I

10. Adho Mukha Svanasana II (right leg lifted)

- Take a large step forward with your right foot into the next pose.

11. Parivrtta Parsvakonasana (right foot forward)

- Take the necessary time to develop this pose. In the first round of the series, you can keep your back knee on the floor and your hands in front of your chest. The second series is the same, but with the back leg straight. During the third series, you can move into the end pose.
- Repeat poses 9 through 11 to the other side and move back into Adho Mukha Svanasana I.

12. Adho Mukha Svanasana I

- Jump forward into the next pose.

13. Malasana I

- Keep breathing into and relaxing your abdomen, so your lower back maintains its cohesion. When you contract your abdominals, they push your lower back backward, and you lose the length you developed in the front of your body.
- Place your hands behind you on the floor, sit down, and lift your legs up into the next pose.

14. Navasana

- Pull your legs in and place your feet on the floor hip-width apart. Push into the floor with your hands behind you to create a fluid movement into the next pose.

15. Utkatasana

- Repeat these poses 14 and 15 three times if you are a beginner. If you want to continue to work on the movement, repeat the following five poses (16 through 20) three times also.
- Keep your movements fluid and light.

16. Navasana

17. Paschimottanasana

- Keep your lower back active by taking hold of your feet (or lower legs) and extending your back with a deep inhalation before moving into the forward bend.

18. Dandasana with the upper body leaning diagonally backward

19. Navasana

20. Utkatasana

- If you are only doing phase 1, stand up in Tadasana and begin again.
- If you are moving into phase 2, jump back into Adho Mukha Svanasana I.

Phase 2

21. Adho Mukha Svanasana I

- Jump into the next pose.

22. Prasarita Padottanasana I

23. Virabhadrasana II (variation)

- Do the pose initially with your knees bent and your lower back extended. Straighten your legs in subsequent repetitions when you are more accomplished.
- Turn your feet outward and push your ankles forward. Place your hands on the insides of your knees and push them outward. After a few breaths, align your upper body by positioning your diaphragm on top of the arch of your lower back, and place your hands in front of your chest. Be certain that your body is not leaning forward but is absolutely straight. Your lower ribs push the weight of your body through the arch of your lower back. From there, the movement divides between your SI joints and hips. Carrying your body weight this way activates the postural muscles in your lower back. This produces a feeling of firmness and flexibility in the stacking of your spine and automatically activates your transverse abdominals.
- If you would like to remain longer in this position, do so.
- Place your hands back on the floor, turn your heels outward, and jump back into the next pose.

24. Adho Mukha Svanasana I

25. Adho Mukha Svanasana II (right leg lifted)

- Take a large step forward with your right foot.

26. Virabhadrasana II

- Move through to the next pose.

27. Parsvakonasana

- Repeat poses 26 and 27 three times, varying the end position of Parsvakonasana. For example, end the first time with your hands in front of your chest in namaskar, the second time with your right arm on the inside of your knee, and the third time with your right arm on the outside of your knee.

· Repeat pose 24, then complete poses 25 through 27 on the other side. Step back to Adho Mukha Svanasana I.

28. Adho Mukha Svanasana I

· Take time to realize higher consciousness.
· If you want to finish your practice here, jump back into Utkatasana and stand up in Tadasana.
· If you are moving into phase 3, step forward with your right foot into Virabhadrasana I.

Phase 3

29. Virabhadrasana I (right)

· Jump from Adho Mukha Svanasana I into the next pose.

30. Prasarita Padottanasana I

31. Complete exercises a through d fluidly and repeat each three times:

a. Backbend from a wide-legged position
b. Wide-legged stance
c. Prasarita Padottanasana I with arms wide
d. Prasarita Padottanasana II

· End in the following pose.

32. Backbend from a wide-legged position

33. Utthita Trikonasana (right)

34. Ardha Chandrasana (right)

35. Virabhadrasana III (right)

· Move back through poses 34 and 35, in reverse order, to Utthita Trikonasana and repeat poses 32 through 35 on the other side.
· Repeat this section, from pose 32 to pose 35, another two times.
· End in a wide-legged stance and jump back to Tadasana.

36. Tadasana

· Repeat the series another two times.
· Do the first repetition from the perspective of stage 5 (connection).
· Do the second repetition from the perspective of stage 6 (turning point).

Inversions

Stage 7: higher consciousness

37. *Salamba Sirsasana with variations (5 to 15 minutes total)*

38. *Halasana (2 to 5 minutes)*

39. *Salamba Sarvangasana with variations (5 to 15 minutes total)*

40. *Savasana (5 to 15 minutes)*

Notes

Chapter 1

1. Patanjali, *Yoga Sutra* 1:2.
2. N. E. Sjoman and H. V. Dattatreya, *Yoga Touchstone* (Calgary, AB: Black Lotus Books, 2004), 7.
3. N. E. Sjoman, *The Yoga Tradition of the Mysore Palace* (New Delhi: Abhinav Publications, 1996), 99.
4. Ibid.
5. Patanjali, *Yoga Sutra* 11:47.

Chapter 2

1. See Leopold Busquet, *Les chaines musculaires,* ed. Roger Frison-Roche (Paris: Frison-Roche, 1992), as well as more recent titles by Leopold Busquet.
2. M. L. Gharote, ed., *Encyclopedia of Traditional Asanas* (Lonavla, India: Lonavla Yoga Institute, 2007).
3. See also G. van Leeuwen, *Stop RSI* (Haarlem, Netherlands: Aramith, 2001).

Chapter 5

1. Hathapradipika 4:4.

Chapter 7

1. Patanjali, *Yoga Sutra* 1:36.

Chapter 13

1. For more information about this, read Clair Davies, *The Trigger Point Therapy Workbook* (Oakland, CA: New Harbinger Publications, 2004).

Asana Index

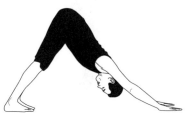

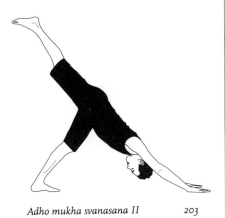

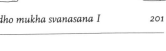

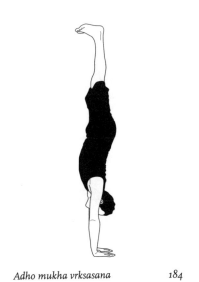

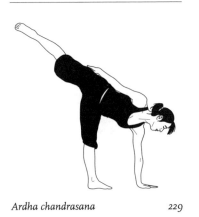

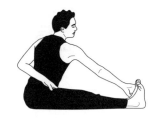

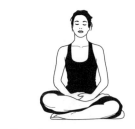

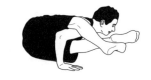

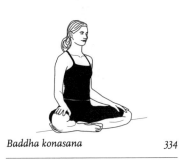

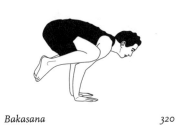

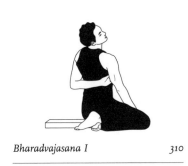

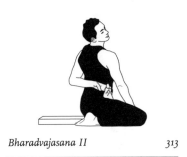

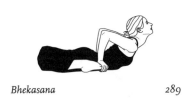

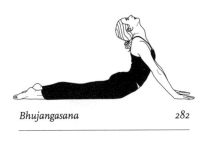

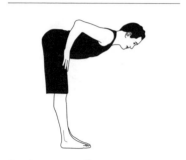

Dandasana (standing)   199

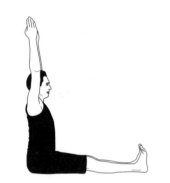

Dandasana (sitting)   254

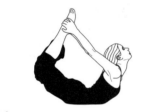

Dhanurasana   288

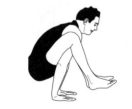

Dvi hasta bhujasana   269

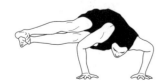

Dvi pada kaundinyasana   322

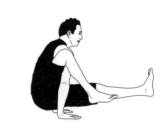

Eka hasta bhujasana   271

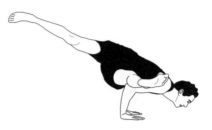

Eka pada kaundinyasana   322

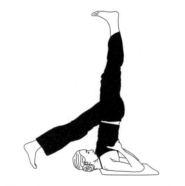

Eka pada sarvangasana   182

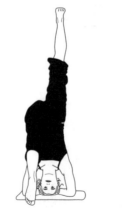

Ekapada sirsasana   165

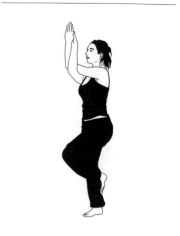

Garudasana (standing)   337

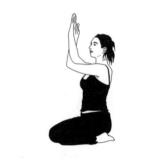

Garudasana (sitting)   337

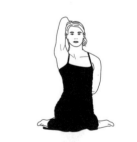

Gomukhasana   336

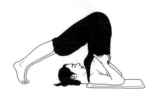

Halasana   174

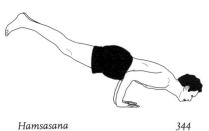

Hamsasana 344

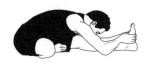

Janu sirsasana 264

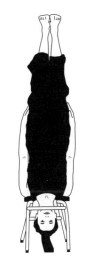

Jatukasana 156

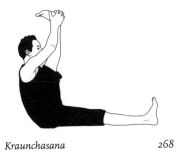

Kraunchasana 268

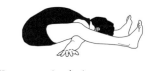

Kurmasana (supine) 269

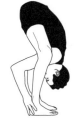

Kurmasana (standing) 269

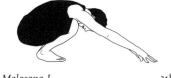

Malasana I 318

Malasana II 319

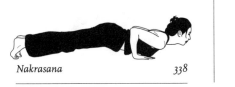

Mayurasana 343

Nakrasana 338

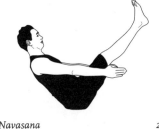

Navasana 251

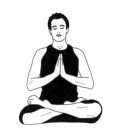

Padmasana 330

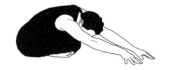

Parivrtta ardha padmasana 313

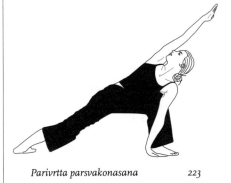

Parivrtta parsvakonasana 223

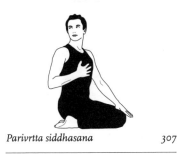

Parivrtta siddhasana 307

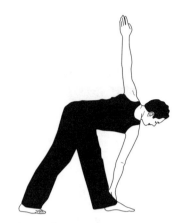

Parivrtta trikonasana   215

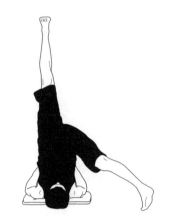

Parsvaika pada sarvangasana   183

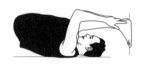

Paschimottanasana (supine)   263

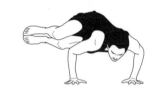

Parsva bakasana   320

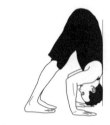

Paschimottanasana (standing)   264

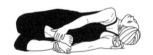

Parsva dhanurasana   289

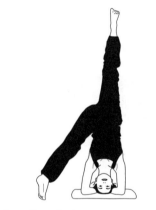

Parsvaika pada sirsasana   166

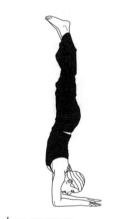

Pincha mayurasana   189

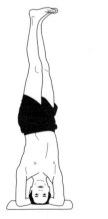

Parsva sirsasana   165

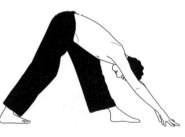

Parsvottanasana   231

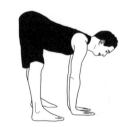

Prasarita padottanasana I   252

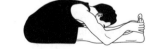

Paschimottanasana   261

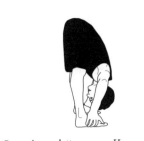

Prasarita padottanasana II 260

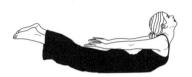

Salabhasana 277

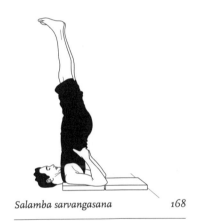

Salamba sarvangasana 168

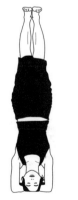

Salamba sirsasana I 157

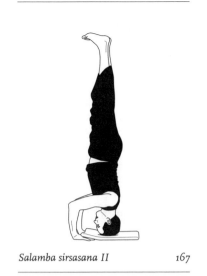

Salamba sirsasana II 167

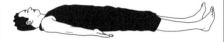

Savasana 344

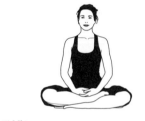

Siddhasana 331

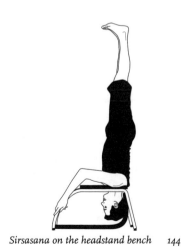

Sirsasana on the headstand bench 144

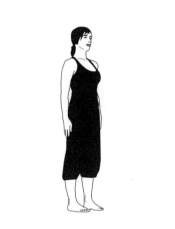

Supta virasana 333

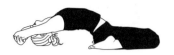

Tadasana 193

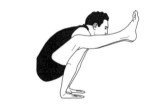

Titibhasana I 270

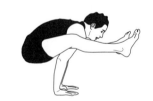

Titibhasana II 270

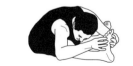

Upavista konasana 266

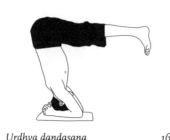

Urdhva dandasana   166

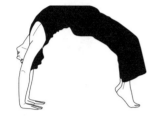

Urdhva dhanurasana   291

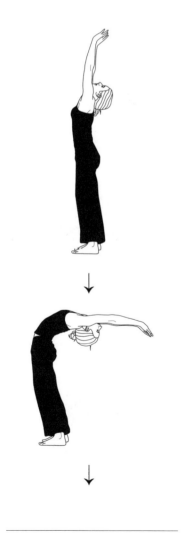

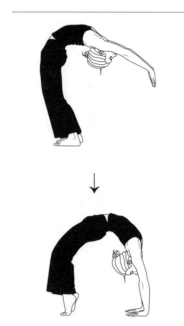

↓

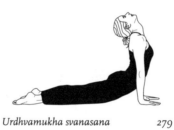

Urdhva dhanurasana from Tadasana
291

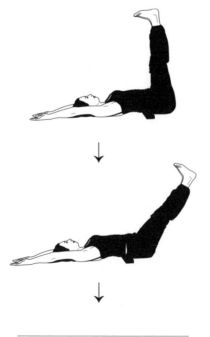

Urdhvamukha svanasana   279

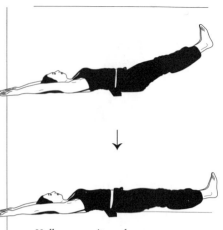

↓

Urdhva prasarita padasana   341

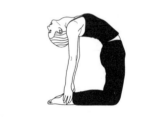

Ustrasana   286

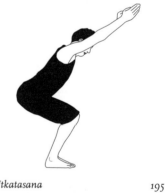

Utkatasana   195

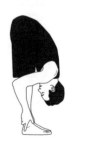

Uttanasana   257

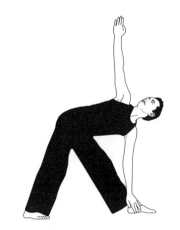

Utthita trikonasana 210

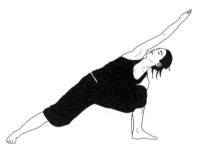

Utthita parsvakonasana 219

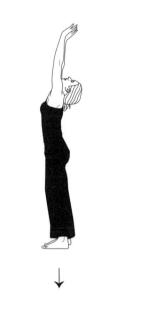

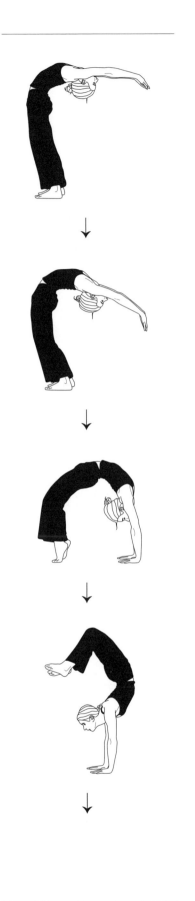

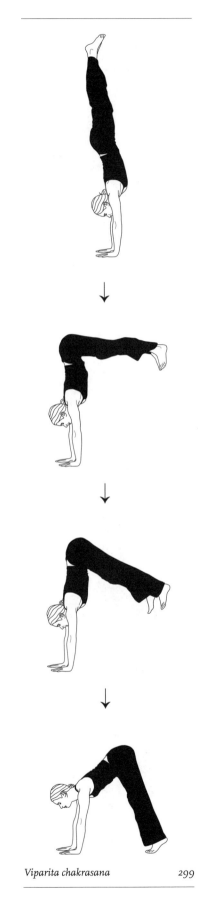

Viparita chakrasana 299

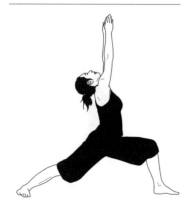

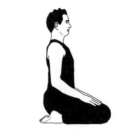

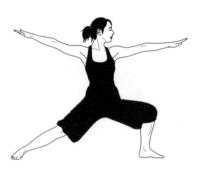

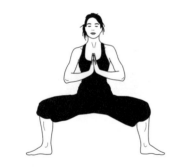

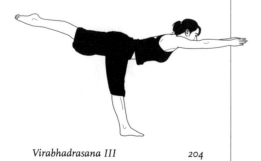

Index

Note: Page numbers followed by *ff* indicate the topic spans several pages following the indicated page.

About the Author

Gert van Leeuwen is the founder of the Critical Alignment Yoga and Therapy studio in Amsterdam. He has been teaching for thirty-five years and is the founder of the Critical Alignment method. He teaches workshops throughout North America and Europe and has established teacher training programs in the Netherlands as well as abroad. He also trains yoga teachers from various backgrounds to become Critical Alignment therapists. Van Leeuwen was a student of Norman Sjoman, who was an early student of B. K. S. Iyengar. Learn more at www.criticalalignment.nl.